Emerging Cancer Therapeutics

Jame Abraham, MD, FACP

Editor-in-Chief

Bonnie Wells Wilson Distinguished Professor and Eminent Scholar
Chief, Section of Hematology-Oncology
Medical Director, Mary Babb Randolph Cancer Center
West Virginia University
Morgantown, West Virginia

Editorial Board

Emerging Cancer Therapeutics

VOLUME 3, ISSUE 3

Melanoma

William H. Sharfman, MD
Guest Editor

Associate Professor of Oncology & Dermatology
Medical Director, Medical Oncology, Johns Hopkins at Green Spring Station
Director of Cutaneous Oncology
The Sidney Kimmel Comprehensive Cancer Center at Johns Hopkins
Lutherville, Maryland

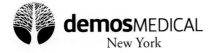
demosMEDICAL
New York

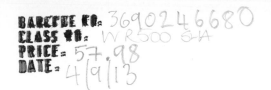

Acquisitions Editor: Richard Winters
Cover Design: Joe Tenerelli
Compositor: Newgen Imaging
Printer: Hamilton Printing

Visit our website at www.demosmedpub.com

Emerging Cancer Therapeutics is published three times a year by Demos Medical Publishing.

Business Office. All business correspondence including subscriptions, renewals, and address changes should be sent to Demos Medical Publishing, 11 West 42nd Street, 15th Floor, New York, NY, 10036.

The ideas and opinions expressed in *Emerging Cancer Therapeutics* do not necessarily reflect those of the Publisher. The Publisher does not assume any responsibility for any injury and/or damage to persons or property arising out of or related to any use of the material contained in this periodical. The reader is advised to check the appropriate medical literature and the product information currently provided by the manufacturer of each drug to be administered to verify the dosage, the method and duration of administration, or contraindications. It is the responsibility of the treating physician or other health care professional relying on independent experience and knowledge of the patient, to determine drug dosages and the best treatment for the patient. Mention of any product in this issue should not be construed as endorsement by the contributors, editors, or the Publisher of the product or manufacturer's claims.

ISSN: 2151-4194
ISBN: 978-1-936287-79-6
E-ISBN: 978-1-617051-61-6

Library of Congress Cataloging-in-Publication Data

Melanoma / William Sharfman, guest editor.
    p. ; cm.—(Emerging cancer therapeutics ; v. 3, issue 3)
  Includes bibliographical references and index.
  ISBN 978-1-936287-79-6—ISBN 978-1-61705-161-6 (e-ISBN)
  I. Sharfman, William. II. Series: Emerging cancer therapeutics; v. 3, issue 3. 2151-4194
  [DNLM: 1. Melanoma—therapy. 2. Skin Neoplasms—therapy. 3. Antineoplastic Agents—therapeutic use. 4. Immunotherapy. 5. Molecular Targeted Therapy. WR 500]

  616.99'477—dc23

             2012042991

Reprints. For copies of 100 or more of articles in this publication, please contact Reina Santana, Special Sales Manager.

Special discounts on bulk quantities of Demos Medical Publishing books are available to corporations, professional associations, pharmaceutical companies, health care organizations, and other qualifying groups. For details, please contact:

Reina Santana, Special Sales Manager
Demos Medical Publishing LLC
11 W. 42nd Street
New York, NY 10036
Phone: 800-532-8663 or 212-683-0072
Fax: 212-941-7842
E-mail: rsantana@demosmedpub.com

Printed in the United States of America
12 13 14 15   5 4 3 2 1

To my dear wife Paula, who has been a constant source of love, support, devotion, and wisdom from the day we first met. She is also the consummate mother of our children, tirelessly striving to bring out the best in each of them. Without her, I could never have brought this project to a successful completion. To my children Mollie, Avi, Chavie, and Arianna: I am so proud of all of you.

Contents

Foreword

Cancer treatment is one of the fastest growing specialties in modern medicine, with better understanding of the disease, improved diagnostic tools, better prognostic information, and ever-changing management options. The most important tool a clinician can have in the fight against cancer is access to current information.

The Emerging Cancer Therapeutics (ECAT) series provides a thorough analysis of key clinical research related to cancer therapeutics, including a discussion and assessment of current evidence, current clinical best practice, and likely near-future developments. The content is in the form of review articles, but the volume format allows for much more in-depth discussion than the typical journal review article. The goal is to provide for the practicing clinician a source of thorough, ongoing analysis and translational assessment of "hot topics" and areas of rapidly emerging new data in cancer therapeutics with significant implications for clinical care.

The ECAT is a valuable tool for practicing cancer specialists of all disciplines and will provide the most comprehensive evidence-based review of pathology, radiology, pharmacology, surgical oncology, radiation oncology, and medical oncology of the topic.

The *Melanoma* volume provides a comprehensive approach to the pathophysiology, epidemiology, clinical features, diagnostic modalities, and current and future treatment options. Experts from around the country have contributed to this volume. This will be a valuable tool for any clinician, researcher, or student of oncology.

Jame Abraham, MD, FACP
Bonnie Wells Wilson Distinguished Professor and Eminent Scholar
Chief, Section of Hematology-Oncology
Medical Director, Mary Babb Randolph Cancer Center
West Virginia University
Morgantown, West Virginia

Preface

Therapy for melanoma has improved dramatically over the past few years. In 2011, the Food and Drug Administration approved two new drugs for the treatment of metastatic melanoma, ipilimumab and vemurafenib, as well as PEG-interferon for adjuvant therapy of stage III patients. These developments are remarkable for many reasons. Most importantly, both ipilimumab and vemurafenib were shown to improve overall survival in metastatic melanoma patients in large, randomized, controlled trials. Despite decades of clinical research in melanoma, involving hundreds of trials with thousands of patients, no treatment had ever shown a survival benefit in metastatic melanoma until now, although high-dose IL-2 has long been known to induce durable remissions. Also remarkable is that none of these recently approved drugs is a cytotoxic chemotherapy. Ipilumumab is a unique immunotherapeutic agent inhibiting CTLA4 on the T cell, and vemurafenib is a targeted therapy turning off mutant BRAF. Clearly, years of research in the immunology and molecular biology of melanoma are beginning to pay off. However, even with these advances, the majority of patients with advanced melanoma will succumb to their disease. There is still a great deal of work to be done to develop more effective and less toxic therapies for our patients.

I have asked an outstanding group of authors to write chapters on important clinical and research topics in melanoma. As much as any cancer, melanoma requires a multidisciplinary approach to treatment, and authors in this volume represent the fields of dermatology, dermatologic surgery, surgical oncology, dermatopathology, and medical oncology.

Drs. Summerer, Kang, and Wang begin with an update on what is known about the prevention of melanoma. Drs. Sharma, Balch, and Balch discuss the change in the melanoma staging system, based on the follow-up of more than 20,000 patients worldwide. Drs. Barnhill, Sarantopoulos, and Gupta discuss variants of melanoma that can present diagnostic challenges and may require different treatment approaches. The mainstay of curing melanoma is still surgery, and Drs. Hatzaras and Lange discuss the ongoing controversies revolving around the sentinel node and regional node dissections. Drs. Gangadhar and Schuchter review adjuvant therapy of high-risk melanoma patients, an area that has not seen any major breakthroughs since 1996, but may be poised for advances in the near future.

The remaining six chapters focus on the treatment of metastatic disease. Drs. Harding and Chapman review the exciting results with single-agent specific V600E mutant inhibitors and discuss future directions that might lead to more durable benefits. Drs. Chae, Patel, and Kim comprehensively review target therapy for patients without BRAF mutations. Dr. O'Day reviews ipilimumab, focusing on its distinctive mechanism of actions, the clinical trials demonstrating its survival benefit, and its unique toxicities. Drs. Hessman, Stewart, Miller, Yang, and Rosenberg review the National Cancer Institute's evolving work on TIL cell therapy.

Dr. Conlon updates us on the enormous potential of new immunotherapeutic agents in metastatic melanoma, and finally, Drs. Amaria and Gonzalez share with us how they approach the advanced melanoma patient in the clinic in this new era of melanoma therapy.

In this rapidly changing field of melanoma therapy, I hope this *Melanoma* volume of Emerging Cancer Therapeutics serves as a valuable reference for physicians and researchers interested in melanoma, elucidating where we are and where the field is going.

William H. Sharfman, MD
Associate Professor of Oncology & Dermatology
Medical Director, Medical Oncology, Johns Hopkins at Green Spring Station
Director of Cutaneous Oncology
The Sidney Kimmel Comprehensive Cancer Center at Johns Hopkins
Lutherville, Maryland

Contributors

Rodabe N. Amaria, MD
Hematology/Oncology Fellow
Department of Medicine
University of Colorado Denver
Aurora, Colorado

Charles M. Balch, MD, FACS
Professor
Department of Surgery
Division of Surgical Oncology
UT Southwestern Medical Center
Dallas, Texas

Glen C. Balch, MD
Assistant Professor
Department of Surgery
Division of Surgical Oncology
UT Southwestern Medical Center
Dallas, Texas

Raymond L. Barnhill, MD
Professor of Pathology
Co-director, Dermatopathology
Director of Melanoma Research
Department of Pathology and Laboratory
  Medicine, and Jonsson Comprehensive
  Cancer Center
University of California, Los Angeles
Los Angeles, California

Young Kwang Chae, MD
Hematology/Oncology Fellow
Division of Cancer Medicine
University of Texas MD Anderson Cancer
  Center
Houston, Texas

Paul B. Chapman, MD
Attending Physician
Department of Medicine
Melanoma Sarcoma Service
Memorial Sloan-Kettering Cancer Center
New York, New York
Professor
Department of Medicine
Weill-Cornell Medical College
New York, New York

Kevin Conlon, MD
Metabolism Branch
Center for Cancer Research
National Cancer Institute
Bethesda, Maryland

Tara C. Gangadhar, MD
Assistant Professor
Department of Medicine
Division of Hematology-Oncology
Abramson Cancer Center of the
  University of Pennsylvania
Philadelphia, Pennsylvania

Rene Gonzalez, MD
Professor
University of Colorado Denver/School of
    Medicine
University of Colorado Cancer Center
Aurora, Colorado

Kapil Gupta, MD
Director of Dermatopathology
Dermatology Group of the Carolinas
Concord, North Carolina

James J. Harding, MD
Medical Oncology Fellow
Department of Medicine
Memorial Sloan-Kettering Cancer Center
New York, New York

Ioannis Hatzaras, MD, MPH
Fellow, Surgical Oncology
Johns Hopkins Medicine
Department of Surgery
Division of Surgical Oncology
Baltimore, Maryland

Crystal J. Hessman, MD
Doctor
Surgery Branch
National Cancer Institute
Bethesda, Maryland

Sewon Kang, MD
Noxell Professor and Chairman
Department of Dermatology
Johns Hopkins School of Medicine
Baltimore, Maryland

Kevin B. Kim, MD
Associate Professor
Department of Melanoma Medical Oncology
University of Texas MD Anderson Cancer
    Center
Houston, Texas

Julie R. Lange, MD, ScM
Associate Professor
Department of Surgery
Johns Hopkins Medicine
Department of Surgery
Division of Surgical Oncology
Baltimore, Maryland

Akemi D. Miller, MD
Doctor
Surgery Branch
National Cancer Institute
Bethesda, Maryland

Steven J. O'Day, MD
Director, The Los Angeles Skin Cancer
    Institute
Department of Medical Oncology
Beverly Hills Cancer Center
Beverly Hills, California

Sapna P. Patel
Assistant Professor
Department of Melanoma Medical Oncology
University of Texas MD Anderson Cancer
    Center
Houston, Texas

Steven A. Rosenberg, MD, PhD
Doctor
Surgery Branch
National Cancer Institute
Bethesda, Maryland

G. Peter Sarantopoulos, MD
Assistant Professor of Pathology
Department of Pathology and Laboratory
    Medicine
UCLA Medical Center
Los Angeles, California

Lynn M. Schuchter, MD
Professor
Department of Medicine
Division of Hematology-Oncology
Abramson Cancer Center of the
    University of Pennsylvania
Philadelphia, Pennsylvania

Rohit R. Sharma, MD
Assistant Professor
Department of Surgery
Division of Surgical Oncology
UT Southwestern Medical Center
Dallas, Texas

Ashley A. Stewart, MD
Doctor
Surgery Branch
National Cancer Institute
Bethesda, Maryland

Barbara Summerer, MD
Research Fellow
Department of Dermatology
Johns Hopkins School of Medicine
Baltimore, Maryland

Timothy Wang, MD
Associate Professor
Director, Cutaneous Surgery and Oncology
    Unit
Department of Dermatology
Johns Hopkins School of Medicine
Baltimore, Maryland

James C. Yang
Doctor
Surgery Branch
National Cancer Institute
Bethesda, Maryland

Emerging Cancer Therapeutics

VOLUME 3, ISSUE 3

Melanoma

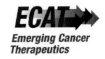

Preventing Melanoma

Barbara Summerer, Sewon Kang, and Timothy Wang*

Department of Dermatology, Johns Hopkins School of Medicine, Baltimore, MD

■ ABSTRACT

Currently, there exists no sure way to prevent melanoma. However, epidemiologic evidence suggests that some melanomas may be prevented by limiting ultraviolet (UV) exposure. Campaigns aimed at educating the public on decreasing UV exposure and the detrimental effects of UV radiation are major tools in reducing the risk of melanoma. General recommendations include wearing sun protective clothing and UV filtering sunglasses, avoiding sun exposure during peak hours, and applying broad spectrum sunscreen. Substances applied to the skin or taken internally as chemoprevention hold potential, but to date none has been proven effective. Until better means of prevention are identified and established, early diagnosis and treatment of melanoma offer the greatest opportunity to reducing its morbidity and mortality. Therefore, much of current work is focused on screening strategies for at-risk and at large populations. Imaging techniques such as dermoscopy and computerized analysis technologies hold promise as useful tools in the evaluation of pigmented lesions. As the worldwide incidence of melanoma continues to rise, public education, prevention and detection strategies can hopefully help to reduce the morbidity and mortality associated with this malignancy.

Keywords: skin cancer, ultraviolet (UV) radiation, sun protection, sunscreen, chemoprevention, screening

*Corresponding author, Department of Dermatology, Johns Hopkins School of Medicine, Baltimore, MD
  E-mail address: twang49@jhmi.edu

Emerging Cancer Therapeutics 3:3 (2012) 391–404.
DOI: 10.5003/2151–4194.3.3.391

demosmedpub.com/ecat

■ INTRODUCTION

The worldwide incidence of melanoma in fair-skinned populations has rapidly been increasing. Over the last 30 years in the United States, melanoma incidence has increased at least three fold. At this rate, it is estimated that one in 36 American males and one in 55 American females will develop invasive melanoma during their lifetime (1). According to data obtained from the National Cancer Institute's Surveillance, Epidemiology, and End Results (SEER) registry, the median age at melanoma diagnosis in the United States is 61 years, with 83% of the cases diagnosed after the age of 45. The median age at death from melanoma is 68 years, with 91.7% dying from melanoma after the age of 45 (2). Patients with ethnic skin types are more likely to have more advanced disease at the time of diagnosis and have lower melanoma-specific survival than Caucasians (3).

Currently, no skin cancer, including melanoma, is entirely preventable. However, recent stability in the incidence of melanoma and melanoma-related mortality in countries where sun avoidance/protections and surveillance strategies were implemented decades ago (4,5) provides epidemiological evidence that at least some melanomas and deaths because of melanoma may be preventable.

Primary prevention describes measures that can be taken to decrease the risk of developing melanoma. These include decreasing exposure to ultraviolet (UV) light and chemopreventative agents. Secondary prevention refers to the reduction of melanoma-related morbidity and mortality through early diagnosis and treatment. Recognizing the genotypic and phenotypic risk factors associated with melanoma will help identify high-risk patients who might benefit most from primary and secondary preventive measures (6).

In this chapter, we will review current thought and research relevant to the prevention of melanoma and reducing its morbidity and mortality through early diagnosis.

■ PRIMARY PREVENTION

The only known preventable factor in the development of melanoma is avoidance of UV radiation (7–9). Campaigns aimed at educating the public on the dangers of UV radiation and reducing UV exposure are major tools in decreasing the risk of developing melanoma.

Ultraviolet Radiation and Skin Cancer

The main source of natural UV radiation is the sun. Although the sun emits electromagnetic (EM) radiation across most of the EM spectrum, the portion that strikes the earth's atmosphere consists of wavelengths ranging from approximately 100 nm to 1 mm. This includes wavelengths that range from the UV through visible light and the infrared spectrums. UV light is most important in the formation of skin cancer, and its spectrum is divided into UVC (100–280 nm), UVB (280–320 nm), and UVA (320–400 nm). Nearly all UV radiation with wavelengths below 290 nm is absorbed in the upper atmosphere; therefore, 6% of the UV radiation that strikes the earth's surface is UVB, and 94% is UVA.

The wavelength of light affects its biologic effect on the skin. UVB penetrates only the epidermis, whereas UVA penetrates into the papillary and upper reticular dermis. UVA is implicated in immediate tanning (minutes) caused by the oxidation of preexisting melanin and/

or redistribution of melanin granules, whereas UVB is more responsible for delayed tanning (days) because of increased production of melanin (10). The energy contained in light is inversely proportional to its wavelength, and UVB is 1,000 times more potent at causing erythema (sunburn) than UVA. UVB can directly damage the DNA, inducing cyclobutane pyrimidine dimers (CPDs) and 6-pyrimidine 4-pyrimidone photoproducts. The CPDs give rise to DNA mutations hallmarked by C to T (C–T) and CC to TT (CC–TT) transitions, the so-called "UVB signature mutations" (11). Frequent detection of CC–TT mutations in nonmelanoma skin cancers supports a major role for UVB radiation in carcinogenesis. UVA, on the other hand, can indirectly damage the DNA by generating reactive oxygen species (ROS), including hydrogen peroxide, hydroxyl radicals, superoxide, singlet oxygen, and peroxyl radicals (11,12). This skin's failure to successfully repair DNA damage can lead to skin cancer. Patients with xeroderma pigmentosum, an autosomal recessive genetic disorder of DNA repair, often develop numerous skin cancers at a young age.

UV light can also affect the local immunity in the skin and cause systemic immunosuppression through mechanisms not fully elucidated. It is known that UV exposure leads to depletion of epidermal dendritic cells (Langerhans cells), thereby interfering with antigen presentation in the skin (13). Keratinocytes damaged by UV exposure can release a number of cytokines, including interleukin (IL)-1β, tumor necrosis factor (TNF)-α, and IL-10, which can activate suppressor T cells (12). Mast cells, fibroblasts, endothelial cells, and dermal dendritic cells have all been shown to be involved in UV-induced immunosuppression (14). The importance of the immune system in preventing cutaneous malignancies

is highlighted by the increased number of skin cancers, including melanoma seen in immunosuppressed transplant patients (15). Inflammation is critical to the production of a tumor-promoting microenvironment. UV-induced damage to cellular membranes can lead to the production of proinflammatory cytokines, and the inflammatory cascade amplifies the production of ROS, resulting in DNA damage (16).

Although the relationship between UV radiation and nonmelanoma skin cancers is well established, the link between UV exposure and melanoma is less robust.

Data that support UV exposure as a causative factor in melanoma carcinogenesis derive from epidemiologic and experimental studies. Epidemiologic studies have demonstrated increased melanoma risk in (a) fair-skinned individuals living in equatorial regions with the most intense UVB radiation (17–19); (b) people with intermittent extreme sun exposure and sunburns (18,20); (c) users of tanning beds (21); and (d) psoriasis patients treated over long periods with oral psoralen plus UVA (PUVA) (22).

Experimental studies linked UV radiation and melanoma genesis in several animal models (23–25), but the mechanisms and the wavelengths responsible have remained elusive. Only recently, it has been demonstrated that UVA can induce melanoma in vivo via oxidative DNA damage in melanocytes but requires the presence of melanin. UVB, on the other hand, promoted melanoma genesis by a melanin-independent pathway with direct DNA damage and seemed to be more effective in inducing gene expression response in melanocytes than UVA (25). In addition, whole-genome and exome sequencing studies have revealed UVB mutational signatures in human melanoma tumors and cell lines (26,27).

In addition to DNA damage, UV can modify the interaction between melanocytes and elements of their microenvironment. Inflammatory mechanisms centered at interferon signaling have been linked to UVB-induced melanoma genesis in vivo (24). Recent studies in a murine melanoma model have indicated the significance of UVB-mediated systemic immunosuppression and tumor progression in a process involving IL-10 and regulatory T cells (28).

Because of UV radiation's effect on nonmelanoma and, possibly, melanoma carcinogenesis, several measures have been implemented to decrease overexposure to UV radiation.

Limiting UV Exposure by Avoidance and Photoprotection

Increased lifetime exposure to excessive sunlight and a history of severe sunburns are associated with an increased risk of melanoma.

Although no study has clearly demonstrated a decrease in melanoma risk by the reduction of UV exposure, interventions to reduce UV exposure are generally endorsed (5,29). Public health measures, including Australia's "Slip! Slop! Slap! Wrap!" and "SunSmart" programs, encourage UV protective behaviors, particularly for minors. Longitudinal multifaceted approaches have been found to be more successful in younger children than in adolescents, who show stronger attitudes against sun-protective behaviors (30). A slight decline in the melanoma incidence rates in Australia's younger cohorts may indicate that their primary prevention programs are successfully shifting attitudes and behaviors related to UV exposure (4,5). Continued evidence of efficacy is likely to encourage other countries to develop and implement melanoma prevention programs tailored to their citizens.

General recommendations for reducing UV exposure include seeking shade, avoiding the sun between peak hours of UV radiation (between 10 a.m. and 4 p.m.), wearing protective clothing, applying sunscreen, putting on a broad-brimmed hat, and wearing UV-filtering sunglasses.

UV Index

Developed by the World Health Organization (WHO), the UV index (UVI) is a measure of the UV radiation striking the earth during peak hours. Numbers range from 0 and 11, where higher numbers denote greater potential for UV-induced damage to the skin and eyes. The UVI is intended to encourage people to use sun protection and to raise awareness of the risk of excess sun exposure. A UVI of 0 to 2 denotes low risk for UV damage; a UVI of 3 to 7 denotes medium to high risk, where wearing UV protective clothing, seeking shade, and the use of sunscreen and UV blocking sunglasses are advised; and a UVI of 8 or higher denotes extreme risk, where avoidance of exposure during peak hours, wearing UV protective clothing, seeking shade, and using sunglasses and sunscreen are strongly advised. In the U.S., the Environmental Protection Agency (EPA) and the National Weather Service publish their forecast UVI daily on the EPA website (http://www.epa.gov/sunwise/uvindex.html).

Sun-Protective Clothing

Clothing is one of the most effective protective measures against UV radiation. Long-sleeved shirts with high necklines, long pants, and brimmed hats offer good protection. In general, tightly woven darker color fabrics offer better protection than loosely woven lighter colors, and dry clothing offers better protection than wet clothing. The degree of protection provided by clothes is defined by the Ultraviolet Protection Factor (UPF), which is now widely used on outdoor wear. There are two methods for determining the UPF. The in vivo method records the minimal erythema dose with and without textiles on test subjects and is an indicator of UVB protection. The in vitro method uses a spectrophotometer to measure the UV (both UVA and UVB) transmission of the fabric and calculates the UPF from this value (31). Clothing can be classified by UPF as providing "good protection" (UPF 15–24), "very good protection" (UPF 25–39), and "excellent protection" (UPF 40 to 50+). A UPF of 15 blocks 93.3% of UV radiation, whereas a UPF of 50+ blocks 98% of UV radiation. To increase their UPF, some fabrics are pretreated with special UV-absorbing chemicals when manufactured or can be washed with UV-absorbing detergents. In general, clothing blocks more UVB transmission than UVA.

Sunscreen

In the 1930s, tanning became fashionable in Western countries, and people began to deliberately expose their skin to the sun. One of the first sunscreens was invented in 1938 by the Austrian chemist Franz Greiter, who, after being sunburned while climbing the glacier Piz Buin, was inspired to develop a sun protection formula that he called "Gletscher Crème" (Glacier Cream). In 1962, Greiter also introduced the term sun protection factor (SPF), which has become a standard used for assessing the effectiveness of sunscreen. As currently used, SPF refers to the amount of UVB radiation required to cause a sunburn on the skin with sunscreen on compared with that required to cause sunburn without sunscreen. Because sunburn is mainly caused by UVB, SPF refers to the amount of protection that the sunscreen offers against UVB only and gives limited information about UVA protection.

Active ingredients in sunscreens either scatter or absorb light energy that reaches the skin.

Agents that scatter radiation contain inorganic opaque particles and are referred to as physical sunscreens. The two major inorganic sunscreens are zinc oxide and titanium dioxide. Both provide protection against UVA and UVB radiation. Zinc oxide offers somewhat greater protection from UVA than titanium dioxide. The activity of inorganic sunscreens also depends on the particle size; larger particles offer broader UVA protection.

Agents that use organic compounds to absorb UV radiation are referred to as chemical sunscreens. Most organic sunscreens absorb UVB; however, several new sunscreens also absorb UVA and have recently been approved for use in the United States.

Both physical and chemical sunscreens are considered over-the-counter drugs and are regulated in the United States by the Food and Drug Administration (FDA). Recognizing the public's confusion with regard to SPF and sunscreen labeling, the FDA issued an updated monograph on sunscreens in 2011 and instituted new regulations with regard to their activity and labeling. Under these new guidelines, SPF continues to describe the amount of UVB protection offered by sunscreen. However, the amount of UVA protection must now be proportional to the SPF. Only sunscreens that offer adequate protection against both UVA and UVB radiation can be labeled as "broad spectrum." Products that contain an SPF of 15 or higher can now state on the label that, if used as directed with other sun protection measures, sunscreen decreases the risk of skin cancer and early skin aging caused by the sun. The FDA specified that shampoos, body washes, towelettes, and powders are currently not acceptable as sunscreen products (32).

Although several trials have shown that sunscreens are effective in preventing squamous cell carcinoma, evidence of their effectiveness in preventing basal cell carcinoma and melanoma is limited. The use of sunscreen plays a major role in skin cancer prevention programs and is endorsed by the American Academy of Dermatology (AAD), which recommends the use of broad spectrum sunscreens with an SPF of 30 during sun exposure and cautions that sunscreens should be used to reduce UV exposure rather than to extend the allowable time spent in direct sunlight.

Vitamin D

Vitamin D is important in calcium homeostasis and bone metabolism and is essential for immune regulation. Cardiovascular disease, diabetes, and certain cancers have also been linked to vitamin D deficiency (33). It is estimated that 40% to 90% of elderly men and women in the United States and Europe are deficient in vitamin D (34–36).

Vitamin D_3 (cholecalciferol) is synthesized in the skin by exposure of 7-dehydrocholesterol to UVB. Vitamin D_3 is then hydroxylated in the liver to 25-hydroxyvitamin D (25-OHD), which is the main circulating and storage form of vitamin D. Further hydroxylation of 25-hydroxyvitamin D occurs in the kidneys to form the active hormone, 1,25-dihydroxycholecalciferol vitamin D (1,25-[OH]$_2$D$_3$) (37). Approximately 90% of the body's total vitamin D is synthesized in the skin during sun exposure, and suberythemal doses of UV exposure are thought to be adequate to satisfy the body's vitamin D requirements; yet, large portions of the population remain vitamin D deficient. The reasons for this paradox are not entirely clear, and balancing the risk of UV induced skin cancer with the risk of vitamin D deficiency is a matter of current debate. There is no scientifically validated, safe threshold level of UV exposure that allows for adequate vitamin D synthesis without increasing skin cancer risk (38). The AAD recommends that vitamin D is obtained from diet (including vitamin D-rich foods such as fish oil and eggs), fortified foods and beverages, and vitamin D supplements. The Institute of Medicine has no recommendation on the use of sun exposure to meet vitamin D requirements.

Indoor Tanning

In 2009, the International Agency for Research on Cancer (IARC), a part of the WHO, concluded that there is sufficient evidence that UV causes cancer in humans and thus classified natural and artificial UV radiation as a group 1 carcinogen (7). A comprehensive meta-analysis conducted by the IARC showed a 75% increase in melanoma incidence for individuals who started using tanning beds before the age of 30 (relative risk 1.75; 95% CI 1.35–2.26) (21). On the basis of these results, the WHO recommends avoiding indoor tanning, particularly in minors (7,9). Several European countries currently restrict the use of tanning beds for people under the age of 18. In the United States, California, Vermont, and Rhode Island prohibit the use of indoor tanning beds by persons under the age of 18 without parental consent (39).

Chemoprevention of Melanoma

Chemoprevention is the use of natural or synthetic agents to prevent, suppress, or delay the progression of premalignant lesions into invasive cancers (40–42). Such an agent would ideally reduce melanoma incidence, mortality, and recurrence rate. Understanding the molecular mechanisms behind melanoma carcinogenesis and the interaction between transformed melanocytes and their microenvironment is critical to designing chemopreventive treatments (40,43). UV radiation may be an initiating event in some melanomas (12), and chemoprevention of these should ideally address events such as apoptosis of cells with DNA damaged by UV light, inhibit adverse oxidative stress and enhance DNA repair, and beneficially influence the local and systemic immune responses (40). Although several agents are currently evaluated, none has yet been proved as effective and further research is needed.

Statins and Fibrates

Case-control studies, animal models, and in vitro experiments have suggested that lipid-lowering drugs such as statins and fibrates may be useful for cancer prevention based on their antiproliferative, proapoptotic, anti-invasive, and immunomodulatory effects (44). Several meta-analyses of clinical trials, however, have so far failed to provide evidence that they reduce the risk of developing melanoma (45,46).

Metformin

The antidiabetes drug metformin inhibits growth in a number of cancer cell lines, including prostate, breast, tobacco-induced lung cancer, and cutaneous squamous cell carcinoma (SCCs) (47). In a recent study, however, metformin failed to inhibit BRAF V600E mutant melanoma cells in vitro and accelerated the growth of BRAF mutant tumors in mice. Therefore, although metformin is promising as a chemopreventative in other cancers, its role in melanoma chemoprevention is less clear at this time.

Retinoids

Retinoids can modulate cell proliferation, differentiation and apoptosis, and the expression of growth factors and inhibit the function of the oncogenic transcription factor activator protein 1 (AP-1) and Wnt/-catenin signaling pathways (48). Systemic retinoids are currently used as chemoprevention for nonmelanoma skin cancer in high-risk patients (49,50). Recently, a novel synthetic retinoid has been shown to induce apoptosis and cell cycle arrest in human melanoma cell lines (51). Currently, however, there is no FDA-approved indication for retinoids in skin cancer prevention.

Nonsteroidal Anti-Inflammatory Drugs

In vitro and animal studies have shown antineoplastic effects of nonsteroidal anti-inflammatory drugs (NSAIDs) in skin cancer (52–54). However, clinical studies investigating the effects of NSAIDs in melanoma prevention have found conflicting results (55,56). Future studies will determine if NSAIDs play a role in melanoma chemoprevention.

Antioxidants

Resveratrol is produced by a variety of plants, such as red grapes, mulberries, peanuts, and cocoa, in response to stress, UV radiation, and fungal infections (57,58). Preclinical studies have shown its antioxidant, anti-inflammatory, and antiproliferative effects (59,60). Resveratrol protected against DNA damage by inhibiting hydroperoxidases and scavenging free radicals and inhibited UV-induced AP-1-mediated activity by interfering with mitogen-activated protein kinase (MAPK) pathways in vitro (61,62). Several clinical trials that assess the chemopreventive properties of resveratrol are ongoing.

Often used as a spice in India and Southeast Asia, *curcumin* is a yellow pigment obtained from the turmeric rhizome (*Curcuma longa*). Curcumin can induce apoptosis in human melanoma cells through the inhibition of several critical pathways, such as the NF-κB cell-survival pathway and the Fas receptor/caspase 8 pathway (42,63).

Numerous other bioavailable antioxidants, such as *epigallocatechin-3-gallate* (EGCG) in green tea or *silymarin* in the milk thistle, are also potential chemopreventive agents (64–67), but data that support their use in melanoma is scarce.

Secondary Prevention

Although melanoma is currently not entirely preventable, early diagnosis and treatment significantly decreases its morbidity and mortality. To promote earlier detection and treatment of melanoma, screening skin exams, public education in melanoma's clinical appearance, and new devices for clinicians have been developed.

Screening

Patient performed self-skin exams (SSE) and physician-performed total-body skin exams (TBSEs) are key components in the early detection of melanoma. Physicians tend to detect thinner melanomas than nonphysicians do (0.68 vs. 0.90 mm) (68), supporting the role of screening skin exams by physicians. In addition, the value of education and SSEs is supported by an Australian study that showed that patients who performed SSEs were diagnosed with thinner melanomas than those who did not (69). Unfortunately, despite education on the importance of SSEs, few patients seem to regularly perform SSEs (68,69). Patient education on the "ABCDEs of melanoma" and the "Ugly duckling sign" can help patients notice suspicious lesions and bring them to the attention of their physicians.

Aitken et al. (70) reported that TBSE reduces the incidence of thick melanomas and suggested that TBSE screening would also reduce melanoma mortality. To date, however, no comprehensive set of data that proves the benefit of mass screening programs in reducing melanoma mortality exists (71,72). Providing some new insight, however, a prospective population-based screening project in Germany demonstrated increased detection of early stage melanomas, with a subsequent decrease in melanoma mortality rate by 50% (73).

Performing TBSEs on all patients can help detect occult skin cancers. The time and cost of such screening programs, however, may make them difficult in a resource-limited environment. Argenziano et al. estimated that, in patients who are not scheduled to undergo skin examination, TBSEs need to be performed on 47 patients for one skin malignancy to be detected and on 400 patients to detect one melanoma. Older patients with focal skin symptoms, a history of previous skin cancer, fair skin type, "skin tumor" as a reason for consultation, and the presence of an equivocal lesion on uncovered areas were found to more likely harbor skin cancer, and thus, TBSEs were recommended in these high-risk patients (74).

Risk Factors for Developing Melanoma
Known risk factors for melanoma include fair skin, blue eyes, a personal or family history of melanoma, excess sun exposure and sunburns, a number of atypical appearing nevi, long-term PUVA therapy, and immunosuppression. Patients with genetic syndromes such as the familial atypical multiple mole-melanoma syndrome (FAMMM) characterized by familial melanoma and multiple atypical nevi in one or more first- or second-

degree relatives are also at elevated risk for melanoma. High-risk members of FAMMM families should closely be followed beginning in adolescence (6,75). Male sex and lower socioeconomic status are also risk factors for later detection of melanoma (76).

In the absence of randomized trials that establish the efficacy of screening for melanoma, recommendations from expert groups vary. The AAD recommends high-risk individuals to seek professional evaluation of the skin at least once per year and to be educated with regard to the need for SSE and sun protection. Outside these risk groups, routine screening is not recommended by the AAD.

Diagnostic Tools

Several imaging technologies are used in clinical practice to identify potential melanoma precursor lesions and to improve diagnostic accuracy.

Dermoscopy

Dermoscopy, also known as skin surface or epiluminescence microscopy, uses a handheld magnifying lens and polarized light source to allow visualization of skin structures and patterns not visible to the naked eye. Structures in the epidermis, dermal-epidermal junction, and superficial dermis can be evaluated. Dermoscopic features of melanoma include asymmetry, the presence of multiple colors, an atypical network, streaks, irregular blood vessels, regression, a blue-white veil, and atypical dots and globules. Studies have demonstrated that the use of dermoscopy by trained and experienced physicians, can lead to earlier detection of featureless melanomas and decrease the number of benign biopsies (77,78). In the hands of experienced users, dermoscopy can be an effective technique to aid in the early recognition of melanoma. However, even for experts, diagnostic challenges will remain for many lesions (79,80).

Automated Analysis Devices

The majority of optical imaging and automated analysis devices used in the detection of melanoma are based on algorithms of dermoscopy. In Australia and Europe, several diagnostic systems have been approved and registered as medical devices. In the United States, diagnostic systems are registered as diagnostic aids and require approval of the FDA (81). In 2011, the first automated multispectral computer imaging system (MelaFind, MELA Sciences, Inc.) for use on atypical pigmented lesions received FDA clearance. The device is approved for use by trained dermatologists to obtain additional information on atypical pigmented skin lesions and help decide on whether to biopsy and is not intended to diagnose melanoma.

Studies have shown that an automated digital dermoscopy system can achieve diagnostic sensitivity and specificity comparable to expert dermatologists when evaluating pigmented lesions (82–84).

Total Body Photography

Total body photography (TBP) can be a useful tool in the identification of new or changing lesions in patients with high risk for melanoma, usually in the context of multiple dysplastic nevi, previous melanoma, or family history of melanoma. The availability of baseline TBP images, including overview pictures of the whole skin surface, selected close-ups of pigmented lesions, and dermoscopic images can be used to track existing pigmented lesions and detect new lesions in high-risk patients (81). With regular follow-up visits, TBP can increase the sensitivity for melanoma detection (85,86).

Other Noninvasive Techniques

Confocal laser scanning microscopy (CLSM) allows for real-time imaging of microanatomic cutaneous structures. Taking advantage of the strong natural contrast of melanin, CLSM can be used for diagnosis of melanocytic lesions, providing high-power morphologic information. A recent study found that CLSM in combination with clinical examination and dermoscopy is a valuable additional tool for noninvasive skin tumor diagnosis and can help reduce unnecessary biopsies. However, CLSM devices are still in the experimental stage and should be reserved to academic institutions in a research setting (80,87).

Aside from CLSM, several noninvasive imaging devices focus on the analysis of morphologic and pathophysiologic changes in melanoma. Examples include multispectral image analysis, optical coherence tomography, high-resolution ultrasound, Raman spectroscopy, and electrical impedance scanning. However, all these methods are not yet fully optimized for melanoma detection and remain under development.

■ CONCLUSION

Currently, no certain way of preventing melanoma exists. Epidemiologic evidence suggests that some melanomas may be prevented by limiting UV exposure; thus, measures of avoiding overexposure to UV radiation are generally recommended. Chemopreventive strategies have the potential to address the heterogeneity of melanoma carcinogenesis and progression; to date, however, no drug has been proved to be effective and safe in melanoma prevention.

Early recognition and treatment of melanoma may offer the greatest opportunity for reducing disease mortality. Several imaging technologies such as traditional dermoscopy and automated digital analysis devices hold promise as useful tools to more objectively evaluate pigmented lesions.

Given the increasing incidence of this disease worldwide, with improved melanoma detection strategies and the development of successful chemopreventive agents, we should seek to significantly reduce melanoma-related morbidity and mortality.

■ REFERENCES

1. Siegel R, Naishadham D, Jemal A. Cancer statistics. *CA Cancer J Clin.* 2012;62:10–29.
2. Howlader N, Noone AM, Krapcho M, et al. (Eds). *SEER Cancer Statistics Review, 1975–2009 (Vintage 2009 Populations).* Bethesda, MD: National Cancer Institute. http://seer.cancer.gov/csr/1975_2009_pops09/, based on November 2011 SEER data submission, posted to the SEER website, April 2012 (accessed July 13, 2012).
3. Wu XC, Eide MJ, King J, et al. Racial and ethnic variations in incidence and survival of cutaneous melanoma in the United States, 1999–2006. *J Am Acad Dermatol.* 2011;65:S26–37.
4. van der Leest RJ, de Vries E, Bulliard JL, et al. The Euromelanoma skin cancer prevention campaign in Europe: characteristics and results of 2009 and 2010. *J Eur Acad Dermatol Venereol.* 2011;25:1455–1456.
5. Erdmann F, Lortet-Tieulent J, Schuz J, et al. International trends in the incidence of malignant melanoma 1953–2008: are recent generations at higher or lower risk? *Int J Cancer.* 2012.
6. Psaty EL, Scope A, Halpern AC, Marghoob AA. Defining the patient at high risk for melanoma. *Int J Dermatol.* 2010;49:362–76.
7. El Ghissassi F, Baan R, Straif K, et al. A review of human carcinogens—part D: radiation. *Lancet Oncol.* 2009;10:751–2.
8. Chang YM, Barrett JH, Bishop DT, et al. Sun exposure and melanoma risk at different latitudes: a pooled analysis of 5700 cases and 7216 controls. *Int J Epidemiol.* 2009;38:814–30.

9. Fisher DE, James WD. Indoor tanning—science, behavior, and policy. *N Engl J Med.* 2010;363:901–3.

10. Gilchrest BA, Park HY, Eller MS, Yaar M. Mechanisms of ultraviolet light-induced pigmentation. *Photochem Photobiol.* 1996; 63:1–10.

11. Black HS, deGruijl FR, Forbes PD, et al. Photocarcinogenesis: an overview. *J Photochem Photobiol B.* 1997;40:29–47.

12. Kanavy HE, Gerstenblith MR. Ultraviolet radiation and melanoma. *Semin Cutan Med Surg.* 2011;30:222–8.

13. Schwarz T. Mechanisms of UV-induced immunosuppression. *Keio J Med.* 2005;54:165–71.

14. Sarchio SN, Kok LF, O'Sullivan C, Halliday GM, Byrne SN. Dermal mast cells affect the development of sunlight-induced skin tumours. *Exp Dermatol.* 2012;21:241–8.

15. DePry JL, Reed KB, Cook-Norris RH, Brewer JD. Iatrogenic immunosuppression and cutaneous malignancy. *Clin Dermatol.* 2011;29:602–13.

16. Nishigori C. Cellular aspects of photocarcinogenesis. *Photochem Photobiol Sci.* 2006;5:208–14.

17. Autier P, Dore JF, Gefeller O, et al. Melanoma risk and residence in sunny areas. *Br J Cancer.* 1997;76:1521–4.

18. Gilchrest BA, Eller MS, Geller AC, Yaar M. The pathogenesis of melanoma induced by ultraviolet radiation. *N Engl J Med.* 1999;340:1341–8.

19. Armstrong BK, Kricker A. The epidemiology of UV induced skin cancer. *J Photochem Photobiol B.* 2001;63:8–18.

20. Garbe C, Leiter U. Melanoma epidemiology and trends. *Clin Dermatol.* 2009;27:3–9.

21. International Agency for Research on Cancer Working Group on Artificial Ultraviolet (UV) Light and Skin Cancer. The association of use of sunbeds with cutaneous malignant melanoma and other skin cancers: a systematic review. *Int J Cancer.* 2007; 120:1116–22.

22. Stern RS. PUVA follow-up study: the risk of melanoma in association with long-term exposure to PUVA. *J Am Acad Dermatol.* 2001;44:755–61.

23. Wood SR, Berwick M, Ley RD, Walter RB, Setlow RB, Timmins GS. UV causation of melanoma in Xiphophorus is dominated by melanin photosensitized oxidant production. *Proc Natl Acad Sci USA.* 2006;103:4111–5.

24. Zaidi MR, Davis S, Noonan FP, et al. Interferon-gamma links ultraviolet radiation to melanomagenesis in mice. *Nature.* 2011; 469:548–53.

25. Noonan FP, Zaidi MR, Wolnicka-Glubisz A, et al. Melanoma induction by ultraviolet A but not ultraviolet B radiation requires melanin pigment. *Nat Commun.* 2012;3:884.

26. Pleasance ED, Cheetham RK, Stephens PJ, et al. A comprehensive catalogue of somatic mutations from a human cancer genome. *Nature.* 2010;463:191–6.

27. Wei X, Walia V, Lin JC, et al. Exome sequencing identifies GRIN2A as frequently mutated in melanoma. *Nat Genet.* 2011;43:442–6.

28. Sahu RP, Turner MJ, Dasilva SC, et al. The environmental stressor ultraviolet B radiation inhibits murine antitumor immunity through its ability to generate platelet-activating factor agonists. *Carcinogenesis.* 2012.

29. Savage P. Malignant melanoma (non-metastatic). *Clin Evid (Online).* 2007;2007:1705.

30. Hart KM, Demarco RF. Primary prevention of skin cancer in children and adolescents: a review of the literature. *J Pediatr Oncol Nurs.* 2008;25:67–78.

31. Majumdar A, Kothari VK, Mondal AK, Hatua P. Effect of weave, structural parameters and ultraviolet absorbers on in vitro protection factor of bleached cotton woven fabrics. *Photodermatol Photoimmunol Photomed.* 2012; 28:58–67.

32. Printz C. Dermatology community applauds new FDA sunscreen regulations: labeling requirements aim to make it easier for consumers to select a sunscreen. *Cancer.* 2012; 118:1–3.

33. Giovannucci E. The epidemiology of vitamin D and cancer incidence and mortality: a review (United States). *Cancer Causes Control.* 2005;16:83–95.

34. Lips P. Vitamin D deficiency and secondary hyperparathyroidism in the elderly: consequences for bone loss and fractures and therapeutic implications. *Endocr Rev.* 2001;22:477–501.

35. Zgaga L, Theodoratou E, Farrington SM, et al. Diet, environmental factors, and lifestyle underlie the high prevalence of vitamin D deficiency in healthy adults in Scotland, and supplementation reduces the proportion that are severely deficient. *J Nutr.* 2011;141:1535–42.

36. Garrett-Mayer E, Wagner CL, Hollis BW, Kindy MS, Gattoni-Celli S. Vitamin D3

supplementation (4000 IU/d for 1 y) eliminates differences in circulating 25-hydroxyvitamin D between African American and white men. *Am J Clin Nutr.* 2012;96:332–6.

37. Gandini S, Raimondi S, Gnagnarella P, Dore JF, Maisonneuve P, Testori A. Vitamin D and skin cancer: a meta-analysis. *Eur J Cancer.* 2009;45:634–41.

38. Ministry of Health and Cancer Society of New Zealand. *Consensus Statement on Vitamin D and Sun Exposure in New Zealand.* Wellington: Ministry of Health; March 2012.

39. AAD Indoor tanning. http://www.aad.org/media-resources/stats-and-facts/prevention-and-care/indoor-tanning (accessed July 16, 2012).

40. Lao CD, Demierre MF, Sondak VK. Targeting events in melanoma carcinogenesis for the prevention of melanoma. *Expert Rev Anticancer Ther.* 2006;6:1559–68.

41. Demierre MF. What about chemoprevention for melanoma? *Curr Opin Oncol.* 2006;18:180–4.

42. Zheng YY, Viswanathan B, Kesarwani P, Mehrotra S. Dietary Agents in Cancer Prevention: An Immunological Perspective (dagger). *Photochem Photobiol.* 2012;88(5):1083–98.

43. Francis SO, Mahlberg MJ, Johnson KR, Ming ME, Dellavalle RP. Melanoma chemoprevention. *J Am Acad Dermatol.* 2006;55:849–61.

44. Demierre MF, Higgins PD, Gruber SB, Hawk E, Lippman SM. Statins and cancer prevention. *Nat Rev Cancer.* 2005;5:930–42.

45. Dellavalle RP, Drake A, Graber M, et al. Statins and fibrates for preventing melanoma. *Cochrane Database Syst Rev.* 2005;(4):CD003697.

46. Kuoppala J, Lamminpaa A, Pukkala E. Statins and cancer: A systematic review and meta-analysis. *Eur J Cancer.* 2008;44:2122–3.

47. Tomic T, Botton T, Cerezo M, et al. Metformin inhibits melanoma development through autophagy and apoptosis mechanisms. *Cell Death Dis.* 2011;2:e199.

48. Tarapore RS, Siddiqui IA, Mukhtar H. Modulation of Wnt/beta-catenin signaling pathway by bioactive food components. *Carcinogenesis.* 2012;33:483–91.

49. Prado R, Francis SO, Mason MN, Wing G, Gamble RG, Dellavalle R. Nonmelanoma skin cancer chemoprevention. *Dermatol Surg.* 2011; 37:1566–78.

50. Lien MH, Fenske NA, Glass LF. Advances in the chemoprevention of non-melanoma skin cancer in high-risk organ transplant recipients. *Semin Oncol.* 2012;39:134–8.

51. Magnussen GI, Ree Rosnes AK, Shahzidi S, et al. Synthetic retinoid CD437 induces apoptosis and acts synergistically with TRAIL receptor-2 agonist in malignant melanoma. *Biochem Biophys Res Commun.* 2012;420:516–22.

52. Bode AM, Dong Z. Signal transduction pathways: targets for chemoprevention of skin cancer. *Lancet Oncol.* 2000;1:181–8.

53. Bair WB,3rd, Hart N, Einspahr J, et al. Inhibitory effects of sodium salicylate and acetylsalicylic acid on UVB-induced mouse skin carcinogenesis. *Cancer Epidemiol Biomarkers Prev.* 2002;11:1645–52.

54. Marks F, Furstenberger G, Neufang G, Muller-Decker K. Mouse skin as a model for cancer chemoprevention by nonsteroidal anti-inflammatory drugs. *Recent Results Cancer Res.* 2003;163:46,57; discussion 264–6.

55. Asgari MM, Maruti SS, White E. A large cohort study of nonsteroidal anti-inflammatory drug use and melanoma incidence. *J Natl Cancer Inst.* 2008;100:967–71.

56. Joosse A, Koomen ER, Casparie MK, Herings RM, Guchelaar HJ, Nijsten T. Nonsteroidal anti-inflammatory drugs and melanoma risk: large Dutch population-based case-control study. *J Invest Dermatol.* 2009; 129:2620–7.

57. Signorelli P, Ghidoni R. Resveratrol as an anticancer nutrient: molecular basis, open questions and promises. *J Nutr Biochem.* 2005;16:449–66.

58. Hurst WJ, Glinski JA, Miller KB, Apgar J, Davey MH, Stuart DA. Survey of the trans-resveratrol and trans-piceid content of cocoa-containing and chocolate products. *J Agric Food Chem.* 2008;56:8374–8.

59. Afaq F, Adhami VM, Ahmad N. Prevention of short-term ultraviolet B radiation-mediated damages by resveratrol in SKH-1 hairless mice. *Toxicol Appl Pharmacol.* 2003;186:28–37.

60. Burkitt MJ, Duncan J. Effects of trans-resveratrol on copper-dependent hydroxyl-radical formation and DNA damage: evidence for hydroxyl-radical scavenging and a novel, glutathione-sparing mechanism of action. *Arch Biochem Biophys.* 2000;381:253–6.

61. Aggarwal BB, Bhardwaj A, Aggarwal RS, Seeram NP, Shishodia S, Takada Y. Role of resveratrol in prevention and therapy of cancer: preclinical and clinical studies. *Anticancer Res.* 2004;24:2783–840.

62. Aziz MH, Reagan-Shaw S, Wu J, Longley BJ, Ahmad N. Chemoprevention of skin cancer by grape constituent resveratrol: relevance to human disease? *FASEB J.* 2005;19:1193–5.

63. Grandjean-Laquerriere A, Gangloff SC, Le Naour R, Trentesaux C, Hornebeck W, Guenounou M. Relative contribution of NF-kappaB and AP-1 in the modulation by curcumin and pyrrolidine dithiocarbamate of the UVB-induced cytokine expression by keratinocytes. *Cytokine.* 2002;18:168–77.

64. Katiyar S, Elmets CA, Katiyar SK. Green tea and skin cancer: photoimmunology, angiogenesis and DNA repair. *J Nutr Biochem.* 2007;18:287–96.

65. Singh T, Katiyar SK. Green tea catechins reduce invasive potential of human melanoma cells by targeting COX-2, PGE2 receptors and epithelial-to-mesenchymal transition. *PLoS One.* 2011;6:e25224.

66. Chen PN, Hsieh YS, Chiou HL, Chu SC. Silibinin inhibits cell invasion through inactivation of both PI3K-Akt and MAPK signaling pathways. *Chem Biol Interact.* 2005;156:141–50.

67. Gharagozloo M, Velardi E, Bruscoli S, et al. Silymarin suppress CD4+ T cell activation and proliferation: effects on NF-kappaB activity and IL-2 production. *Pharmacol Res.* 2010;61:405–9.

68. Carli P, De Giorgi V, Palli D, et al. Dermatologist detection and skin self-examination are associated with thinner melanomas: results from a survey of the Italian Multidisciplinary Group on Melanoma. *Arch Dermatol.* 2003;139:607–12.

69. Aitken JF, Janda M, Lowe JB, et al. Prevalence of whole-body skin self-examination in a population at high risk for skin cancer (Australia). *Cancer Causes Control.* 2004;15:453–6.

70. Aitken JF, Elwood M, Baade PD, Youl P, English D. Clinical whole-body skin examination reduces the incidence of thick melanomas. *Int J Cancer.* 2010;126:450–8.

71. Wolff T, Tai E, Miller T. Screening for skin cancer: an update of the evidence for the U.S. Preventive Services Task Force. *Ann Intern Med.* 2009;150:194–8.

72. Greinert R, Boniol M. Skin cancer—primary and secondary prevention (information campaigns and screening)—with a focus on children and sunbeds. *Prog Biophys Mol Biol.* 2011;107:473–6.

73. Breitbart EW, Waldmann A, Nolte S, et al. Systematic skin cancer screening in Northern Germany. *J Am Acad Dermatol.* 2012;66:201–1.

74. Argenziano G, Zalaudek I, Hofmann-Wellenhof R, et al. Total body skin examination for skin cancer screening in patients with focused symptoms. *J Am Acad Dermatol.* 2012;66:212–9.

75. Argenziano G, Kittler H, Ferrara G, et al. Slow-growing melanoma: a dermoscopy follow-up study. *Br J Dermatol.* 2010;162:267–73.

76. Geller AC, Swetter SM, Brooks K, Demierre MF, Yaroch AL. Screening, early detection, and trends for melanoma: current status (2000–2006) and future directions. *J Am Acad Dermatol.* 2007;57:555,72; quiz 573–6.

77. Altamura D, Avramidis M, Menzies SW. Assessment of the optimal interval for and sensitivity of short-term sequential digital dermoscopy monitoring for the diagnosis of melanoma. *Arch Dermatol.* 2008; 144:502–6.

78. Menzies SW, Emery J, Staples M, et al. Impact of dermoscopy and short-term sequential digital dermoscopy imaging for the management of pigmented lesions in primary care: a sequential intervention trial. *Br J Dermatol.* 2009;161:1270–7.

79. Argenziano G, Zalaudek I, Ferrara G, et al. Dermoscopy features of melanoma incognito: indications for biopsy. *J Am Acad Dermatol.* 2007;56:508–13.

80. Wang SQ, Hashemi P. Noninvasive imaging technologies in the diagnosis of melanoma. *Semin Cutan Med Surg.* 2010;29:174–8.

81. Menzies SW. Cutaneous melanoma: making a clinical diagnosis, present and future. *Dermatol Ther.* 2006;19:32–9.

82. Boldrick JC, Layton CJ, Nguyen J, Swetter SM. Evaluation of digital dermoscopy in a pigmented lesion clinic: clinician versus computer assessment of malignancy risk. *J Am Acad Dermatol.* 2007;56:417–21.

83. Baldi A, Murace R, Dragonetti E, et al. Definition of an automated Content-Based Image Retrieval (CBIR) system for the comparison of dermoscopic images of pigmented skin lesions. *Biomed Eng Online.* 2009;8:18.

84. Fruhauf J, Leinweber B, Fink-Puches R, et al. Patient acceptance and diagnostic utility of automated digital image analysis of pigmented skin lesions. *J Eur Acad Dermatol Venereol.* 2012;26:368–72.

85. Kittler H, Binder M. Risks and benefits of sequential imaging of melanocytic skin lesions in patients with multiple atypical nevi. *Arch Dermatol.* 2001;137:1590–5.

86. Salerni G, Carrera C, Lovatto L, et al. Characterization of 1152 lesions excised over 10 years using total-body photography and digital dermatoscopy in the surveillance of patients at high risk for melanoma. *J Am Acad Dermatol.* 2012.

87. Eichert S, Mohrle M, Breuninger H, Rocken M, Garbe C, Bauer J. Diagnosis of cutaneous tumors with in vivo confocal laser scanning microscopy. *J Dtsch Dermatol Ges.* 2010;8:400–1.

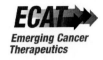

Evolution of the Melanoma Staging System

Rohit R. Sharma, Glen C. Balch, and Charles M. Balch*

*Department of Surgery, Division of Surgical Oncology,
UT Southwestern Medical Center, Dallas, TX*

■ ABSTRACT

The American Joint Committee on Cancer (AJCC) Melanoma Database consists of nearly 40,000 patients with stages I to IV melanoma. Critical analysis of this database has led to the publication of the seventh edition of the Melanoma Staging System, which went into effect in January 2010. It reflects an evidence-based evolution in our understanding of the natural history of melanoma biology. The Melanoma Staging and Classification System identifies and assigns significance to the most important clinical and pathologic factors that can be used to determine outcomes and guide the selection of therapy. The important melanoma-related prognostic factors identified from this database are primary tumor thickness, ulceration, mitotic rate, intralymphatic disease, regional nodal metastasis, and an elevated lactic dehydrogenase. The purpose of this chapter is to review the historical evolution of the melanoma staging system and to discuss the role of prognostic factors in the clinical management of this disease.

Keywords: cancer staging, prognostic factors, tumor thickness, level of invasion, mitotic rate, ulceration

*Corresponding author, Department of Surgery, Division of Surgical Oncology, UT Southwestern Medical Center, 5323 Harry Hines Blvd., Dallas, TX 75390
   E-mail address: charles.balch@utsouthwestern.edu

Emerging Cancer Therapeutics 3:3 (2012) 405–420.
© 2012 Demos Medical Publishing LLC. All rights reserved.
DOI: 10.5003/2151–4194.3.3.405

■ INTRODUCTION

Melanoma staging and classification have evolved since the original publications of Clark and Breslow elucidated the use of level of microinvasion through the skin and a measured depth of melanoma invasion using a micrometer, respectively, as important prognostic factors (1,2). Investigators have since attempted to identify additional clinical and prognostic factors that enable outcome prediction for melanoma patients and stratification within a cohesive staging system. The seventh edition of the melanoma staging system that is currently in effect represents an evidence-based approach that incorporates these advances in our understanding of the natural history of melanoma. The purpose of this chapter is to briefly present the historical evolution of the melanoma staging system and to discuss the role of important clinical and pathologic factors that determine prognosis and guide therapy.

■ HISTORICAL PERSPECTIVE

The first *Cancer Staging Manual* was published by the American Joint Committee on Cancer (AJCC) in 1977 and included a set of rules used for classifying malignant melanoma (Table 1) (3). This initial publication established the foundation on which subsequent versions of melanoma staging would be based. The classification system was controversial, because emerging research was beginning to show that the measured depth of invasion may have greater importance than the level of invasion for predicting melanoma prognosis. The authors decided at that time to include both prognostic factors until it could be demonstrated that one of these or another parameter was most accurate. As will be evident later, controversy was not limited

to the first edition of the melanoma staging system.

The subsequent four editions of the melanoma staging system continued to incorporate tumor thickness and level of invasion to characterize the primary tumor (3–7). Regional disease was described by the gross dimensions of involved lymph nodes and the number of intransit lesions. Distant metastatic disease was subcategorized by skin/subcutaneous or visceral involvement based on survival differences between these two groups.

During the time interval between the publication of the first and fifth editions of the melanoma staging system, accumulated data from single institution studies assisted in the elaboration of additional important prognostic factors for melanoma (e.g., ulceration, age, gender, site of melanoma, and primary tumor mitotic rate). Although these prognostic factors were incorporated into ongoing clinical trials, they had not yet been included in the melanoma staging system. This criticism led physicians to question the appropriateness of the melanoma staging system in effect at the time. Several publications have highlighted the controversial areas of melanoma staging published in the fifth edition of the *Cancer Staging Manual*, which included (a) defining optimal cutoffs for tumor thickness and the relevance of level of invasion; (b) recognizing the importance of ulceration as a prognostic factor; (c) acknowledging the prognostic implications of satellite lesions and local recurrences; and (d) eliminating the size of nodal metastases as a component of the N category (8–11).

To address the shortcomings of the fifth edition of the melanoma staging system, the AJCC assembled an international group of melanoma experts and formed the Melanoma Staging Committee in

TABLE 1   First edition of the melanoma staging system

Primary Tumor		
T1	Invasion of papillary dermis and/or less than 0.75 mm thickness	
	T1a	Satellite(s) within immediate or regional area of the primary lesion
	T1b	Intransit metastasis directed toward lymph node-draining basin
T2	Papillary-reticular dermis interface and/or 0.75 to 1.5 mm thickness	
	T2a	Satellite(s) within immediate or regional area of the primary lesion
	T2b	Intransit metastasis directed toward lymph node-draining basin
T3	Reticular dermis and/or 1.51 to 3.0 mm thickness	
	T3a	Satellite(s) within immediate or regional area of the primary lesion
	T3b	Intransit metastasis directed toward lymph node-draining basin
T4	Subcutaneous tissue and/or greater than 3 mm thickness	
	T4a	Satellite(s) within immediate or regional area of the primary lesion
	T4b	Intransit metastasis directed toward lymph node-draining basin

Nodal Involvement:	
N0	No regional lymph node involvement
N1	Regional lymph node involvement of first station nodes only
N2	Lymph node involvement other than first station nodes

Distant Metastasis:	
MX	Not assessed
M0	No known distant metastases
M1	Distant metastasis present: Specify site (pulmonary, osseous, hepatic, brain, lymph nodes, bone marrow, pleura, skin, eye, other)

Stage Grouping:	
Stage I	Any T N0 M0
Stage II	Any Ta, Tb, N0 or N1, M0
Stage III	Any T, Ta, or Tb, Any N, M1, or M2; Any T, Ta, or Tb, N1; N2, Any M

Source: Adapted from Ref. (3). Used with permission of the American Joint Committee on Cancer (AJCC), Chicago, Illinois. The original source for this material is the *AJCC Manual for Staging Cancer,* 1st edition (1977), published by Whiting Press.

1998. Their goal was to amalgamate the many clinical and pathologic factors reflecting the true biology of melanoma published in single institution studies into a cohesive melanoma staging system. This group included experts from 13 major melanoma centers and cooperative study groups spanning North America, Europe, and Australia. This was an unprecedented collaborative effort where the members agreed to merge their individual prospectively collected melanoma patient data into a single unified database to develop and validate a new evidence-based melanoma staging system. A statistical subcommittee developed the guidelines for standardized data submission from the 13 individual prospective databases. Survival analysis results from this unified database consisting of 17,600 patients led to the proposal of major changes to the melanoma staging system incorporated into the sixth edition of the *Cancer Staging Manual,* published in 2002 (12).

The new staging system emphasized melanoma tumor thickness as the primary factor for determining prognosis and assessing risk for metastases over level of invasion, which had been incorporated into earlier versions. This decision was not initially straightforward. Vollmer et al. (13) reported a meta-analysis of melanoma prognostic factors, concluding that "the majority (42 of 54 studies) of studies published until 1988 showed tumor thickness to be a more powerful prognostic factor than level of invasion (8 of 48 studies)." After publication of this study, the AJCC revised its staging recommendations for the third edition of the melanoma staging system, stating that tumor thickness should supersede the level of invasion in cases of prognostic discrepancy. This decision was then reversed at the time of publication of the fourth edition of the melanoma staging system to select the less favorable finding (i.e., thickness or level of invasion) when determining the T category. This reversal in the T category recommendations was likely influenced by a case series of 3,323 patients from the John Wayne Cancer Center, which demonstrated that both tumor thickness and level of invasion had prognostic significance when survival rates were analyzed in thickness groups of <1.5 mm or ≥1.5 mm (14). A subsequent study by Büttner et al. (15) swung the pendulum back again in favor of tumor thickness. Using a multivariate statistical analysis, they concluded that T category cutoff points of 1, 2, and 4 mm had a more powerful prognostic value than the existing system and worked well because of its simplicity. The level of invasion in this study was only significant for melanomas ≤1 mm in thickness. Results published from the analysis of a combined database from the University of Alabama (UAB) and the Sydney Melanoma Unit (SMU) of 4,568 melanoma patients added further

confirmation to the results in the study by Büttner et al. (11). The UAB/SMU group concluded that the best cutoffs for stratifying melanoma based on univariate analyses of survival curves were 1, 2, and 4 mm. When the previously accepted tumor thickness thresholds of 0.75, 1.5, and 4 mm were compared with the proposed strata, the older cutoffs poorly predicted survival. The level of invasion, once again, was statistically significant for melanomas ≤1 mm in thickness, but the absolute 10-year survival difference between levels was small and inconsistent (94.8% level II, 84.7% level III, and 88.6% level IV). They concluded that the level of invasion contributed little additional prognostic information beyond what was ascertainable from tumor thickness alone. Further weakening the case for using the level of invasion for melanoma staging was the presence of interobserver variability among pathologists when histologically determining this parameter (16,17). For these reasons, the T classification cutoffs were changed to whole-integer thresholds (1, 2, and 4 mm) and no longer as strongly influenced by the level of invasion. Clark's level of invasion now had a more limited role in identifying a subgroup of T1 melanomas at higher risk for metastases.

The changes to the sixth edition of the Melanoma Staging System extended beyond clarifying the role of primary tumor thickness and Clark's level of invasion as prognostic factors. Ulceration was now defined as the second most important prognostic factor after primary tumor thickness and, when present, identified a locally advanced lesion. Satellite lesions, previously included in the T category, were now grouped with intransit lesions in the N category. Stage III disease was modified to represent regional metastases from melanoma and no longer included melanomas >4 mm in thickness. The dimensions of nodal metastases were no longer considered to have prognostic significance. This was supplanted by the number of involved lymph nodes (1 vs. 2–3 vs. ≥4 positive nodes) and further subcategorized based on the presence of microscopic or macroscopic disease within the regional nodes. Stage IV disease was restructured to include an elevated lactic dehydrogenase (LDH) as an adverse prognostic indicator and a separate category for pulmonary metastases. Finally, data from sentinel lymph node biopsy procedures were included in the pathologic staging of melanoma. Clinical staging alone did not account for the prognostic information gleaned from this procedure, which has been performed with increasing frequency since the original description of the technique by Dr. Donald Morton (18).

Since the publication of this major revision to the melanoma staging system in 2002, the unified melanoma database used by the AJCC has grown to include 30,946 stage I, II, and III melanomas and 7,972 patients with stage IV melanoma. Critical analysis of this data has led to the publication of the seventh edition of the *AJCC Melanoma Staging and Classification System* in 2009, which went into effect in 2010 (Table 2 and Figure 1) (19). This seventh edition reflects the current state of knowledge in melanoma biology and our understanding of prognostic factors affecting patient outcomes. It is the syntheses of nearly 35 years of ongoing melanoma clinical and basic science research. Three important changes were included in the seventh edition of this classification system: (a) the mitotic rate was used to identify T1b melanomas was used; (b) immunohistochemistry (at least one positive melanoma-specific marker—HMB-45, Melan-A, or MART-1) was now an acceptable means for diagnosing nodal metastases, even when hematoxylin and eosin (H&E) staining

was negative; and (c) a lower threshold for lymph node tumor burden to diagnose regional nodal metastases was eliminated.

■ PROGNOSTIC FACTORS

According to the AJCC Melanoma Staging Committee, there are five criteria that guide the selection of prognostic factors for inclusion in the melanoma staging system (8,9). "First, the staging system must be practical, reproducible, and applicable to the diverse needs of all medical disciplines. Second, the criteria must accurately reflect the biology of melanoma based on consistent outcome results of patients treated at multiple institutions from multiple countries. Third, the criteria must be evidence-based and reflect the dominant prognostic factors consistently identified in Cox multivariate regression analyses. Fourth, the criteria must be relevant to current clinical practice and regularly incorporated in clinical trials. Lastly, fifth, the required data must be sufficiently easy for tumor registrars to identify in medical records to code staging information."

Tumor Thickness and Level of Invasion

The recommendations for using tumor thickness when staging melanoma are unchanged with the seventh edition of the melanoma staging system that is currently in effect (19). Ten-year survival is inversely related to increasing melanoma primary tumor thickness (92% T1, 80% T2, 63% T3, and 50% T4). The level of invasion is no longer a part of the current melanoma staging guidelines, particularly for melanomas ≤1 mm in thickness. It has been replaced by the primary tumor mitotic rate described as follows. Primary tumor characteristics continue to guide the selection of excision margins and the use of regional lymph node

TABLE 2   Seventh edition of the melanoma staging system

Primary Tumor (T)

TX	Primary tumor cannot be assessed
TO	No evidence of primary tumor
Tis	Melanoma in situ
T1	melanoma ≤1.00 mm in thickness
	T1a Without ulceration and mitosis $<1/mm^2$
	T1b With ulceration and/or mitoses $≥1/mm^2$
T2	melanoma 1.01 to 2.00 mm thick
	T2a Without ulceration
	T2b With ulceration
T3	melanoma 2.01 to 4.00 mm thick
	T3a Without ulceration
	T3b With ulceration
T4	melanoma >4 mm thick
	T4a Without ulceration
	T4b With ulceration

Regional Lymph Nodes (N)

N1	1 node involved with melanoma
	N1a Micrometastasis
	N1b Macrometastasis
N2	2 to 3 nodes involved with melanoma
	N2a Micrometastasis
	N2b Macrometastasis
	N2c intransit/satellite lesions without metastatic nodes
N3	≥ 4 nodes, or matted nodes, or intransit/satellite lesions with metastatic nodes

Distant Metastases (M)

M0	No detectable evidence of distant metastases
M1a	Distant skin, subcutaneous, or nodal metastases with normal lactic dehydrogenase (LDH)
M1b	Lung metastases with normal LDH
M1c	All other visceral metastases (normal LDH) or any distant metastases (elevated LDH)

	Clinical Staging	Pathologic Staging	
Stage 0	TisN0M0	TisN0M0	
Stage IA	T1aN0M0	T1aN0M0	
Stage IB	T1b-T2aN0M0	T2aN0M0 T1b-T2aN0M0	
Stage IIA	T2b-T3aN0M0	T2b-T3aN0M0	
Stage IIB	T3b-T4aN0M0	T3b-T4aN0M0	
Stage IIC	T4bN0M0	T4bN0M0	
Stage III	Any T ≥N1 M0	Stage IIIA	T1–4a,N1aorN2a, M0
		Stage IIIB	T1–4b, N1a or N2a, M0
			T1–4a, N1b or N2b or N2c, M0
		Stage IIIC	T1–4b, N1b or N2b or N2c, M0
			Any T, N3, M0
Stage IV	Any T, Any N, M1	Any T, Any N, M1	

Source: Adapted from Ref. (19). Used with the permission of the American Joint Committee on Cancer (AJCC), Chicago, Illinois. The original source for this material is the *AJCC Cancer Staging Manual*, 7th edition (2010), published by Springer Science and Business Media LLC; www.springer.com.

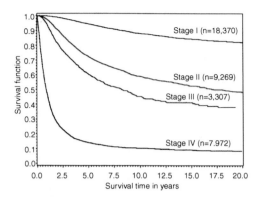

FIGURE 1

Survival rates for patients with AJCC stages I-IV melanoma.

Source: Adapted from Ref. 19, figure 31.1. Used with the permission of the American Joint Committee on Cancer (AJCC), Chicago, Illinois. The original source for this material is the *AJCC Cancer Staging Manual*, 7th edition (2010), published by Springer Science and Business Media LLC; www.springer.com.

staging procedures. Consensus guidelines recently published jointly by the Society of Surgical Oncology and the American Society for Clinical Oncology recommend that primary melanomas ≥1 mm in thickness, in the absence of clinically detectable regional nodal disease, should be offered a sentinel lymph node staging procedure (20,21). The routine use of a sentinel lymph node staging procedure for all melanomas <1 mm in thickness cannot be supported by the current evidence. The consensus guidelines recommend, instead, that a sentinel lymph node biopsy procedure may be considered for individuals with high-risk primary melanomas (associated with ulceration and/or a mitotic index of ≥1/mm^2) measuring <1 mm in thickness when the benefits of the procedure outweigh its risks. In contrast, the National Comprehensive Cancer Network (NCCN) recommends that a sentinel lymph node biopsy procedure should be discussed and offered to these individuals with high-risk primary melanomas measuring 0.76 to 0.99 mm in thickness (22). Our practice currently follows the recommendations of the NCCN.

Primary Tumor Ulceration

Ulceration was recognized as the second most important prognostic factor after tumor thickness at the time of publication of the sixth edition of the melanoma staging system and remains an important component of the seventh edition currently in effect (23,24). It is histologically characterized by the absence of an intact epidermis overlying the primary melanoma. The incidence of ulceration is 6% for melanomas ≤1 mm in thickness and increases to 63% for melanomas >4 mm in thickness (10). When ulceration is present, it identifies a locally advanced melanoma with a higher metastatic potential and is associated with worse survival relative to its nonulcerated counterpart (23–26). In fact, survival for ulcerated melanoma is nearly the same as that for nonulcerated melanoma of the next highest thickness category (Table 3).

Mitotic Rate

The proliferation of cells within the primary melanoma is expressed by the mitotic rate and denoted as the number of mitoses per square millimeter. An elevated mitotic rate identifies a more rapidly growing melanoma with the potential for earlier metastases and worse survival than a tumor with little or no mitotic activity. The adverse effect of mitotic rate on melanoma survival was first described in 1953 (27). More recently, mitotic rate has been identified as an independent prognostic factor in melanoma (28–40).

Multivariate evaluation of the primary tumor mitotic rate using the AJCC melanoma database has shown this parameter to be an independent adverse predictor of survival (19). Ten-year survival ranges from 97% for melanomas ≤0.5 mm in thickness and mitotic rate <1/mm^2

TABLE 3 Five-year survival rates of pathologically staged patients (from the 2008 AJCC Melanoma Staging Database)

	IA	IB	IIA	IIB	IIC	IIIA	IIIB	IIIC
Nonulcerated	T1a 97%	T2a 91%	T3a 79%	T4a 71%		N1a, N2a 78%	N1b, N2b 48%	N3 47%
Ulcerated		T1b 94%	T2b 82%	T3b 68%	T4b 53%		N1a, N2a 55%	N1b, N2b, N3 38%

Source: Adapted from Ref. (19) table 31.2. Used with the permission of the American Joint Committee on Cancer (AJCC), Chicago, Illinois. The original source for this material is the *AJCC Cancer Staging Manual,* 7th edition (2010), published by Springer Science and Business Media LLC; www.springer.com with permission.

to 28% for melanomas >6 mm in thickness and a mitotic rate >10/mm² (Table 4) (40). It ranks second only to tumor thickness in predicting survival in the setting of localized melanoma (40,41). When micrometastatic regional nodal disease from melanoma is present, mitotic rate ranks fourth after the number of metastatic lymph nodes, age, and ulceration in its ability to predict survival.

Mitotic rate is a continuous variable, and no lower threshold could be identified in the AJCC melanoma database to serve as a predictor for survival. Patient prognosis was worse in the presence of any elevation of the mitotic activity ($\geq 1/mm^2$) than if none was detected. Therefore, a mitotic rate of $\geq 1/mm^2$ was selected to identify primary melanomas with an increased metastatic risk. When this prognostic factor was examined for T1 melanomas, it was found to be the most powerful predictor of survival (19). When ulceration and mitotic rate were both included in this analysis, Clark's level was no longer a statistically significant predictor of survival. On the basis of these results, the AJCC has required mitotic rate to be a part of the histologic assessment of the primary melanoma and incorporated this into the current staging system. In addition to the presence of primary tumor ulceration, an elevated mitotic rate is used for identifying the higher risk subset of T1 melanomas that may be considered for a sentinel lymph node biopsy procedure.

Intralymphatic Disease

Satellite lesions, previously included in the T category, were grouped with intransit lesions in the N category as stage III disease with the issuance of the sixth edition of the melanoma staging system. The seventh edition continues to retain this staging convention. A study form the M. D. Anderson Cancer Center demonstrated that the distinction of satellite versus intransit lesions based on the distance from the primary tumor had no prognostic significance, because both represented intralymphatic dissemination of melanoma (42). Survival is nearly the same for individuals with satellite, intransit, and lymph node metastases, supporting the proposal that these should be grouped as stage III disease (43–53). When satellite/intransit and lymph node disease are concurrently present, the survival for this group is worse than when intralymphatic disease is present in the absence of regional nodal metastases (28–35% versus 41–56%, respectively) (54,55). The melanoma staging committee therefore recommended

TABLE 4 Ten-year survival rate by tumor thickness and mitotic rate

Mitotic Rate (mitoses/mm²)

Tumor Thickness (mm)	No. of Patients	<1.00			1.00 to 1.99			2.00 to 4.99			5.00 to 9.99			10.00 to 19.99			>20.00			Overall		
		No.	%	SE	No.	%	SE	No.	%	SE	No.	%	SE	No.	%	SE	No.	%	SE	No.	%	SE
0–0.50	1,521	1,194	97.1	0.9	207	97.1	1.7	89	93.2	3.9	27	87.7	8.6	4*						0*	96.7	0.8
0.51–1.0	3,340	1,472	92.5	1.1	895	87.4	1.8	775	86.4	2.0	161	82.2	4.6	36*						1*	89.3	0.8
1.01–2.0	3,367	488	90.9	1.8	188	83.1	2.2	1,351	79.4	1.7	577	76.5	2.6	205	70.1	4.7		73.8	8.7	43	80.9	1.0
2.01–3.0	1,520	78	77.2	6.6	100	75.8	4.2	555	65.3	3.0	397	70.8	3.1	241	58.2	4.6		47.7	9.8	61	67.0	1.7
3.01–6.0	1,459	58	78.8	8.2		56.7	7.8	381	57.1	4.0	477	58.5	3.2	33	55.2	3.8		34.3	8.7	110	56.8	1.9
>6.00	414	11*			18*	53.0	8.7	89	52.6	6.0	135	52.6	6.0	119	28.1	7.6		28.1	7.6	42*	48.0	3.8

Abbreviation: SE = standard error.

*10-year survival rates cannot be accurately calculated in these subgroups because of small patient numbers, short follow-up duration, and/or insufficient number of events (deaths).

Source: Adapted from Ref. (40), table 2. Reprinted with permission.

that, whenever possible, the status of the regional lymph nodes should be included in the staging system in the presence of satellite/intransit disease.

Regional Nodal Metastases

The dimensions of lymph nodes, with either a 5 cm (fourth edition) or a 3 cm cutoff (fifth edition), were once considered significant factors in categorizing the nature of regional metastases. Several series have evaluated melanoma prognosis relative to the clinical or pathologic dimensions of nodal disease (10,11,43,47,56–58). Multivariate analysis of the data from these studies showed that size was not a significant prognostic factor. The most powerful prognostic factor was the number of positive lymph nodes (Figure 2) (46,47,56,59–61). Five-year survival decreased with the increasing number of involved lymph nodes, with the best grouping defined by the cutoffs of 1 versus 2–3 versus ≥4 nodes (49,62–65).

Increased melanoma awareness, intensive screening efforts, and the early use of sentinel lymph node staging procedures have resulted in a gradual shift in the clinical presentation of regional nodal melanoma metastases from predominantly macroscopic to microscopic disease. Concurrent advances in the histologic detection of melanoma within these lymph nodes have also taken place. With the introduction of the seventh edition of the melanoma staging system, melanoma can be diagnosed within the regional nodes by either H&E staining or immunohistochemistry (66–68). Melanoma-specific markers (e.g., HMB-45, Melan-A, or MART-1) and the presence of malignant cell morphology are required to make this diagnosis when relying on immunohistochemistry alone. Overall, immunohistochemistry increases the likelihood of detecting even the smallest aggregates of melanoma cells. This enhanced detection of

melanoma has led to the redefining of what is considered clinically significant disease within the regional lymph nodes. In the current system, there is no minimum volume threshold of metastatic tumor within the lymph node required to diagnose regional metastases. Small-volume (≤0.1 mm) lymph node metastasis is associated with worse outcomes compared with the negative node (69,70). These modifications are a significant departure from the prior melanoma staging system, which required H&E detection of melanoma by microscopic evaluation of the regional lymph nodes and a minimum volume of disease to diagnose stage III disease.

Lymph node staging has also evolved to further subcategorize the status of regional nodes based on the presence of microscopic or macroscopic disease determined by their method of detection. Examination of 2,313 patients from the AJCC melanoma database with stage III melanoma demonstrated a 5-year survival of 67% and 43% in patients with micrometastases versus

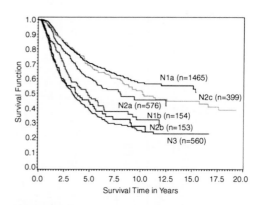

FIGURE 2

AJCC Collaborative Melanoma Database: Stage III survival curves by N classification.

Source: Adapted from Ref. (19), figure 31.3. Used with the permission of the American Joint Committee on Cancer (AJCC), Chicago, Illinois. The original source for this material is the *AJCC Cancer Staging Manual,* 7th edition (2010), published by Springer Science and Business Media LLC; www.springer.com.

macrometastases, respectively (71). Within the group of patients with micrometastases, there was marked variation in 5-year survival, which ranged from 87% for single nodal micrometastasis arising from a non-ulcerated melanoma ≤2 mm in thickness to 23% for four or more nodal micrometastases in the presence of an ulcerated, >6 mm thick primary melanoma. The most significant independent predictor of survival in patients with nodal micrometastases was the number of positive lymph nodes (Figure 3). Additional factors, in rank order, that affect survival in this group included primary tumor thickness, age, ulceration, anatomic site of the primary tumor, and gender. When the mitotic rate of the primary tumor was incorporated into the model for micrometastatic nodal disease, it was the second most powerful predictor of survival, next to the number of positive lymph nodes. Age differences in the 5-year survival were also noted in the micrometastatic group, with rates of 74%, 65%, and 47% in patients aged <50, 50–69, and ≥70 years, respectively. In the setting of macroscopic nodal disease, age, the number of positive lymph nodes,

primary tumor ulceration, and anatomic site of the primary melanoma independently predicted survival. In the setting of either micrometastatic or macrometastatic disease, Clark's level was not a significant predictor of survival.

Lactic Dehydrogenase

Evaluation of the Melanoma Staging Database demonstrated that an elevated LDH is an adverse prognostic indicator in patients with distant metastases from melanoma. Two-year survival was 40% and 18% in patients with distant melanoma metastases having a normal or elevated LDH level, respectively (9,72).

■ DISCUSSION

The Melanoma Staging System currently in effect reflects an evidence-based evolution in our understanding of the natural history of melanoma biology. It serves to identify and assign significance to the most important clinical and pathologic factors that can be used to determine outcomes and

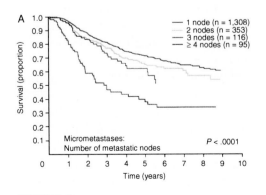
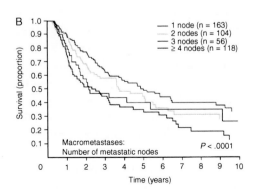

FIGURE 3

Kaplan–Meier survival curves of patients with regional node metastasis. (A) number of nodes containing micrometastases. (B) Number of nodes containing macrometastases.

Source: Adapted from Ref. (71), figure 1. Reprinted with permission. © 2010 American Society of Clinical Oncology. All rights reserved.

guide the selection of therapy. The seventh edition of the melanoma staging system identifies primary tumor thickness, ulceration, mitotic rate, intralymphatic disease, regional nodal metastases, and an elevated LDH as important prognostic factors.

Historically, increasing primary tumor thickness has been recognized as the most important prognostic factor for identifying individuals with melanoma who are at increased risk for regional lymph node metastases. A sentinel lymph node staging procedure has been recommended for patients with melanomas ≥1 mm in thickness and no clinical evidence of regional nodal metastases. Since tumor thickness is a continuous variable, it is implied that a subset of melanomas <1 mm in thickness may also be at increased risk for lymph node metastases. According to the current melanoma staging system, thin melanomas with an increased potential for regional lymph node dissemination may be identified by the presence of either primary tumor ulceration or an elevated mitotic rate ($\geq 1/mm^2$). Although a sentinel lymph node staging procedure is not routinely recommended for all individuals possessing thin primary melanomas with these high-risk features, select individuals may be considered for regional nodal staging if the benefits of the procedure outweigh the potential risks. These recommendations have recently been set forth in guidelines jointly established by the Society of Surgical Oncology and the American Society of Clinical Oncology (20,21). In contradistinction to this recently published consensus guideline, the NCCN recommends that a sentinel lymph node staging procedure be discussed and offered to patients with high-risk melanomas ranging from 0.76 mm to 0.99 mm in thickness (22). Our practice follows the recommendations of the NCCN.

Knowing the status of the sentinel lymph node has additional important implications for the patient. In the presence of a positive sentinel lymph node, the treating physician now has the opportunity to consider and discuss the roles for both regional lymphadenectomy and adjuvant systemic therapies with the patient. In some cases, knowing the status of the sentinel lymph node is a requirement for enrollment in melanoma clinical trials. Not having this information may exclude some patients from availing themselves of this treatment option.

Detection of regional nodal disease by immunohistochemistry is a significant departure from the prior melanoma staging system. Not only does this technique increase the sensitivity of detecting melanoma metastases within the regional lymph nodes but it also reflects the enhanced understanding that all micrometastatic melanoma within the lymph node is clinically significant. This idea is further supported by data from the Multicenter Selective Lymphadenectomy Trial-I, which showed that micrometastatic lymph node disease eventually progresses to become clinically significant, and when detected at that advanced stage, it portends a worse survival than if it was recognized earlier (73). The recognition of micrometastatic versus macrometastatic disease also has implications in the selection of adjuvant therapy. The EORTC 18991 study examined the role of adjuvant therapy with pegylated interferon alfa-2b in 1,256 patients with resected stage III melanoma (74). With a median follow-up of 3.8 years, the study concluded that adjuvant pegylated interferon alfa-2b resulted in an improved recurrence-free and distant metastasis-free survival in the subset of patients with micrometastases within the regional lymph nodes. Furthermore, substage and the presence of primary tumor ulceration were important correlates of improved recurrence-free survival (75). This survival advantage was not realized in the group of patients with macroscopic lymph node disease. These data suggests that the diagnosis of micrometastases within the regional lymph nodes (regardless of the size of the tumor volume) by immunohistochemistry could be a separate indication for selecting specific adjuvant systemic therapies for melanoma.

Although the implementation of the revised melanoma staging system may seem like it is an endpoint, it is really only a beginning. The rigorous evidence-based approach used for arriving at the current staging system has identified important prognostic factors for use in managing the care of patients with melanoma. However, the data on which this resource is predicated are constantly evolving. New evidence through clinical and basic science research supporting the use of current, putative, or as yet unrecognized prognostic factors for melanoma will continue to grow. The prognostic modeling used in the melanoma staging system needs to easily be adaptable to compelling new evidence. To address this ever-changing need, the AJCC Melanoma Staging Committee has released a web-based application (http://www.melanomaprognosis.org) that can be used in real time to create individualized patient prognostic models (1-, 2-, 5-, and 10-year survival) for stages I, II, and III melanoma. This powerful tool has the potential to incorporate additional predictive covariates even before they can formally be adopted into the next melanoma staging system. The potential future applications of this resource are even greater when one considers the knowledge gained from identification of morphogenetic correlates from molecular-based profiling studies that have occurred in recent years.

■ REFERENCES

1. Breslow A. Thickness, cross-sectional areas and depth of invasion in the prognosis of cutaneous melanoma. *Ann Surg.* 1970; 172:902–8.
2. Clark WH, Jr., From L, Bernardino EA, Mihm MC. The histogenesis and biologic behavior of primary human malignant melanomas of the skin. *Cancer Res.* 1969;29:705–27.
3. Ketcham AS, Christopherson WM, Anderson WAD, et al. Staging of malignant melanoma. In: Beahrs OH, Carr DT, Rubin P, eds. *AJCC Manual for Staging of Cancer.* 1st ed. Chicago, IL: Whiting Press; 1977.
4. Melanoma of the skin. In: Beahrs OH, Myers MH, eds. *AJCC Manual for Staging of Cancer.* 2nd ed. Philadelphia, PA: Lippincott Raven, 1983.
5. Melanoma of the Skin. In: Beahrs OH, Henson DE, Hutter RVP, eds. *AJCC Manual for Staging of Cancer.* 3rd ed. Philadelphia, PA: Lippincott Raven, 1988.
6. Malignant melanoma of the skin. In: Beahrs OH, Henson DE, Hutter RVP, Kennedy BJ, eds. *AJCC Manual for Staging of Cancer.* 4th ed. Philadelphia, PA: Lippincott Raven, 1992.
7. Malignant melanoma of the skin. In: Fleming ID, Cooper JS, Henson DE, et al, eds. *AJCC Cancer Staging Manual.* 5th ed. Philadelphia, PA: Lippincott Raven, 1997.
8. Balch CM, Buzaid AC, Atkins MB, et al. A new American Joint Committee on Cancer staging system for cutaneous melanoma. *Cancer.* 2000;88:1484–91.
9. Balch CM, Buzaid AC, Soong SJ, et al. Final version of the American Joint Committee on Cancer staging system for cutaneous melanoma. *J Clin Oncol.* 2001;19:3635–48.
10. Balch CM, Soong SJ, Gershenwald JE, et al. Prognostic factors analysis of 17,600 melanoma patients: validation of the American Joint Committee on Cancer melanoma staging system. *J Clin Oncol.* 2001;19:3622–34.
11. Buzaid AC, Ross MI, Balch CM, et al. Critical analysis of the current American Joint Committee on Cancer staging system for cutaneous melanoma and proposal of a new staging system. *J Clin Oncol.* 1997;15:1039–51.
12. Melanoma of the skin. In: Greene FL, Page DL, Fleming ID, Fritz A, Balch CM, Haller DG, Morrow M, eds. *AJCC Cancer Staging Manual.* 6th ed. New York, NY: Springer; 2002.

13. Vollmer RT. Malignant melanoma: a multivariate analysis of prognostic factors. *Pathol Annu.* 1989;24 Pt 1:383–407.

14. Morton DL, Davtyan DG, Wanek LA, Foshag LJ, Cochran AJ. Multivariate analysis of the relationship between survival and the microstage of primary melanoma by Clark level and Breslow thickness. *Cancer.* 1993;71:3737–43.

15. Buttner P, Garbe C, Bertz J, et al. Primary cutaneous melanoma. Optimized cutoff points of tumor thickness and importance of Clark's level for prognostic classification. *Cancer.* 1995;75:2499–506.

16. Lock-Andersen J, Hou-Jensen K, Hansen JP, Jensen NK, Sogaard H, Andersen PK. Observer variation in histological classification of cutaneous malignant melanoma. *Scand J Plast Reconstr Surg Hand Surg.* 1995;29:141–8.

17. Scolyer RA, Shaw HM, Thompson JF, et al. Interobserver reproducibility of histopathologic prognostic variables in primary cutaneous melanomas. *Am J Surg Pathol.* 2003;27:1571–6.

18. Morton DL, Wen DR, Wong JH, et al. Technical details of intraoperative lymphatic mapping for early stage melanoma. *Arch Surg.* 1992; 127:392–9.

19. Melanoma of the skin. In: Edge SB, Byrd DR, Compton CC, eds. *AJCC Cancer Staging Manual.* 7th ed. New York, NY: Springer; 2010.

20. Wong SL, Balch CM, Hurley P, et al. Sentinel lymph node biopsy for melanoma: American Society of Clinical Oncology and Society of Surgical Oncology joint clinical practice guideline. *Ann Surg Oncol.* 2012; 19(11):3313–24.

21. Wong SL, Balch CM, Hurley P, et al. Sentinel lymph node biopsy for melanoma: american society of clinical oncology and society of surgical oncology joint clinical practice guideline. *J Clin Oncol.* 2012;30:2912–8.

22. Coit DG, Thompson JA, Andtbacka R, Anker CJ. Melanoma: NCCN clinical practice guidelines in oncology. In *NCCN Guidelines.* 3.2012 ed. Fort Washington, MD; 2012.

23. Balch CM, Wilkerson JA, Murad TM, Soong SJ, Ingalls AL, Maddox WA. The prognostic significance of ulceration of cutaneous melanoma. *Cancer.* 1980;45:3012–7.

24. McGovern VJ, Shaw HM, Milton GW, McCarthy WH. Ulceration and prognosis in cutaneous malignant melanoma. *Histopathology.* 1982;6:399–407.

25. Cascinelli N, Marubini E, Morabito A, Bufalino R. Prognostic factors for stage I melanoma of the skin: a review. *Stat Med.* 1985;4:265–78.

26. Thorn M, Ponten F, Bergstrom R, Sparen P, Adami HO. Clinical and histopathologic predictors of survival in patients with malignant melanoma: a population-based study in Sweden. *J Natl Cancer Inst.* 1994;86:761–9.

27. Allen AC, Spitz S. Malignant melanoma: a clinicopathological analysis of the criteria for diagnosis and prognosis. *Cancer.* 1953;6:1–45.

28. Attis MG, Vollmer RT. Mitotic rate in melanoma: a reexamination. *Am J Clin Pathol.* 2007;127:380–4.

29. Azzola MF, Shaw HM, Thompson JF, et al. Tumor mitotic rate is a more powerful prognostic indicator than ulceration in patients with primary cutaneous melanoma: an analysis of 3661 patients from a single center. *Cancer.* 2003;97:1488–98.

30. Barnhill RL, Katzen J, Spatz A, Fine J, Berwick M. The importance of mitotic rate as a prognostic factor for localized cutaneous melanoma. *J Cutan Pathol.* 2005;32:268–73.

31. Francken AB, Shaw HM, Thompson JF, et al. The prognostic importance of tumor mitotic rate confirmed in 1317 patients with primary cutaneous melanoma and long follow-up. *Ann Surg Oncol.* 2004;11:426–33.

32. Gimotty PA, Elder DE, Fraker DL, et al. Identification of high-risk patients among those diagnosed with thin cutaneous melanomas. *J Clin Oncol.* 2007;25:1129–34.

33. Gimotty PA, Guerry D, Ming ME, et al. Thin primary cutaneous malignant melanoma: a prognostic tree for 10-year metastasis is more accurate than American Joint Committee on Cancer staging. *J Clin Oncol.* 2004;22:3668–76.

34. Kesmodel SB, Karakousis GC, Botbyl JD, et al. Mitotic rate as a predictor of sentinel lymph node positivity in patients with thin melanomas. *Ann Surg Oncol.* 2005;12:449–58.

35. Kruper LL, Spitz FR, Czerniecki BJ, et al. Predicting sentinel node status in AJCC stage I/II primary cutaneous melanoma. *Cancer.* 2006; 107:2436–45.

36. Paek SC, Griffith KA, Johnson TM, et al. The impact of factors beyond Breslow depth on predicting sentinel lymph node positivity in melanoma. *Cancer.* 2007;109:100–8.

37. Retsas S, Henry K, Mohammed MQ, MacRae K. Prognostic factors of cutaneous

melanoma and a new staging system proposed by the American Joint Committee on Cancer (AJCC): validation in a cohort of 1284 patients. *Eur J Cancer.* 2002;38:511–6.

38. Scolyer RA, Thompson JF, Shaw HM, McCarthy SW. The importance of mitotic rate as a prognostic factor for localized primary cutaneous melanoma. *J Cutan Pathol.* 2006;33:395–6; author reply 7–9.

39. Sondak VK, Taylor JM, Sabel MS, et al. Mitotic rate and younger age are predictors of sentinel lymph node positivity: lessons learned from the generation of a probabilistic model. *Ann Surg Oncol.* 2004;11:247–58.

40. Thompson JF, Soong SJ, Balch CM, et al. Prognostic significance of mitotic rate in localized primary cutaneous melanoma: an analysis of patients in the multi-institutional American Joint Committee on Cancer melanoma staging database. J *Clin Oncol.* 2011;29:2199–205.

41. Balch CM, Gershenwald JE, Soong SJ, Thompson JF. Update on the melanoma staging system: the importance of sentinel node staging and primary tumor mitotic rate. *J Surg Oncol.* 2011;104:379–85.

42. Singletary SE, Tucker SL, Boddie AW, Jr. Multivariate analysis of prognostic factors in regional cutaneous metastases of extremity melanoma. *Cancer.* 1988;61:1437–40.

43. Buzaid AC, Tinoco LA, Jendiroba D, et al. Prognostic value of size of lymph node metastases in patients with cutaneous melanoma. *J Clin Oncol.* 1995;13:2361–8.

44. Callery C, Cochran AJ, Roe DJ, et al. Factors prognostic for survival in patients with malignant melanoma spread to the regional lymph nodes. *Ann Surg.* 1982;196:69–75.

45. Cascinelli N, Bufalino R, Marolda R, et al. Regional non-nodal metastases of cutaneous melanoma. *Eur J Surg Oncol.* 1986;12:175–80.

46. Cascinelli N, Vaglini M, Nava M, et al. Prognosis of skin melanoma with regional node metastases (stage II). *J Surg Oncol.* 1984;25:240–7.

47. Coit DG, Rogatko A, Brennan MF. Prognostic factors in patients with melanoma metastatic to axillary or inguinal lymph nodes. A multivariate analysis. *Ann Surg.* 1991;214:627–36.

48. Haffner AC, Garbe C, Burg G, Buttner P, Orfanos CE, Rassner G. The prognosis of primary and metastasising melanoma. An evaluation of the TNM classification in 2,495 patients. *Br J Cancer.* 1992;66:856–61.

49. Karakousis CP, Seddiq MK, Moore R. Prognostic value of lymph node dissection in malignant melanoma. *Arch Surg.* 1980;115:719–22.

50. Karakousis CP, Temple DF, Moore R, Ambrus JL. Prognostic parameters in recurrent malignant melanoma. *Cancer.* 1983;52:575–9.

51. Roses DF, Karp NS, Oratz R, et al. Survival with regional and distant metastases from cutaneous malignant melanoma. *Surg Gynecol Obstet.* 1991;172:262–8.

52. Singletary SE, Shallenberger R, Guinee VF, McBride CM. Melanoma with metastasis to regional axillary or inguinal lymph nodes: prognostic factors and results of surgical treatment in 714 patients. *South Med J.* 1988;81:5–9.

53. Sutherland CM, Mather FJ, Krementz ET. Factors influencing the survival of patients with regional melanoma of the extremity treated by perfusion. *Surg Gynecol Obstet.* 1987;164:111–8.

54. Cavaliere R, Cavaliere F, Deraco M, et al. Hyperthermic antiblastic perfusion in the treatment of stage IIIA-IIIAB melanoma patients: comparison of two experiences. *Melanoma Res.* 1994;4 Suppl 1:5–11.

55. Stehlin JS, Jr., Giovanella BC, Gutierrez AE, de Ipolyi PD, Greeff PJ. 15 years' experience with hyperthermic perfusion for treatment of soft tissue sarcoma and malignant melanoma of the extremities. *Front Radiat Ther Oncol.* 1984;18:177–82.

56. Drepper H, Biess B, Hofherr B, et al. The prognosis of patients with stage III melanoma: prospective long-term study of 286 patients of the Fachklinik Hornheide. *Cancer.* 1993;71:1239–46.

57. Bevilacqua RG, Coit DG, Rogatko A, Younes RN, Brennan MF. Axillary dissection in melanoma: prognostic variables in node-positive patients. *Ann Surg.* 1990;212:125–31.

58. Karakousis CP, Goumas W, Rao U, Driscoll DL. Axillary node dissection in malignant melanoma. *Am J Surg.* 1991;162:202–7.

59. Balch CM. Cutaneous melanoma: prognosis and treatment results worldwide. *Semin Surg Oncol.* 1992;8:400–14.

60. Morton DL, Wanek L, Nizze JA, Elashoff RM, Wong JH. Improved long-term survival after lymphadenectomy of melanoma metastatic to regional nodes: analysis of prognostic factors in 1134 patients from the John Wayne Cancer Clinic. *Ann Surg.* 1991;214:491–9; discussion 9–501.

61. Roses DF, Provet JA, Harris MN, Gumport SL, Dubin N. Prognosis of patients with pathologic stage II cutaneous malignant melanoma. *Ann Surg.* 1985;201:103–7.

62. Balch CM, Soong SJ, Murad TM, Ingalls AL, Maddox WA. A multifactorial analysis of melanoma—part III: prognostic factors in melanoma patients with lymph node metastases (stage II). *Ann Surg.* 1981;193:377–88.

63. Cohen MH, Ketcham AS, Felix EL, et al. Prognostic factors in patients undergoing lymphadenectomy for malignant melanoma. *Ann Surg.* 1977;186:635–42.

64. Slingluff CL, Jr., Vollmer R, Seigler HF. Stage II malignant melanoma: presentation of a prognostic model and an assessment of specific active immunotherapy in 1,273 patients. *J Surg Oncol.* 1988;39:139–47.

65. Calabro A, Singletary SE, Balch CM. Patterns of relapse in 1001 consecutive patients with melanoma nodal metastases. *Arch Surg.* 1989;124:1051–5.

66. Ohsie SJ, Sarantopoulos GP, Cochran AJ, Binder SW. Immunohistochemical characteristics of melanoma. *J Cutan Pathol.* 2008;35:433–44.

67. Spanknebel K, Coit DG, Bieligk SC, Gonen M, Rosai J, Klimstra DS. Characterization of micrometastatic disease in melanoma sentinel lymph nodes by enhanced pathology: recommendations for standardizing pathologic analysis. *Am J Surg Pathol.* 2005;29:305–17.

68. Gibbs JF, Huang PP, Zhang PJ, Kraybill WG, Cheney R. Accuracy of pathologic techniques for the diagnosis of metastatic melanoma in sentinel lymph nodes. *Ann Surg Oncol.* 1999;6:699–704.

69. Scheri RP, Essner R, Turner RR, Ye X, Morton DL. Isolated tumor cells in the sentinel node affect long-term prognosis of patients with melanoma. *Ann Surg Oncol.* 2007;14:2861–6.

70. van Akkooi AC, de Wilt JH, Verhoef C, et al. Clinical relevance of melanoma micrometastases (<0.1 mm) in sentinel nodes: are these nodes to be considered negative? *Ann Oncol.* 2006;17:1578–85.

71. Balch CM, Gershenwald JE, Soong SJ, et al. Multivariate analysis of prognostic factors among 2,313 patients with stage III melanoma: comparison of nodal micrometastases versus macrometastases. *J Clin Oncol.* 2010;28:2452–9.

72. Balch CM, Gershenwald JE, Soong SJ, et al. Final version of 2009 AJCC melanoma staging and classification. *J Clin Oncol.* 2009;27:6199–206.

73. Morton DL, Thompson JF, Cochran AJ, et al. Sentinel-node biopsy or nodal observation in melanoma. *N Engl J Med.* 2006;355:1307–17.

74. Eggermont AM, Suciu S, Santinami M, et al. Adjuvant therapy with pegylated interferon alfa-2b versus observation alone in resected stage III melanoma: final results of EORTC 18991, a randomised phase III trial. *Lancet.* 2008;372:117–26.

75. Eggermont AM, Suciu S, Testori A, et al. Ulceration and stage are predictive of interferon efficacy in melanoma: results of the phase III adjuvant trials EORTC 18952 and EORTC 18991. *Eur J Cancer.* 2012;48:218–25.

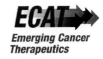

Emerging Cancer
Therapeutics

Less Common Variants of Cutaneous Melanoma

Raymond L. Barnhill*[1], G. Peter Sarantopoulos[1], and Kapil Gupta[2]

[1]*Department of Pathology and Laboratory Medicine, University of California, Los Angeles, CA*

[2]*Dermatology Group of the Carolinas, Concord, NC*

■ ABSTRACT

Melanoma is among the most diverse neoplasms affecting man. Herein we will review the clinical and histologic features of some of the less common subtypes of cutaneous melanoma which clinicians and pathologists may encounter. There will be a disproportionate focus on the histopathology and prognosis, as the clinical presentation of these lesions is, in most cases, elusive and, in some cases, frankly deceptive. The discussion will include the following entities: desmoplastic melanoma, nevoid melanoma, spitzoid melanocytic neoplasms and spitz-like melanoma, angiotropic melanoma, blue nevus-like melanoma, and melanomas combined with basal or squamous cell carcinoma.

Keywords: melanoma, melanocytic nevus, Spitz tumor, blue nevus, angiotropism

*Corresponding author, Department of Pathology and Laboratory Medicine, University of California, Los Angeles, CA
   E-mail address: rbarnhill@mednet.ucla.edu

Emerging Cancer Therapeutics 3:3 (2012) 421–460.
© 2012 Demos Medical Publishing LLC. All rights reserved.
DOI: 10.5003/2151–4194.3.3.421

■ INTRODUCTION

Cutaneous melanoma is one of the most heterogeneous and complex human neoplastic systems. Consequently, on a regular basis one encounters melanomas that are difficult to categorize as one of the four major subtypes."[1](1). If there is difficulty in classifying an individual lesion as a "conventional" subtype of melanoma, there is clearly even greater difficulty in establishing whether less common variants of melanoma can be recognized based on objective evidence. In practical terms, the recognition and description of additional legitimate variants of melanoma must have some particular biological significance or relevance, and there must be objective criteria for their recognition and distinction from other presentations of melanoma. It is evident that this has not been achieved for many entities and much more basic research is needed.

The recognition and delineation of both conventional and less common variants of melanoma correspond to a wide range of clinical, microscopic, genetic, and molecular phenotypic characteristics. Clinical considerations for classification of melanoma subtype may include: 1) age of melanoma onset, e.g., birth, childhood and adolescence, and adulthood, 2) anatomic sites such as skin subject to continuous or intermittent sun exposure, acral and mucosal surfaces, 3) associations with precursor lesions such as congenital, dysplastic, or blue nevi, and 4) association with hereditary melanoma and atypical nevus kindreds.

A number of histological and cytological attributes have provided the basis for current melanoma classification: 1) intraepidermal arrangement (or growth pattern) of melanoma cells: lentiginous, pagetoid, nested, or absence of an intra-epidermal component, 2) epidermal surface configuration, e.g., verrucous, polypoid surface topography; 3) stromal alterations, e.g., desmoplasia, mucin deposition; 4) morphologic resemblance or mimicry of benign melanocytic neoplasms, i.e., "nevoid" melanoma, "spitzoid" melanoma, blue nevus-like melanoma (malignant blue nevus), resemblance to plexiform spindle cell nevus; 5) peculiar cytological characteristics, e.g., small cell, spindle cell, epithelioid cell, balloon cell, signet ring cell, rhabdoid cell, clear cell variants of melanoma, etc.; 6) other morphologic properties, e.g., neurotropism, neural differentiation, angiotropism, and adnexotropism; 7) pigmentary characteristics, e.g., amelanotic, pigment-synthesizing, or "animal-type" melanoma; and 8) host response and regression. Increasingly, molecular advances are providing new insights into the pathogenesis of melanoma. Thus, for example, particular mutations in the mitogen-activated protein (MAP) kinase, such as *BRAF,* and the phosphatidylinositol 3 (PI3) signaling have suggested that there are different pathways for melanoma development.

This chapter will outline the clinical and histologic features of some of the less common variants or presentations of cutaneous melanoma which clinicians and pathologists are likely to encounter in clinical practice. There will be a disproportionate focus on the histopathology and prognosis, as the clinical presentation

---

[1]According to the current WHO classification, there are four major subtypes of melanoma: 1) Lentigo maligna melanoma, (2) Superficial spreading melanoma, 3) Acral lentiginous melanoma, and 4) Nodular melanoma. Although the latter classification has generally been accepted by many over the years, the artificiality and limitations of this classification have clearly been recognized. However, based on recent basic advances, it is increasingly evident that there are melanomas with different developmental origins owing to an interplay of intrinsic host factors such as molecular genotype and the environment, e.g., sun exposure.[1] Thus, some refinements in the classification of melanoma are beginning to appear.

of these lesions is, in most cases, elusive and, in some cases, frankly deceptive when compared to conventional lesions of cutaneous melanoma. The discussion will include the following entities: desmoplastic melanoma, nevoid melanoma, spitzoid melanocytic neoplasms and spitz-like melanoma, angiotropic melanoma, blue nevus-like melanoma (malignant blue nevus), and melanomas combined with non-melanoma skin cancer.

■ DESMOPLASTIC MELANOMA AND DESMOPLASTIC NEUROTROPIC MELANOMA

Desmoplastic melanoma (DM) is a variant of spindle cell melanoma and is probably more appropriately termed a "desmoplastic melanocytic or neurocristic sarcoma" because of its phenotypic characteristics and biological behavior (1,3–14). As with "nevoid" melanoma (see below), DM harbors as perhaps its greatest significance, its accurate identification as cutaneous melanoma. The issue is compounded by the fact that the lesion is often amelanotic and highly infiltrative with a propensity for perineurial spread, which may contribute to its hallmark capacity for local recurrence—a feature that distinguishes it from other types of melanoma. Furthermore, DM often appears deceptively indolent initially with a very low frequency of regional lymph node metastases; however, particularly if not adequately excised and after local recurrence, often multiple, DM may become aggressive with a sarcoma-like clinical course, sometimes with rather prototypic metastases to the lungs.

DM is among the most heterogenous variants of melanoma (4,6–14). With the characterization of larger numbers of DM, it has become increasing appreciated that DM constitutes a spectrum of melanomas,

rather than a single entity. This spectrum encompasses: 1) pure DM which is typified by a pauci-cellular spindle cell nodule with desmoplastic stromal matrix; 2) desmoplastic-neurotropic melanoma (DNM), i.e., DM with associated neurotropism and/or neural differentiation; 3) pure neurotropic melanoma, i.e., a spindle cell melanoma with neurotropic phenotype and showing little or no desmoplasia; 4) "mixed" or "combined" variants of DM/DNM which may exhibit an additional more cellular component of conventional melanoma, e.g., comprised of epithelioid and/or spindle cells (constituting about 10 to 50% or more of the DM) (12). The importance of recognizing the latter variants of DM is reflected in differences in biological behavior, prognosis, and management.

Clinical Features

The demographics of DM have been characterized by a predominance of males in the sixties and seventies, with the majority of reported lesions involving sun-damaged areas of the head and neck, although not at the exclusion of other body sites, including acral and mucosal surfaces (3–13). They present as nodules or plaques, sometimes depressed, which are very often amelanotic. However, in those cases that demonstrate pigmentation, it is often in the form of a conventional melanoma (often lentigo maligna) component, which happens to be congruent on a histologic level, as these lesions often represent the invasive component of melanomas involving chronically sun-exposed skin. (For purposes of this discussion, the conventional historical terms "lentigo maligna" and "lentigo maligna melanoma" are used to represent lentiginous in situ and invasive melanomas arising in chronically sun-damaged skin). However, desmoplastic melanoma can also arise de novo, and it is this situation in which it poses the greatest diagnostic challenge. The lesion may also appear scar-like clinically, which is appropriate given the histologic profile. Rare variants of de novo DM appear to arise in melanocytic nevus remnants suggesting an additional pathway to DM.

Histopathologic Features

The histologic hallmark of DM is that of an ill-defined spindle cell neoplasm of varying concern with regard to density and cytologic atypia, that often demonstrates a highly infiltrative pattern of growth amidst sclerotic collagen fibers. In fact, the collagen density on scanning magnification resembles a scar, with the embedded cellularity being reminiscent of an accompanying fibroblastic component (Figure 1). Other variants of DM may demonstrate a more conspicuous spindle cell proliferation in which the degree of sclerosis is less ubiquitous throughout the lesion (Figure 2). The spindle cells may be present as single, markedly atypical, infiltrating cells (Fig. 3) or as a predominant arrangement of fascicles that sweep through dense collagen bundles in a manner reminiscent of a neural or smooth muscle proliferation. There is nuclear hyperchromasia and contour irregularity of the spindle cell forms (Figure 3), often with the added histologic features of lymphoid aggregates and solar elastosis. In fact, these latter two features in the setting of a sclerotic lesion, even with minimal or almost no cytologic atypia and inconspicuous mitotic activity, are often instrumental in arriving at the correct diagnosis. This is particularly important in those cases which are deceptively benign in appearance. The mitotic count in most tumors is relatively modest, adding to the diagnostic confusion. It is also of the utmost importance to always examine the dermal-epidermal junction in such cases for a subtle lentiginous melanocytic component possibly representative of an overlying atypical lentiginous melanocytic proliferation or melanoma in situ/lentigo maligna.

Neurotropic melanoma is often associated with atypical lentiginous melanocytic proliferation or lentiginous forms of melanoma. However, some NM may arise with any type of intraepidermal component, e.g., pagetoid involvement, or de novo without an intraepidermal component (13).

The term neurotropism refers to both the involvement of perineurium and endoneurium of cutaneous nerves by melanoma spindle cells and neural differentiation (Figure 4) (13). There may be considerable thickening of the perineurium and expansion of the endoneurial space by the tumor involvement. Extension of tumor along the cutaneous nerves may, however, be extensive and subtle. Histological clues to nerve involvement include the presence of hyperchromatic spindle cells in the perineurium or endoneurium and mucinous alteration of the nerve. Melanoma spindle cells involving cutaneous nerves usually show nuclear enlargement, hyperchromatism, and pleomorphism.

The term neurotropism also describes neural or Schwannian differentiation in a pattern resembling peripheral nerve sheath tumors such as neurofibromas or neuromas ("malignant neuroma") and the recapitulation of perineurium and endoneurium. The tumor cells in such areas are characterized by serpiginous or wavy nuclear configurations and filamentous cytoplasmic processes. However, the tumor cells demonstrate loose fascicular arrangements, cytologic atypia, and occasional mitotic figures. Some tumors may

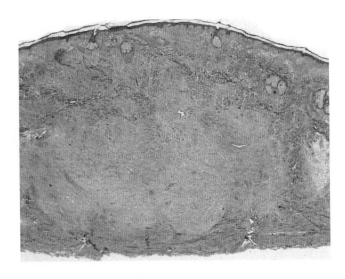

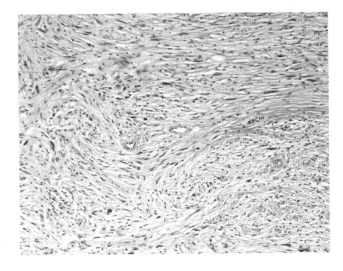

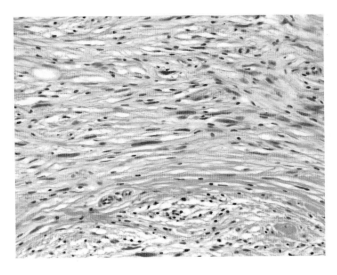

FIGURE 1
Desmoplastic melanoma: scanning magnification discloses a large dermal fibrotic nodule.

FIGURE 2
Desmoplastic melanoma: fascicles of atypical spindle cells with stromal desmoplasia.

FIGURE 3
Desmoplastic melanoma: note the nuclear enlargement and pleomorphism of spindle cells.

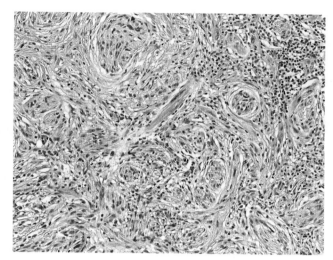

FIGURE 4

Neurotropic melanoma: pure invasive neurotropic component associated with lentigo maligna. Dermal invasive component is comprised of spindle cells arranged in fascicles resembling cutaneous nerves. There is little or no desmoplasia present. Higher magnification showing spindle cells with nuclear enlargement and pleomorphism.

be indistinguishable from a malignant peripheral nerve sheath tumor without observation of an atypical intraepidermal melanocytic proliferation.

Special Techniques

The immunohistochemical profile in most lesions of DM is characterized by S-100, Sox10, p75 neurotrophin receptor, and Vimentin positivity (4,9,10,14,15). Smooth muscle actin positivity indicative of myofibroblastic differentiation may be present in many cases. Melan A/Mart-1, HMB45, tyrosinase, and microphthalmia transcription factor (MITF) immunostains are almost always not expressed by the invasive spindle cell component. As a practical aside, it is important to exercise caution with regard to the S-100 stain in biopsy and re-excision specimens of DM, as there is almost invariably some degree of S-100 staining within the native dermis, and in the setting of non-melanocytic proliferations. These may be indicative of dermal antigen presenting cells. Such cells have also been documented in scars, where the

nature of these cells have been postulated by different researchers as being representative of Langerhans cells (16), fibroblasts (17), and Schwann cells or regenerating nerve twigs (18). It is important to note that such cells do normally exist in the dermis as they represent a common pitfall that may contribute to an erroneous diagnosis of DM, particularly in the setting of scars that mimic DM, and also in the setting of re-excision specimens where they may be misinterpreted as being representative of residual DM.

The pathogenesis of DM remains unresolved. Some investigators, by way of immunohistochemical and ultrastructural analysis, have suggested that bidirectional differentiation is at play in these tumors (14). In one sense, DM and DNM, represent a spectrum of primitive neurocristic neoplasms with lines of differentiation including melanocytic with melanin synthesis, fibrocytic as evidenced by collagen and mucin production, myofibroblastic because of the expression of myogenic markers, and neurosustentacular, i.e., neurotropism and neural differentiation.

Differential Diagnosis

The histologic differential diagnosis of DM includes: scar, desmoplastic or sclerosing nevus, desmoplastic Spitz tumor, sclerosing blue nevus, dermatofibroma, dermatofibrosarcoma protuberans (DFSP), peripheral nerve sheath tumors, sarcomas, spindle cell squamous cell carcinoma, and atypical fibroxanthoma. Perhaps the most important initial step in distinguishing a DM is an examination of the dermal-epidermal junction for the presence of a suspicious junctional melanocytic component and the lesion for the presence of melanin within tumor cells.

DM can quite incredibly mimic a scar. It is important to beware of "scars" that demonstrate (1) conspicuous cellularity, (2) solar elastosis, (3) lymphoid aggregates, (4) retained adnexal structures, and (5) a lack of horizontal fibrosis, vertically oriented vessels, and erythrocyte extravasation. Greater scrutiny should be applied to the cytomorphology in such cases, with regard to plump spindled cells with nuclear hyperchromasia and mitotic activity.

Desmoplastic/sclerosing nevi are usually well-circumscribed and show features of benign nevomelanocytes, only embedded in an inordinately sclerotic stroma. Aside from this sclerotic stroma, there is little resemblance in most instances, both architecturally and cytomorphologically, to DM.

Desmoplastic Spitz tumors often impart the appearance of a dermatofibroma, both clinically and histologically. Examination of the cytomorphology may raise some concern given the plumpness of the cells that is typical of spitzoid lesions. However, there is not a dominant spindled cytomorphology with wide dermal involvement. The lesions are usually relatively well-circumscribed and the cells are usually identifiable as being spitzoid. There is perhaps more chance for confusion with an atypical Spitz tumor rather than with a DM.

Sclerosing blue nevus, once again, resembles DM only by way of the dermal sclerosis. Dermal sclerosis is a relatively consistent feature of common blue nevi and sclerosing blue nevi. The presence of relatively bland epithelioid and fusiform cells with delicate to prominent cytoplasmic melanization dominates the histologic appearance.

Dermatofibromas, conventional and cellular, have been known to mimic DM, as some dermatofibromas indeed show a plump spindled cytomorphology with, in some cases, significant cytologic atypia and apparently increased mitotic activity. However, there is usually evidence of peripheral collagen trapping, no junctional melanocytic component, and, in most cases, a relatively bland cytomorphology. In addition, the heterogeneity of the cellular populace, in the form of multinucleate and xanthomatized histiocytes, and a mixed inflammatory cell element, help to distinguish dermatofibroma from DM. This applies, even to those cases of cellular dermatofibroma and atypical fibrous histiocytoma which show dense dermal cellularity and bizarre cells. In the vast majority of cases, dermatofibroma variants can be distinguished from DM on routine staining.

DFSP demonstrates a highly cellular and diffuse dermal proliferation of spindled cells that involves the dermis and subcutis. The primary arrangement is storiform in most cases. Furthermore, the cytomorphology of DFSP is characteristically monotonous. In fact, it is more monotonous and homogeneous than dermatofibromas. The spindled nuclei are delicate and betray their malignant nature largely by way of architecture, rather than cytomorphology, in the form of diffuse involvement of the dermis and subcutis with entrapment of subcutaneous adipocytes. Diagnostic confirmation is achieved via positive staining for CD34, and lesional negativity for S-100, allowing for histologic distinction from DM.

Neural proliferations such as malignant peripheral nerve sheath tumor (MPNST) pose a significant challenge, for in the absence of a junctional melanocytic component, there is histologic and immunohistochemical overlap with regard to S-100. However, a potentially useful discriminating feature in this setting is the patchy positivity of S-100 in MPNST as opposed to the diffuse lesional positivity for S-100 in most cases of DM. In addition, some MPNST's may be associated with a background of neurofibroma. Further, MPNST arising in the skin is a distinctly uncommon phenomenon. However, distinguishing between these two conditions can pose a serious diagnostic challenge.

Sarcomas such as fibrosarcoma and leiomyosarcoma can show significant histologic overlap with DM. However, immunohistochemistry allows consistent differentiation from DM.

Spindle cell squamous cell carcinoma also shows considerable histologic overlap with DM. Scrutiny of the dermal-epidermal junction can be instrumental in such cases, should either keratinocyte atypia or a junctional melanocytic proliferation be identified. If this does not prove useful, immunohistochemistry is a reliable arbitrator in these cases.

Atypical fibroxanthoma can show spindle cell features. Once again, the immunohistochemical profile serves to resolve the diagnostic confusion.

The biological behavior of DM has been a subject of some controversy, largely due to the relatively low number of cases, and the increasing recognition of the fact that the natural history of this lesion appears to differ from that of conventional melanomas. Firstly, diagnostic delay, by virtue of the subtlety of the clinical and histologic findings, contributes significantly to the advanced Breslow depth that this lesion often demonstrates at diagnosis. Furthermore, even in those cases that are biopsied, limited lesional sampling may, in some cases, preclude the comprehensive histologic analysis that is required to diagnose these lesions. The mean Breslow depths, according to a large review of the literature, ranged from 2.0 to 6.5 mm (6). Most cases present with at least a Clark level IV. Also, local recurrence, more so than distant metastasis, distinguishes this tumor from other types of melanoma. Perineurial and endoneurial invasion in DNM and the ill-defined nature of these lesions, likely plays a significant role in this regard. It is held that distant spread is less common despite the advanced tumor thickness that is characteristic of DM (7). One study involving 129 patients and a mean tumor thickness of 4.2 mm reported recurrence in 39.5% of the cases, with 14% recurring locally. (8). A review of the literature, encompassing a total of 703 patients, documented a local tumor recurrence rate of 27.2%, a nodal metastatic rate of 7.1%, and a rate of systemic metastasis of 19.8% (6). A more recent study addressing the issue of nodal metastasis in DM reported one nodal metastasis in their cohort of 18 cases that underwent lymph node biopsy (7).

The prognosis of DM is generally regarded as being more favorable than that of conventional melanomas for a given tumor thickness. One study of 129 patients with a mean tumor thickness of 4.2 mm reported 76% and 64% respective 5 and 10-year rates of survival (12). In addition, a study performed at the Sydney Melanoma Unit in which they evaluated 280 patients with a mean tumor thickness of 2.5 mm reported a 5-year survival of 75%. Ninety of these 280 patients represented cases of the neurotropic variety of desmoplastic melanoma. The researchers failed to demonstrate that perineural invasion affected rates of survival in DM. Further, they reported fewer lymph node metastases in DM as compared to those associated with conventional melanomas (9). It has further been reported that DM lesions greater than 4 mm in thickness demonstrate a 60% 5-year survival compared to 40% in non-desmoplastic melanomas (10). These findings contrast with those of a study involving 89 patients in which investigators reported rates of survival that were similar to those of non-desmoplastic melanoma of similar thickness (11). A more recent study engaged in a nuanced examination of the histologic features insofar as their prognostic contribution. They subdivided cases of DM into "pure" and "mixed" subtypes, being respectively representative of lesions with prominent stromal desmoplasia and those in which the desmoplastic component was simply an element of what was otherwise a more conventional melanoma. They reported that those patients classified as pure DM showed a significantly lower incidence of lymph node metastasis, and a lower 5-year melanoma-specific mortality as compared to the mixed DM patients. Further, they discovered that the melanoma-specific mortality was equal among the pure DM and conventional melanoma patients, despite a 3-fold higher median tumor depth in the former. Interestingly, they also reported that the lymph node metastases in the mixed DM patients were characterized by the non-desmoplastic component of the primary mixed DM lesions (12). It may, therefore, be reasonable, as Hawkins et al. suggest, to subclassify these lesions, and designate the pure forms of DM as *Spindle Cell* melanomas.

There exists, therefore, reasonable evidence to support the notion that DM's maintain a prognostic advantage when compared to conventional lesions of cutaneous melanoma. However, the question that is perhaps more intriguing relates to the pathobiology of this neoplasm. Specifically, should a lesion that deviates, on a morphologic, immunohistochemical, and behavioral basis, from melanoma, continued to be classified as a melanoma versus a "primitive melanocytic or neurocristic spindle cell sarcoma" (one can recall the use of the historical term "melanosarcoma")? Perhaps future studies will seek to address this issue.

Management

DM carries a high risk for local recurrence which is directly related to its frequent amelanotic appearance, often advanced stage at the time of diagnosis, Breslow thickness > 4.0 mm, and neurotropic and angiotropic properties, as mentioned above. Thus, resection of DM with clear surgical margins as early as possible in its development is crucial to its successful clinical management. Although not systematically studied, most surgeons recommend a minimum clearance of at least 1 to 3 cm. As already discussed, there is increasing evidence that SLNB) may not be indicated for "pure" variants of DM because of their low incidence of regional lymph node metastases

■ NEVOID MELANOMA

It is well established that melanoma may show differentiation along the lines of almost every variant of benign melanocytic nevus or tumor. Thus, *a priori* a subset of melanomas closely resembles melanocytic nevi. Hence the rubric "nevoid" melanoma has appeared in the literature as a direct result of this fundamental diagnostic problem of differentiating melanoma from nevus. In this article "nevoid" melanoma (NM) is defined as a tentative group of melanomas that more or less recapitulate the architectural configuration and cytomorphology of melanocytic nevi, yet concomitantly demonstrate histologic criteria for, and the biological behavior of, melanoma (1,13,19–24). However one can make the case that until a series of "NMs" have been characterized at the clinical, histologic and molecular levels with long-term follow-up, there is no scientific basis that NMs exist as a legitimate entity. Since many such lesions are not diagnosed initially and are detected only in retrospect, the histologic diagnosis of NM remains controversial and consensus criteria have not been established. Suffice to say that nevoid melanoma remains a subject of ongoing research. In any case, this problem of the distinction of melanoma from nevus is among the most treacherous diagnostic problems in all of dermatopathology, and as such, carries significant medicolegal implications.

Clinical Features

Although more rigorous studies are needed, from the NMs reported thus far in the literature, they seem generally comparable to conventional melanomas in terms of demographic characteristics. Most cases have been reported in women, with some degree of predilection for the legs and trunk (1, 13, 19, 20). This condition has no clinically distinctive features. In fact, it most often imparts the appearance of a nevus, which stands to reason when one understands the nature of the histopathology.

Histopathologic Features

The histologic diagnosis of "nevoid" melanoma is notoriously difficult since important standard criteria for melanoma are usually absent. For example, many such lesions are often less than 5 to 7 mm in greatest diameter; asymmetry, poor circumscription, and pagetoid melanocytosis are absent or minimal; apparent "maturation" may be present; and the constituent melanocytes may be smaller and less atypical than the usual high-grade melanoma cells (1, 13,19–24). Thus scanning magnification, in most cases, reveals a relatively small-diameter, predominately or purely dermal nevomelanocytic proliferation that shows symmetry and sharp circumscription with even an element of maturation by virtue of the diminution of the cellular density with lesional descent (Figs. 5–7). The extent to which the overall size and configuration of the individual lesion resembles or deviates from that of a nevus compromises or reinforces the histopathologist's suspicion for melanoma. Some cases may be verrucous or polypoid in configuration and, importantly, some proportion of cases are amelanotic.

The common denominators among many nevoid melanomas that should alert the pathologist to the diagnosis include: 1) dermal mitoses, 2) a sheet-like appearance, i.e., hypercellularity and crowding of dermal melanocytes, 3) a monomorphous appearance of melanocytes, 4) subtle but definite cytologic atypia as evidenced by nuclear enlargement, nuclear pleomorphism, irregularity of nuclear membranes, coarsening of nuclear chromatin, and often distinct nucleoli (Figure 8), 5) the lack of conventional maturation and presence of irregular infiltrating features at the base, and 6) angiotropism. Perhaps the minimal essential criteria needed for (nevoid) melanoma are dermal mitoses, a

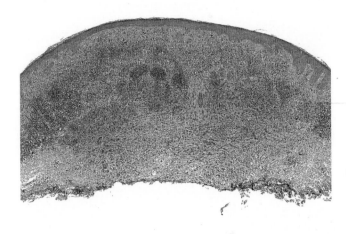

FIGURE 5
Nevoid melanoma: scanning magnification demonstrating a symmetrical and well-circumscribed dermal melanocytic proliferation.

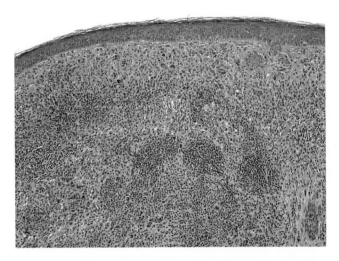

FIGURE 6
Nevoid melanoma: note diminished cellular size and density with lesional descent suggesting maturation. There are discreet dermal nests of melanocytes suggesting a nevus.

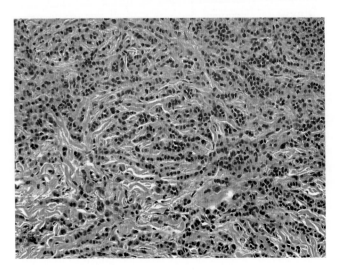

FIGURE 7
Nevoid melanoma: note cords of melanocytes with infiltrative pattern in deeper dermis.

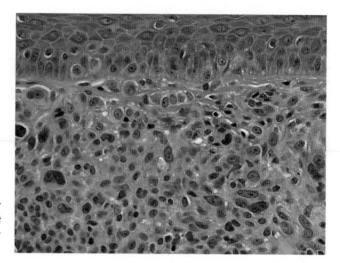

FIGURE 8
Nevoid melanoma: high power view demonstrating prominent nuclear enlargement and nuclear pleomorphism.

sheet-like pattern, and cytologic atypia. It is clear that the greater the number of criteria present the greater the certitude of the diagnosis of melanoma. In terms of cytomorphology, the melanocytes vary from relatively small cuboidal cells to enlarged round, ovoid or spindled cells. Typically, melanoma cells of the same size are present throughout the lesion and at the base, albeit with, in some cases, the added element of decreased cellular density suggesting maturation. In some instances, cellular and nuclear sizes of melanocytes are slightly diminished with depth. This is accompanied by increased mitotic activity in most lesions. Mitotic activity is particularly contributory to the diagnosis when it involves the lower third of the dermal melanocytic populace. The intraepidermal component, if present, may be subtle or limited in nature. One may observe melanocytes arranged as single cells and /or in junctional nests along the dermal-epidermal junction. The nesting may result in confluence of nested aggregates of melanocytes replacing the basilar portion of the epidermis. The epidermis is frequently effaced, thinned, and associated with dermal-epidermal separation. Pagetoid spread may be

present in a proportion of cases and is an important finding in confirming a diagnosis of melanoma; however it is often not a conspicuous feature. Inflammation and necrosis are less conspicuous than in conventional melanomas, or may be altogether absent. In some proportion of cases, the proliferation can assume a perineural and angiotropic pattern of spread.

Differential Diagnosis

The differential diagnosis of NM includes: 1) various types of melanocytic nevi with atypical features, and 2) metastatic melanoma. The difficulty with this diagnosis, as already mentioned, is directly related to the distinction of melanoma from nevus and that any individual melanocytic lesion may show a spectrum of features shared by both melanoma and nevi. As in all things, a comprehensive analysis and a high index of suspicion and sensitivity to certain subtle clues often leads one to the correct diagnosis. A melanocytic lesion may raise definite diagnostic suspicion for melanoma on an almost visceral level at scanning magnification. Such suspect lesions often impart a sheet-like or crowded configuration and monomorphous appearance of the dermal component. In addition, the lesional base is usually ill-defined with hyperchromatic cells infiltrating the dermis in a single-cell and cord-like fashion. Higher magnification often reveals round, ovoid or spindled melanocytes resembling nevus cells but also showing some cellular enlargement, nuclear enlargement, irregularity of nuclear contours, thickening of nuclear membranes, and commonly subtle but distinct nucleoli. Further examination reveals the presence of variable mitotic activity, sometimes limited in number. Mitoses located in the lower third of the lesion, in this setting, provide additional support for melanoma.

Certain variants of melanocytic nevi that are especially difficult to distinguish from ("nevoid") melanomas include polypoid cellular compound or dermal nevi, congenital and congenital-pattern nevi, melanocytic nevi with halo reactions, traumatized and inflamed nevi, acquired and congenital melanocytic nevi with atypical dermal nodule formation, melanocytic nevi removed from pregnant women, and melanocytic nevi from particular anatomic sites such as the vulva, breast, or scalp. The characteristics suggesting melanoma are the very same that have been emphasized above: dermal mitoses, the appearance of dermal hypercellularity, a monomorphous quality of dermal melanocytes, cytologic atypia, and perhaps diminished maturation. As with all melanocytic lesions one must have certain essential clinical information including age, gender, anatomic site, and history of melanoma, pregnancy, trauma or other pertinent factors before definitively interpreting melanocytic lesions. Likewise, the histopathologist must have at least the essential histologic criteria present and, optimally, additional abnormal features to assure a confident diagnosis of melanoma. Thus, in general the diagnosis of melanoma cannot be based on a single abnormal finding. For example, mitotic figures can be seen in nevi, especially in certain contexts such as nevi in young individuals, polypoid cellular nevi, nevi with halo reactions, and atypical dermal nodules associated with nevi, and traumatized nevi. Often such mitoses are noted only in the superficial half of such nevi and the mitotic rates are usually about 1 to 4 per mm^2. The mere presence of such mitotic activity, in and of itself, does not and should not prompt a more serious diagnosis. However more significant mitotic rates, mitoses observed at the base of a lesion, and atypical forms should prompt careful scrutiny for other features supporting melanoma. Hypercellularity also occurs in nevi with some frequency; however such hypercellular nevi usually display diminished cellularity and maturation with depth. Cytologic "atypia", depending upon one's threshold, is seen in most nevi in the form of senescent atypia, characterized by nuclear enlargement with some contour irregularity and multinucleation. However, the degree of consistent nuclear enlargement, nuclear irregularity, thickening of nuclear membranes, and distinctively enlarged and multiple nucleoli observed in melanoma are usually lacking in nevi. Maturation is a variable phenomenon in ordinary nevi, depending upon the depth of dermal extension, involvement of adnexal structures, and the like.

Some advocate the employment of Ki-67 and HMB45 as adjunctive diagnostic measures; however, in the authors' opinion, such ancillary studies are limited in their diagnostic utility.

It is important to note that the spectrum of NM is clearly on a continuum with conventional "nodular" melanoma and the distinction of the two is probably artificial and not reproducible in many cases. It should be emphasized that as with nodular melanoma one should always consider metastatic melanoma in the differential diagnosis of "nevoid" melanomas. Although criteria have been suggested for distinguishing metastatic from primary melanoma, often clinical information is crucial to establishing a lesion as primary vs. metastatic.

The outcome from reviewing many such lesions raising suspicion for nevoid melanoma results in the major groupings of 1) controversial lesions including many atypical nevi that lack unequivocal criteria for melanoma and 2) lesions interpreted as nevoid melanoma by a consensus of observers or based on an adverse event such as metastasis. Thus, one will encounter lesions lacking sufficient criteria for melanoma. Such lesions should be reported descriptively as atypical melanocytic neoplasms and possibly as biologically indeterminate for some tumors, with the additional qualification that a melanoma cannot be entirely excluded. Further, if the lesion approaches one millimeter in depth, the dilemma is further compounded with regard to the inclusionary criteria for sentinel lymph node biopsy. There is as yet no viable solution to this dilemma. However, the most sound approach is likely an honest discussion of the situation with the patient, and possibly the surgical oncologist, with a presentation of all facts in hopes of arriving at a mutually agreeable course of action.

The prognosis of nevoid melanomas, if established as melanoma, appears indistinguishable from that of conventional melanomas in the studies thus far published. Thus, the standard prognostic factors including clinical stage and Breslow thickness are the major determinates of clinical outcome. However, the prognosis of such lesions in general requires more rigorous study.

Management

Patients with melanocytic lesions established as nevoid melanoma should be managed as conventional melanomas.

■ SPITZOID MELANOCYTIC NEOPLASMS AND SPITZ-LIKE MELANOMA

Spitzoid melanocytic neoplasms have occupied a special niche in the melanocytic neoplastic system for many years, and there is increasing evidence that they are a biologically unique melanocytic neoplasm (13, 25–53). Yet there are still many unresolved questions with respect to the biological nature, natural history, and biological potential of spitzoid melanocytic lesions in general (32–35). For example, do malignant spitzoid lesions exist as such; do they exist in particular age groups such as prepubertal children or even in older individuals; do they have a unique molecular genotype; do they have a different biological potential, possibly less aggressive, than conventional melanomas? Are Spitz tumors in general (or a subset of Spitz tumors) capable of spreading or metastasizing beyond the primary site yet not constitute a conventional malignant neoplasm and metastasis?

As with "nevoid" melanoma the term "spitzoid" melanoma has surfaced in the medical literature as a direct result of the difficulty or impossibility in some cases of distinguishing melanoma from Spitz tumors. One particular source for the use of the term "spitzoid" melanoma (SM) has come about from the retrospective diagnoses of melanocytic lesions (as cutaneous melanoma) which had been initially interpreted as "Spitz nevus" and have subsequently shown clearly documented adverse events such as lymph node metastases, more distant metastases, and/or death. Thus, although the term SM would seem to have merit, in fact "SM" has been used with such imprecision in the literature that the term itself has become almost meaningless in the authors' view (32,53). The essential problem is the indiscriminate application of this term to a heterogeneous group of spitzoid-appearing lesions that differ considerably in terms of many phenotypic and genotypic characteristics and biological potential (Figure 9) (32–35, 39–53). For example, the term has been applied to:

(1) lesions originally interpreted as Spitz nevi and following an adverse event are in retrospect diagnosed as melanoma;

(2) conventional (or "typical"), atypical or controversial spitzoid tumors in children, adolescents, and adults with or without clinical lymph node metastases and no apparent progression of disease;

(3) atypical or controversial spitzoid tumors in children and adolescents or adults with clinical lymph node metastases, no apparent progression of

disease, and with or without genotypic aberrations;

(4) atypical or controversial spitzoid tumors in children and adolescents and adults with positive sentinel lymph node involvement and no apparent disease progression (54–57);

(5) atypical or controversial spitzoid tumors with chromosomal aberrations associated with conventional melanoma;

(6) conventional melanomas having some resemblance to Spitz tumors.

For the time being, the authors recommend that the use of the term "spitzoid" melanoma should be curtailed until rigorous guidelines regarding its usage are formulated.

Spitzoid lesions, like other melanocytic lesions, occur along a histologic continuum of benign, atypical, and malignant, perhaps low-grade and high-grade, and must be evaluated utilizing all clinical, histopathologic, and other criteria available (32,33, 36–38, 41–51). After examination, one can usually assign a given lesion to one of three categories: (1) Spitz tumors without appreciable

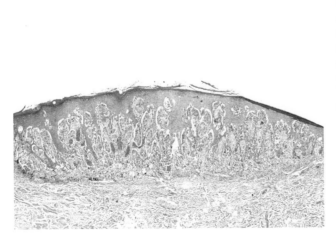

FIGURE 9
Compound spitzoid melanocytic neoplasm: this field demonstrates a small-diameter, well-circumscribed, and symmetrical compound melanocytic proliferation. This lesion was interpreted independently as both a "Spitz nevus" and a "spitzoid melanoma," illustrating the difficulty posed by many spitzoid melanocytic proliferations. Note vertical orientation of spindled melanocytes and clefting between junctional melanocytic nests and surrounding epidermis. Dermal mitoses are not observed in this lesion.

abnormality, (2) Spitz tumors with one or more atypical features (atypical Spitz tumor) including those with indeterminate biological or malignant potential, possibly including a percentage of low-grade malignant lesions, and (3) cutaneous melanoma, potentially low-grade and high-grade (32).

The authors believe that it is overly simplistic to impose an (often arbitrary) interpretation of either 'Spitz's nevus' or melanoma on every spitzoid lesion (32). This approach is not satisfactory for patient care and does not provide a realistic methodology for dealing prospectively with such a difficult problem. Such an exercise undoubtedly results in both the overdiagnosis of melanoma and underrecognition of atypical or ambiguous lesions requiring more medical attention. Patients may unfairly suffer the psychological burden of a grave diagnosis and be subjected to overly aggressive and potentially harmful therapies. Conversely, some proportion of patients will have the false and unjustified assurances of a benign diagnosis and may not receive appropriate treatment and follow-up.

Clinical Features

The majority of Spitz tumors occur in young individuals particularly under the age of 10–20 years (25–32). The older the patient, especially individuals beyond the age of 40 years, the greater the likelihood of malignancy. However, Spitz tumors may occur with greater frequency in older adults than has been appreciated owing to the propensity of many pathologists to *a priori* interpret them as melanoma.

Other clinical factors such as the location of the tumor, clinical appearance, history of recent changes in a long-standing stable lesion, and family history of melanoma should be considered carefully. Spitz tumors commonly involve the extremities and face. The location of atypical tumors on sites less commonly involved by Spitz tumor, such as the back, is also another factor suggesting careful scrutiny of the lesion for melanoma.

In general, Spitz tumors are relatively small (often < 5 to 6 mm in diameter), symmetrical, and well-defined, dome-shaped nodules or plaques with uniform pink or reddish coloration. Roughly 10% are pigmented. Atypical variants show larger diameters (i.e., > 5 mm), particularly greater than 1 cm and increasingly abnormal gross morphologic features including irregular borders, irregular topography, ulceration, and irregular coloration.

Histopathologic Features

The histological interpretation of spitzoid melanocytic neoplasms, as with all melanocytic lesions, first of all involves a qualitative (or gestalt) assessment as to whether the lesion of interest is obvious melanoma or not. Even if considered unequivocal conventional melanoma, the histopathologist should be able to systematically analyze the lesion with a battery of fairly standardized histological criteria and other techniques in order to objectively corroborate his/her interpretation of melanoma, or, alternatively, a spitzoid melanocytic neoplasm with or without atypical properties (see Figs. 10–16) (32,33 52,53). These principal microscopical attributes include the following:

Size (diameter in mm): Most typical Spitz nevi/tumors measure less than 5–6 mm. Size beyond 5 to 6 mm, especially > 10mm is generally considered abnormal. This is a continuous variable and there are obvious exceptions to this criterion.

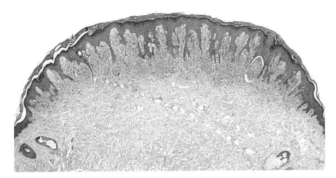

FIGURE 10
Compound Spitz tumor: scanning magnification demonstrates a prototypic conventional Spitz tumor. This lesion is characterized by small-diameter, sharp circumscription, symmetry, and absence of the following: ulceration, effacement of the epidermis, dermal mitoses, and extension into subcutaneous fat.

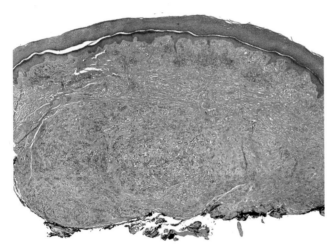

FIGURE 11
Atypical compound spitzoid melanocytic neoplasm: biopsy sampling of lesion from the foot of a 17-year-old female demonstrating a compound melanocytic neoplasm with asymmetry of the junctional and dermal components and lack of maturation. Note nodular portion of the lesion in the deep dermis. FISH testing revealed loss of 6q23.

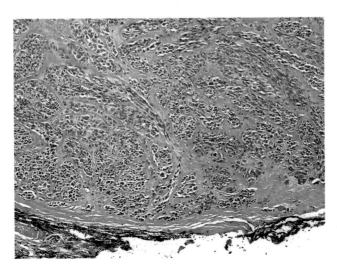

FIGURE 12
Atypical compound spitzoid melanocytic neoplasm: higher magnification of deep dermal nodule.

FIGURE 13
Atypical compound spitzoid melanocytic neoplasm: higher magnification of deep dermal nodule. Note large atypical epithelioid melanocytes with conspicuous nucleoli and mitotic figures. The mitotic rate was 3 per mm^2.

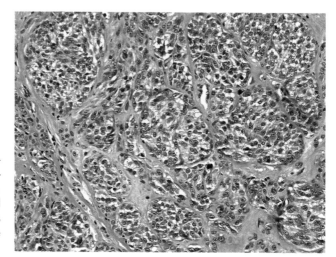

FIGURE 14
Melanoma resembling a Spitz tumor: scanning magnification shows a poorly circumscribed, asymmetric and ulcerated atypical melanocytic proliferation measuring 8 mm in diameter and 6.1 mm in thickness.

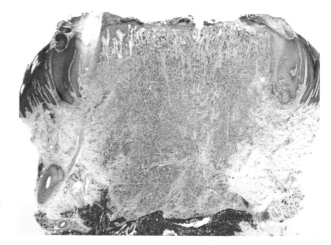

FIGURE 15
Melanoma resembling a Spitz tumor: higher magnification of dermal component demonstrating high cellular density and confluence of melanocytes. The mitotic rate was 7 per mm^2.

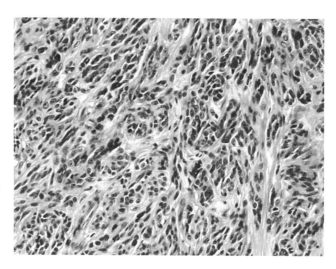

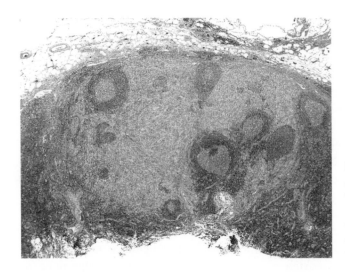

FIGURE 16
Melanoma resembling a Spitz tumor: sentinel lymph node (SLN) biopsy from the groin. The SLN contains a large nodule of atypical melanocytes replacing most of the lymph node.

Tumor thickness (measured in mm): Significant (Breslow) depth and involvement of the subcutaneous fat are considered abnormal.

Asymmetry: Increasing asymmetry is abnormal as in all melanocytic lesions.

Epidermal configuration: Most typical Spitz nevi/tumors show a prototypic symmetrical and crescent-shaped or plaque-type pattern of epidermal hyperplasia without effacement or disruption of the epidermis by the spitzoid melanocytic elements. In fact, the relationship between junctional nests and fascicles of melanocytes and the epidermis is unique: the nests and especially the fascicles of melanocytes insinuate between keratinocytes in a serpiginous and nondisruptive fashion quite unlike the consumptive and obliterative effects of melanoma. Even with pagetoid melanocytosis and transepidermal elimination of nests of melanocytes the epidermis generally remains rather surprisingly undisturbed. Another characteristic feature is the clefting between the epidermis and the superficial aspects of junctional nests of melanocytes (Figs. 22, 23). Unfortunately, many spitzoid lesions are traumatized and consequently they do not often maintain the orderly and symmetrical properties described above to the degree ideally one may expect.

Ulceration: Ulceration is an abnormal finding; however, ulceration is often at least partially induced by trauma and its significance may vary.

Poor circumscription: The most banal Spitz nevi/tumors tend to be sharply circumscribed at their peripheries whereas atypical lesions are often less well-circumscribed. This parameter obviously correlates with asymmetry and other organizational attributes.

Pagetoid melanocytosis: Pagetoid spread may be observed not infrequently in Spitz tumors. However, such pagetoid spread should be limited to the lower half of epidermis, should not extend peripherally, should be only focal, and sparsely cellular. More extensive pagetoid spread involving the upper half of the epidermis, a large segment of the lesion (one or more high-power fields), and in a single-cell or small nested pattern is distinctly abnormal. External trauma may be a factor leading to excessive pagetoid spread in benign lesions.

Prominent confluence and high cellular density of melanocytes: These two parameters are closely correlated and are among the most important criteria for assessing melanocytic lesions. Unfortunately, these characteristics are subjective and therefore difficult to recognize reliably and reproducibly. These two parameters are also often closely linked to diminished or absent maturation (see below). Confluent cellular aggregates or nodules of considerable size and with crowded appearance in the dermal component, particularly replacing the dermis, and extending deep without maturation are also decidedly atypical. Breslow thickness obviously may capture the significance of such expansile dermal nodules. One caveat is the occurrence of such nodules in Spitz tumors of young children, which may take on less importance in the latter context.

Lack of zonation and maturation: Zonation refers to the side-to-side homogeneity often observed in typical Spitz tumors. Whereas maturation is the progressively diminished sizes of nests of melanocytes and gradual dispersion of melanocytes to smaller nests and single cells with depth. The latter phenomenon, in its most developed state, involves a nondisruptive infiltration of melanocytes among collagen bundles and involution of melanocytes to smaller cells with smaller nuclei with depth. Therefore, the non-uniformity (heterogeneity of organization) of a lesion when scanned from side to side and the continued presence of nests and fascicles of similar sizes deep indicate potentially aggressive properties.

Few or no dull pink (Kamino) bodies: Although this feature may be seen in both Spitz tumors and melanomas, the presence of clear cut aggregates of Kamino bodies may be a marker suggesting a more typical Spitz tumor.

Mitotic rate per mm^2: The mitotic rate of the dermal component is one of the most important parameters for evaluating spitzoid lesions as increasing proliferative rate seems to correlate with likelihood of aggressive behavior or malignancy. Furthermore, this parameter is quantifiable. Mitoses observed in the deepest parts of the dermal or subcutaneous component—that is, near the deep margin, also seem to have greater significance than more superficially located mitoses. There are clearly no absolute thresholds for the mitotic rate being indicative of benignancy or malignancy, and the authors caution against using mitotic rate alone (or any single criterion alone) for the interpretation of a melanocytic lesion. It is important in almost all instances to have several distinctly abnormal parameters present to confirm malignancy. Every lesion must be systematically assessed on a case-by-case basis. In any event, high mitotic rates, particularly beyond six mitoses per mm^2 raise concern for malignancy. Unusual circumstances that may confound the importance of high mitotic rate include: (1) developing Spitz tumors may be in a growth phase and mitotic rate may have less significance, (2) Spitz tumors in very young individuals may have somewhat higher mitotic rates, and (3) external trauma and significant inflammation may be factors leading to higher mitotic rates.

Cytologic attributes suggesting a more atypical spitzoid lesion and possibly melanoma include heterogeneity of cell type throughout the lesion, particularly in an asymmetrical or haphazard pattern; high-nuclear-to-cytoplasmic ratios; granular or 'dusty' cytoplasm vs the ground glass cytoplasm of Spitz melanocytes; absence of delicate or dispersed chromatin patterns with thickening of nuclear membranes; a large proportion of melanocytes with hyperchromatic nuclei; and the presence of large eosinophilic nucleoli.

Ancillary Techniques

Immunohistochemistry

Spitzoid lesions have been evaluated with a variety of bio-markers. S-100 protein and Melan-A/Mart-1 show diffuse expression throughout both Spitz tumors and melanoma in contrast to the characteristic diminished expression of HMB45, tyrosinase, and other markers toward the base of Spitz tumors. In addition, there is a gradient of diminished proliferation with increasing depth of the dermal component paralleling mitotic rate and cyclin D1 expression in Spitz tumors. Although requiring much more study for standardization, Ki-67 expression may be useful in the risk stratification of Spitz tumors (33, 36–38, 48). For example, in one study atypical Spitz tumors had a mean Ki-67 labeling index of 10% relative to 0.53% in ordinary nevi, 5.04% in conventional Spitz tumors, and 36.83% in conventional melanomas (37); whereas in another study a Ki-67 proliferation index less than 2% favored a conventional Spitz tumor, one greater than 10% melanoma, and indices between 2 and 10% were equivocal (36). The qualitative loss of Ki-67 expression vs continued labeling with depth as with other markers such as HMB-45 also correlates with maturation and a less atypical lesion.

Spitz tumors also appear to exhibit lower rates of p53, bcl-2, and fatty acid synthase expression compared to melanoma (37, 38).The loss of p16 expression in atypical spitzoid melanocytic neoplasms also may favor melanoma (48). Although many of the latter markers are of interest, they require rigorous assessment with greater numbers of cases and long term follow-up in order determine whether they have any predictive value in the evaluation of spitzoid lesions.

Comparative Genomic Hybridization and Fluorescence In Situ Hybridization

From the small number of studies thus far published, it seems that a relatively large proportion of Spitz tumors including a significant percentage of atypical or controversial variants fail to show chromosomal or genetic aberrations by comparative genomic hybridization (CGH) and fluorescence in situ hybridization (FISH) (39–47). That is to say, in general, the lesions studied do not show chromosomal aberrations, as are usually observed in conventional melanomas. In an early study of Spitz tumors, about 15% of the lesions demonstrated an increased copy number of chromosome 11p, generally correlating with Spitz tumors which were often larger in size, dermal-based, desmoplastic, with vesicular nuclei in melanocytes, dermal infiltrating features, and were associated with *HRAS* mutation; whereas 85% showed no chromosomal aberrations (39, 40). A recent small series of spitzoid melanocytic neoplasms analyzed by array CGH has shown that among 16 atypical Spitz tumors, 44% showed chromosomal aberrations, whereas 56% showed none (41). The chromosomal aberrations documented in these 7 ASTs were unusual and not observed to date in conventional melanomas. Another recent investigation of 75 atypical Spitz tumors utilizing six FISH probes targeting major melanoma chromosomal loci, has suggested that gains in 6p25 and 11q13 and homozygous deletion of 9p21 may correlate with increased risk for aggressive behavior and potentially death, respectively (45,46). However, another comprehensive analysis of FISH results has shown almost comparable rates of FISH positivity in "atypical Spitz tumors" (62% FISH positive) and "Spitzoid melanomas" (71% FISH positive) (47). From this information spitzoid melanocytic lesions may be categorized as: 1) spitzoid melanocytic lesions without any apparent genotypic aberrations, perhaps corresponding to conventional or typical Spitz tumors; 2) spitzoid lesions with various genotypic aberrations, some newly-described and not associated with conventional melanoma, and not having clearly established biological significance, perhaps corresponding to atypical Spitz tumors including possibly some low-grade neoplasms; and 3) spitzoid lesions with genotypic aberrations usually associated with conventional melanoma, perhaps corresponding to both low-grade spitzoid melanocytic neoplasms and some high-grade neoplasms (probably including conventional melanoma). The latter scheme is not new but may potentially have greater predictive value for disease progression and outcome but still requires rigorous validation (32–34, 47).

Therefore, it is certain that there must be much more detailed and objective clinical, histologic, and molecular characterization of spitzoid melanocytic lesions, correlation with natural history, particularly with rare cases manifesting distant metastases and death, and long-term follow-up, perhaps of at least 15 years, in order to clearly define distinct patient subgroups (32, 34, 47, 53).

Loss of Heterozygosity
Two independent studies have recently demonstrated loss of heterozygosity on chromosome 9p with DNA polymorphic markers in two of 27 and five of five 'Spitz nevi' (49,50). The latter findings corroborate the loss of chromosomal 9p with CGH and homozygous deletion of 9p21 observed with FISH.

Analysis of Gene Mutations
Recent work has shown that a series of conventional Spitz tumors and the so-called spitzoid melanomas in prepubescent children failed to show any hotspot activating mutations in the B-raf, N-ras, or H-ras genes (51). The general absence of B-raf mutations in spitzoid lesions contrasts with a high rate of mutation (53–80%) in conventional melanomas and (70–90%) in melanocytic nevi and suggests a different and perhaps yet to be characterized developmental pathway for spitzoid lesions (33).

Sentinel Lymph Node Biopsy
The application of SLNB to atypical spitzoid melanocytic lesions potentially provides a means of obtaining more information about the biological characteristics of such lesions (54–57). However, upon closer scrutiny there are several fundamental questions that must be addressed before one can begin to have any meaningful data on this issue: one must have a much better understanding of the metastatic process in general versus non-malignant cellular migration and spread, and other possible explanations for the presence of ectopic cells in lymph nodes and other sites; the nature and significance of SLN deposits associated with all melanocytic lesions requires much more rigorous study and analysis; and finally, only the study of sufficient numbers of cases with long-term follow-up will provide the data to definitively know the biological nature of many SLN deposits associated with various spitzoid lesions, if they are inherently different from conventional melanomas, and if they potentially have better prognoses. Thus without such data it is impossible to know, in general, the true biological significance of spitzoid deposits in SLN. However, there are accumulating data available from the literature. Among these studies, mostly in children and adolescents, who have undergone sentinel lymph biopsy for spitzoid melanocytic tumors (probably a heterogeneous group of typical and atypical spitzoid lesions and possibly some true

melanomas), up to about 50% of patients have shown positive SLNB (57). In most instances, the tumor deposits have been microscopic and generally have involved the parenchyma or subcapsular sinuses of the SLN. With completion lymphadenectomy, only a small of percentage of patients have showed any further nodal involvement— usually only a single additional node being involved. None of the patients thus far have shown any further disease progression with follow-up ranging from months to several years (57). Although these data are preliminary and not yet conclusive due to lack of consensus interpretation of the primary spitzoid neoplasms and sufficient long-term follow-up, the patients appear to show no progression of disease and thus the positive SLN does not correlate with risk of further metastatic disease. As a result, the data suggest that many SLN deposits from spitzoid tumors appear indolent and possibly some are benign or, at least, biologically indeterminate. Consequently, atypical Spitz tumor deposits in SLNs may possibly have a different biology or significance than metastases from conventional melanoma (32–35).

Differential Diagnosis

Since we lack objective data and sufficient follow-up, the significance or weighting of the various features already mentioned has not been established. However, at present the final interpretation of a Spitzoid lesion remains almost entirely histopathologic with important consideration given to clinical information. Almost all other parameters have not yet been sufficiently studied as to have any significant impact on the final interpretation. However, some indices such as the Ki-67 labeling, CGH, and FISH may provide additional useful information in the final deliberation about

a lesion. In the future, such ancillary data may take on much greater importance.

Some may point out that such an approach seems to render many or most Spitz tumors atypical. In the process of evaluating Spitz tumors common sense must prevail, and one must keep in mind that one is most likely dealing with a biological continuum with many or most Spitz tumors at the 'benign' or 'less aggressive' end of the spectrum. There is little question that as these various parameters progressively accumulate in number and severity, the probability of an aggressive phenotype or malignancy increases. It is apparent that certain parameters take on more significance than others (*represents most helpful features) (32). Potentially aggressive tumors or melanomas thus often have large size* (>5–6mm, often >10mm*); may have significant depth*; demonstrate distinct asymmetry*; poor circumscription; heterogeneity of cellular populations*; more disordered intraepidermal proliferative patterns of melanocytes without clefting; extensive pagetoid spread; irregular epidermal alterations including thinning and effacement; significant melanocytic density and confluence*; and the lack of zonation or diminished cellular density with depth (maturation)*. The lack of uniformity or homogeneity of cell type along comparable strata (from side to side) of the tumor cannot be overemphasized as a major criterion favoring melanoma. Similarly, the failure of a tumor to show progressive dispersion of melanocytes to smaller aggregates and particularly to single melanocytes (among apparently unaffected collagen bundles) in the deepest part of the lesion also suggests melanoma. Usually concurrent with depth is the uniform diminution of cellular and nuclear sizes and regular spacing of melanocytes in a Spitz nevus/tumor; the failure to observe the latter feature should prompt consideration of melanoma. Cytologic features favoring melanoma include alterations that are a distinct departure from what is considered acceptable for a Spitz tumor*: heterogeneity of cell type throughout the lesion, particularly in an asymmetrical or haphazard pattern; high-nuclear-to-cytoplasmic ratios; granular or 'dusty' cytoplasm vs the ground glass cytoplasm of Spitz melanocytes; absence of delicate or dispersed chromatin patterns with thickening of nuclear membranes; a large proportion of melanocytes with hyperchromatic nuclei; and large eosinophilic nucleoli. As discussed above, the greater the absolute rate (per mm^2)* and number of deeply located (dermal) mitoses*, the more evidence one has for favoring melanoma. Atypical mitoses and necrotic cells suggest melanoma, but are not absolute.

Acknowledging that this differential diagnosis is perhaps the most difficult one in melanoma pathology, there are circumstances that make it even more exasperating, if not impossible. In particular, trauma and significant host response often introduce abnormal features such as ulceration, asymmetry, heterogeneity, dermal mitoses, and cytologic abnormality suggesting the greater likelihood of melanoma. It must be kept in mind that the nuclei in Spitz tumors are delicate and that any artifact such as tissue compression or overstaining or significant host response may introduce alterations suggesting greater cytologic atypicality. In the latter circumstances, the pathologist must consider carefully all of the criteria available before rendering an interpretation. When entertaining the possibility of melanoma, one must always consider a Spitz tumor with overlapping features of pigmented spindle cell nevus/tumor and one with phenotypic heterogeneity ('combined nevus'). Pigmented spindle cell tumors show considerable overlap

with Spitz tumors and may introduce features suggesting melanoma such as greater pagetoid melanocytosis, expansile papillary dermal nests, and the absence "ground glass" cytoplasm. Spitz tumors with phenotypic heterogeneity ('combined nevus') may exhibit asymmetry and heterogeneity, two attributes suggesting melanoma. One must assess each component of such a lesion individually with the criteria already mentioned, and it will usually be possible to resolve the issue.

Management

All spitzoid melanocytic neoplasms should be fully resected if possible in order to facilitate complete histopathologic examination and also to diminish the risk of recurrence (32). It is clear that it will not be possible to completely resect all Spitz tumors, especially some occurring in difficult anatomic sites in children. Clinical judgment must come into play, and the risks and benefits of surgery and optimal patient care prudently assessed. Atypical spitzoid neoplasms obviously require comparable excision for the same reasons but with greater clearance (up to 1 cm) in order to provide even greater assurance that they are completely resected. The reasons for recommending excision with margins free of the tumor are that (1) Spitz tumors not completely excised have persisted (recurred) at the same site and eventuated in metastases and/or death, and (2) some persistent/recurrent Spitz tumors may be more atypical than the original lesions and even more difficult to distinguish from melanoma and some have resulted in metastases. Spitzoid melanocytic tumors assigned an indeterminate biological potential probably merit surgical margins of approximately 1 cm since this is considered the minimum standard of care for melanoma. The place of SLNB in the management of atypical spitzoid melanocytic lesions remains controversial as discussed above. Further, accumulating data suggest that the outcome from SLN biopsy may not provide any meaningful prognostic information for spitzoid lesions even if positive (32, 34, 35, 41, 54–57). Patients should be carefully monitored by regular examinations for recurrence (and metastasis in the case of atypical Spitz tumors). All patients should be managed on an individual basis and efforts made to avoid both overly aggressive and suboptimal management strategies.

■ ANGIOTROPIC MELANOMA

The importance of angiotropism as a biological phenomenon and prognostic factor in localized melanoma and the microscopic correlate of *extravascular migratory metastasis* (see below) has recently been emphasized (58,59). Angiotropic melanoma is defined as the close apposition of melanoma cells to the abluminal surfaces of either blood or lymphatic channels (in a *pericyte-like location*), or both (Figure 17). By definition, there is no tumor present within vascular lumina. Angiotropic foci must be located either at the advancing front of the tumor or at some distance (usually within 1 to 2 mm) from the main tumoral mass. Although angiotropism is likely to be present within the mass of an invasive melanoma, there is no specific means at present to differentiate simple entrapment of vessels by tumor from angiotropism. Immunohistochemistry with markers such as S-100 protein or Melan-A/Mart-1 (Fig. 18) may aid in the identification or confirmation of angiotropism. Angiotropism is observed with greater frequency in melanomas also demonstrating neurotropism and adnexotropism

suggesting closely related mechanisms. Angiotropism is observed much more frequently than vascular invasion; for example, in a series of 650 consecutive invasive melanomas, the frequency of vascular/lymphatic invasion was 1.4 percent.

Lugassy and Barnhill have proposed that an important mechanism of melanoma metastasis may be the migration of tumor cells along the *abluminal* surfaces of vascular channels or *extravascular migratory metastasis (EVMM)*, a mechanism by which some tumor cells spread to nearby or more distant sites (58, 59) This mechanism of tumor spread appears to have a convincing developmental basis because of its striking similarity to the abluminal vascular migration of neural crest stem cells from the neural crest to distant sites in the embryo. Evidence for EVMM has also been based on ultrastructural, immunopathologic, and laboratory studies; in the latter, melanoma cells are closely apposed to the external surfaces of the endothelial cells of blood vessels in a *pericyte-like location* without evidence of intravasation (60,61). Ultrastructurally, the melanoma cells are linked to endothelium by an amorphous matrix containing laminin (not organized in basement membranes) as confirmed by immunohistochemistry (60–62) The latter morphologic structure has been termed the "Angio-tumoral Complex". According to this proposed mechanism, tumors cells begin the process of local spread by competing with pericytes for the periendothelial position or pericyte-like location for migration along the external surfaces of vessels (58).

Clinical and Histopathologic Features

The clinical and histologic features of primary angiotropic melanoma have been delineated in a series of thirty-six cases

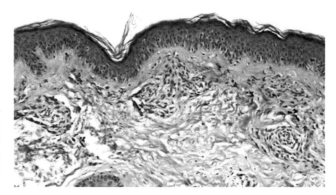

FIGURE 17
Angiotropic melanoma: thin lentigi-nous melanoma with angiotropism of melanoma cells. Melanoma cells show close apposition to abluminal surfaces of superficial microvascular channels.

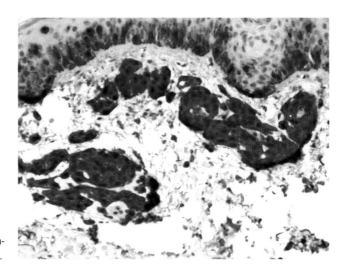

FIGURE 18
Angiotropic melanoma: Mart-1 high-lights the angiotropic melanocytes.

(Table 1). The clinical findings did not differ significantly from those in a large population-based study of melanoma. All conventional types of cutaneous melanoma were observed with pagetoid, lentiginous, and nested intraepidermal components, or "nodular" morpholo-gies. The 35 cutaneous tumors ranged in Breslow thickness from 0.46 to 8.25 mm with a mean of 1.64 mm. One patient had a mucosal melanoma involving the uter-ine cervix with lentiginous intraepithelial melanoma component and an extensive invasive component measuring 35 mm in thickness. All cutaneous melanomas (31/35) were level IV with the exception of two that were level II and two that were level V. Six (17%) of the tumors also showed neurotropism (58).

The prognostic significance of angi-otropism as a qualitative variable, i.e., one that is simply recorded as present or absent, has recently been reported (63). A series of patients with primary cutaneous

TABLE 1 Clinical and histopathologic characteristics of 36 patients with angiotropic melanoma

Case	Age	Sex	Site	Thick-ness	Level	SLN	Metastases	Follow-Up (Months)
1	38	F	R. UPPER ARM	0.61	IV			18
2	69	M	R. EAR	1.60	IV	SLN-		18
3	17	F	L. CHEEK	2.20	IV			16
4	31	F	R. POST ARM	1.0	IV			15
5	47	F	R. ANT THIGH	1.61	IV	SLN-		18
6	51	M	KNEE	0.71	IV			16
7	42	M	R. SHOULDER	0.75	IV			20
8	49	M	BUTTOCK	1.58	IV	SLN-		16
9	14	M	L. CHEST	3.13	IV	SLN-		18
10	34	F	L. FOOT	2.31	IV			18
11	16	M	R.CHEST	1.25	IV			23
12	43	F	LOWER LEG	1.47	IV	SLN-		24
13	55	M	R. ARM	0.46	II			26
14	81	F	R. ARM	1.0	IV	SLN-		15
15	37	F	LOW BACK	1.31	IV			16
16	66	M	ARM	0.92	IV			15
17	21	F	L.THIGH	2.62	IV	SLN-		24
18	18	F	L. SCAPULA	0.54	IV			15
19	52	M	L. LEG	0.84	IV			24
20	49	F	CENTRAL BACK	3.21	IV	SLN-	Widespread	24
21	89	M	R. SIDE FACE	1.44	IV			16
22	54	M	NECK	1.41	IV	SLN-		16
23	60	M	L. BACK	1.00	IV	SLN-		18
24	69	M	L. HEEL	0.88	IV			25
25	52	F	R. POST SHOULDER	0.68	IV			21
26	71	M	L. FOREARM	0.88	IV			21
27	39	M	BACK	1.76	IV	SLN+		24
28	33	F	R. LOW.BACK	0.84	IV			16
29	13	M	BACK	2.33	IV	SLN+		24
30	71	M	L. TEMP SCALP	2.11	IV		Lungs	16
31	56	F	R. ARM	0.78	II		In-transit	2
32	27	F	R. LEG	0.84	IV			3
33	89	F	UTERUS	35	NA		Micromet	1
34	48	F	L. HEEL	8.25	V		Regional LN	14
35	75	F	NOSE	3.95	V			12
36	23	M	L. TEMP SCALP	1.16	IV	SLN-		11

melanoma and documented metastasis were matched for Breslow thickness, age, gender, and site, with a similar group of patients with non-metastasizing primary melanoma and long-term follow-up. Angiotropism as defined above was found exclusively in patients with metastasizing melanoma, and vascular/lymphatic invasion was absent. These preliminary results strongly suggest that angiotropism is an important prognostic factor correlating with metastasis, even beyond that of tumor thickness. A recent investigation has independently confirmed the importance of angiotropism as a prognostic factor in loco-regional metastasizing melanomas (64).

The prevalence of angiotropism and EVMM in melanoma metastases has been investigated in 26 patients with metastatic melanoma. Among the 26 melanoma metastases studied, angiotropism of melanoma cells was observed in some portion of the metastasis in 23 cases (65) Thirteen out of 16 in-transit metastases, all seven epidermotropic metastases, and two of three satellite metastases showed angiotropism. In general, the in transit metastases were small and some were epidermotropic while others involved solely the reticular dermis and possibly the subcutaneous fat. Melanoma cells cuffed the external surfaces of microvessels within the metastasis, at the peritumoral interface of the metastasis, or in immediate proximity to the main portion of the metastasis, in a pattern analogous to the angio-tumoral complex. The melanoma cells were present in one or more layers and occasionally in small aggregates juxtaposed to the external vascular wall. There was no evidence of intravascular involvement (intravascular invasion) in any of the 26 human melanoma metastases. Simultaneous (double) immunostaining of five specimens with S 100 protein and CD31 highlighted melanoma cell angiotropism, i.e., melanomas cells expressing S 100 were observed along the external surfaces of microvessels labeling with CD31 (65).

Management

At present there are no definitive data to suggest that melanomas demonstrating angiotropism should be managed any differently than conventional melanomas. However, with the acquisition of new research findings in large patient cohorts this may change in the future. Continued investigations are underway to define the molecular basis of EVMM and potential therapeutic avenues for intervention in the metastatic process (66–70).

■ BLUE NEVUS-LIKE MELANOMA (MELANOMA ARISING IN OR RESEMBLING A BLUE NEVUS; MALIGNANT BLUE NEVUS)

Cutaneous melanoma originating from or associated with a preexisting blue nevus, commonly a cellular blue nevus (CBN), or closely resembling a blue nevus was first delineated by Allen and Spitz under the term "malignant blue nevus"(71–83) The term has not been without controversy and many have called for its abandonment. Nonetheless, this appelation continues to be used in the literature since this variant of melanoma has a unique developmental basis, i.e., origin from or resemblance to a BN, a rather distinctive clinicopathologic phenotype, and unique somatic mutations of guanine nucleotide-binding protein (GNAQ) in common with or blue nevi and uveal melanoma (82). Blue nevus-like melanoma (BNLM) are extremely rare, as less than two hundred cases have thus far been reported.

Clinical Features

The average age of patients at diagnosis is in the mid-forties, about two-thirds of patients are men, and there is no predilection for any particular anatomic site, such as the scalp as was previously thought (78, 79, 81). Blue nevus-like melanomas most frequently present as blue or blue-black plaques or nodules ranging from about 1 to 4 cm (mean: 2.9 cm) which are often multinodular. There is usually a history of recent enlargement or change in a previously stable blue nevus. Recent evidence suggests that BNLM are not more aggressive than other forms of conventional melanoma, as was previously believed; rather they are commonly diagnosed at a more advanced stage (81).

Histopathologic Features

In the most common presentations, BNLMs are often large (usually > 2 to 3 cm, range 0.5 to > 6 cm) asymmetrical nodular or multinodular tumors comprised of aggregations of spindled cells in tightly packed fascicles in the dermis and often the subcutis (Figs. 19–23) (71–75,78,79,81). In a recent large series of cases, the median Breslow thickness was 5.5 mm with a range from 1.1 to 15 mm) (81). Median Clark level was V and 26% of the BNLMs were ulcerated. By definition, there is usually sparing of the epidermis (Figure 19). Epithelioid malignant melanocytes are often a conspicuous component and useful for the recognition of BNLM. Multinucleate giant cells are also occasionally encountered. Melanin pigment and nuclear vacuolization are noted in approximately two-thirds of cases (74) Necrosis, a feature previously thought characteristic of BNLM, is observed in only about one-third of cases (74). In general, there is striking cytologic atypia, prominent nuclear pleomorphism, infrequent mitotic figures (approximately 1 to 2 but often > 5 to 6 mitoses/mm^2) and, uncommonly, atypical mitoses. Most BNLM have a component of CBN, but elements of common blue nevus

(pigmented dendritic melanocytes, fibrosis, and melanophages) and rarely nevus of Ota or nevus of Ito may be observed.

BNLM usually presents in one of three patterns: (1) a lesion with an overtly malignant component juxtaposed to a benign blue nevus component, usually a CBN; (2) a more subtle sarcoma-like presentation (without florid benign and malignant components) initially suggesting CBN but exhibiting large densely cellular fascicles or nodules of spindle cells that on closer inspection have sufficient atypicality for malignancy and are distinctly more abnormal than the usual small fascicular or alveolar patterns in CBN; or (3) a lesion suggesting a benign CBN with additional atypical features such as large diameter, asymmetry, prominent cellular density, nuclear pleomorphism, and some mitotic activity at least focally, but not obviously malignant, that subsequently results in malignant behavior (the authors' term such lesions biologically indeterminate) (80).

Ancillary Techniques

Comparative Genomic Hybridization and Fluorescence In Situ Hybridization

The recently developed molecular techniques CGH and FISH appear to hold promise for their application to the difficult diagnostic problem of histologically ambiguous cellular blue nevoid melanocytic neoplasms (79, 82, 47). In particular, the distinction of CBN and atypical variants from BNLM can be one of the greatest challenges faced by histopathologists. In a recent study of cellular blue nevoid lesions assessed by CGH, all seven BNLMs showed multiple chromosomal aberrations with an average of eight per lesion as compared to none observed in 11 CBN (79). Interestingly, among 11 lesions considered to be atypical CBN, three of 11 cases

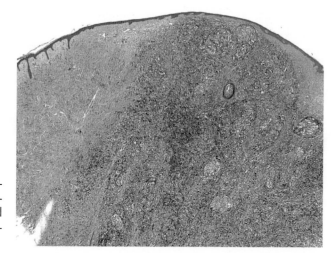

FIGURE 19
Blue nevus-like melanoma (malignant blue nevus): scanning magnification showing relatively small diameter biphasic nodular melanocytic neoplasm.

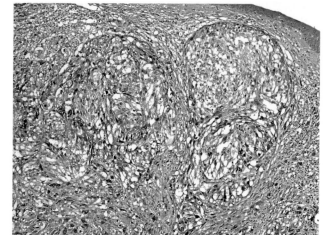

FIGURE 20
Blue nevus-like melanoma (malignant blue nevus): high magnification demonstrating hypercellular nests of heavily-melaninized atypical spindled to epithelioid melanocytes in superficial dermal portion of melanoma.

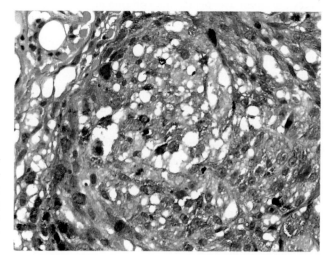

FIGURE 21
Blue nevus-like melanoma (malignant blue nevus): higher magnification of Figure 20 showing nodular component containing severely atypical spindled to epithelioid melanocytes with prominent nucleoli.

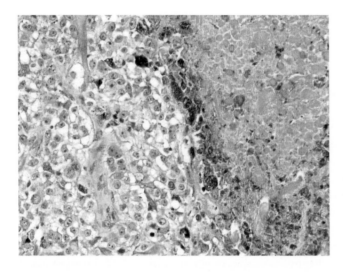

FIGURE 22
Blue nevus-like melanoma (malignant blue nevus) (scalp): high magnification demonstrating severely atypical melanocytes abutting zone of tissue necrosis.

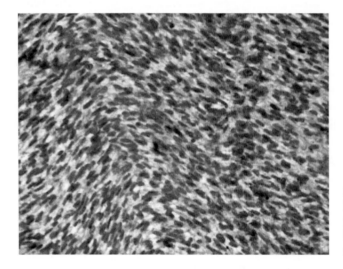

FIGURE 23
Blue nevus-like melanoma (malignant blue nevus): higher magnification demonstrating severely atypical spindled melanocytes.

(27%) showed one to three chromosomal abnormalities, paralleling their intermediate status between conventional CBN and BNLM. The recent application of FISH with four probes targeting the chromosomal loci 6p25, 6q23, 11q23, and the centromere of chromosome 6 (Cep6) has shown relatively comparable findings (83). Five of five BNLMs demonstrated FISH abnormalities compatible with melanoma versus none observed in 12 conventional CBN. However, a recent comprehensive analysis of 575 melanocytic lesions by FISH revealed that both conventional and atypical CBNs may show comparable rates of positivity (40 to 50%) as BNLM (50%) (47).

Differential Diagnosis

The differential diagnosis of blue nevus-like melanoma includes CBN and its atypical variants, primary or metastatic melanoma, and clear cell sarcoma (76–81, 84). The difficulty of CBN and closely-related lesions showing features that seem to deviate from the stereotypic image of CBN conceived in the literature stems from several factors: cellular blue neoplasms as a group are rare and consequently inadequate information is currently available about these lesions in general, both benign (and atypical) and malignant forms show a continuum of overlapping features; CBN may show regional (including sentinel) lymph node involvement suggesting metastatic melanoma (but not definitive evidence of malignancy); and finally, metastases may develop after the passage of long disease-free intervals, e.g., up to fifteen years in one instance. In any case, histopathologic criteria for the distinction of BNLM from CBN have been proposed in the literature. For example, as outlined above, an unquestionably malignant component often with large epithelioid malignant melanocytes juxtaposed to a bland CBN component is the single most reliable histologic criterion. Other important criteria include large size, i.e., > 1 cm, especially > 2 to 3 cm, asymmetry, multinodular configuration, mitotic rate > 2 to 3, especially > 5 to 6 per mm², atypical mitoses, zonal necrosis, nodule formation, infiltrating features, significant cytologic atypia, location on the scalp, and age beyond 45 years. Outside of exceptionally rare lesions showing overt malignant characteristics with or without a benign blue nevus remnant, the following attributes appear to lack specificity for discriminating CBN from BNLM: size, presence of mitoses (both may have fairly low mitotic rates of approximately 2/mm²), necrosis, hypercellularity, cytologic atypia, and regional lymph node involvement. Consequently, it has been difficult to define the limits of atypicality acceptable in some percentage of CBN on the one hand and the minimal essential criteria for malignancy on the other (Figs. 41–43). As

a result, an intermediate category of tumors termed "atypical blue or atypical cellular blue nevi" often with the additional qualification of indeterminate biological potential has been introduced to accommodate these controversial or borderline neoplasms (80).

Because there are no histologic features specific for BNLM, a contiguous remnant of blue nevus should be identified or a history of an antecedent blue nevus documented to distinguish BNLM from either nodular or metastatic melanoma.

Clear cell sarcoma (CCS) is distinguished by the typical clinical presentation in young adults, involvement of distal extremities, deep soft tissue involvement, typical histology, and immunohistochemistry. However, rarely CCS may present as a primary dermal neoplasm (84). If necessary, the Ewing sarcoma-cyclic AMP-dependent transcription factor (EWS-ATF-1) fusion gene in CCS can be identified through the use of RT-PCR or FISH testing.

Prognosis

The authors of most reported series of BNLM in the literature contend that BNLM is an aggressive neoplasm perhaps with a less favorable prognosis versus that of conventional melanoma (74). However, recent evidence from Australia argues against this commonly held belief (81). After adjustment for a more advanced stage, BNLMs appear to be no more aggressive than conventional melanomas. In this case-control study, 23 patients with BNLM were matched with a control population of conventional melanoma patients. The latter two groups were matched for age, gender, anatomic site, Breslow thickness, and ulceration. An analysis of outcomes showed that there were no significant differences between the two groups with respect to melanoma-specific mortality or overall mortality. Further, the two groups demonstrated comparable rates (43%) of loco-regional recurrences; and, interestingly, patients with BNLMs manifested a slightly lower frequency of distant metastases compared to conventional melanoma patients. One must consider that most BNLM have been reported from large tertiary care centers with significant referral biases, most BNLM are diagnosed at an apparently advanced stage, many BNLM involve the scalp which is considered a relatively high-risk anatomic site, and it may not be possible to apply the Breslow method for measuring thickness to BNLM for comparison with conventional melanomas. Further, it is possible that pathologists have failed to recognize a subset of more indolent BNLM, i.e., those that have not shown aggressive behavior early on in their course and thus are never recognized or are diagnosed only in retrospective after the development of metastases several years later.

Management

With respect to the management of patients with MBN, there is growing evidence that the same therapeutic measures as for conventional melanoma are applicable.

■ COMPOSITE MELANOMAS: MELANOMAS ASSOCIATED WITH OTHER MALIGNANT EPITHELIAL NEOPLASMS

The occurrence of cutaneous melanoma in close proximity to or within other epithelial malignant tumors is a rare and poorly-understood phenomenon which has reported in the literature over the past 30 years (85–90). The two entities most commonly associated with melanoma have been basal cell carcinoma and squamous cell carcinoma. The nature of this relationship has been the source of considerable confusion and the lack of standardized terminology. A critical analysis of the cases reported thus indicates that these tumors can more or less be categorized into four principal categories (89): 1) Collision tumors: the collision of melanoma with either squamous or basal cell carcinoma. By definition, the two neoplasms are in close proximity but maintain distinct physical boundaries; 2) Colonization of an epithelial neoplasm by melanocytes: The most common example of this is the colonization of an epithelial tumor, such as a seborrheic keratosis (melanoacanthoma), poroma, squamous cell carcinoma, basal cell carcinoma, Paget disease, etc., by benign pigmented dendritic melanocytes resulting in an appearance which simulates melanoma in situ. On the other hand, melanomas in situ may directly colonize tumors such as basal cell carcinoma, and this represents a true manifestation of composite melanoma in situ and basal cell carcinoma. 3) Combined tumors: In this circumstance, two distinct neoplasms, i.e., cutaneous melanoma, usually invasive, and another such as squamous cell carcinoma exhibit intimate intermingling of the two phenotypically different tumor cells populations. 4) Biphenotypic tumors: A malignant neoplasm comprised of tumor cells with biphenotypic differentiation, i.e., individual tumor cells show evidence of both melanocytic and epithelial differentiation (in the case of a malignant neoplasm with melanocytic and keratinocytic differentiation). To date, only extremely rare tumors have been documented to show such apparent biphenotypic differentiation in individual tumor cells by either immunohistochemistry or electron microscopy (86). The pathogenesis for such dual or biphenotypic differentiation has not been clearly elucidated.

Clinical and Histopathological Features

Since so few cases have been reported, there are no distinctive clinical or histological features apparent in the literature. As illustrated in Figs. 24 and 25, one of the most common presentations is an admixture of two distinct tumor cell populations. Immunohistochemistry is critical for the elucidation of the relationship between the two tumor cell components in such composite neoplasms (Figure 25). However, the phenotypic nature of many such unusual neoplasms may still defy easy classification. On may suspect a single line of differentiation or potentially the association of two distinct tumor cell populations as outlined in the classification above. Without sophisticated ancillary techniques such as dual immunolabeling, electron microscopy, cell culture, and molecular techniques, it may be virtually impossible to confirm whether biphenotypic malignant neoplasms with melanocytic differentiation actually exist.

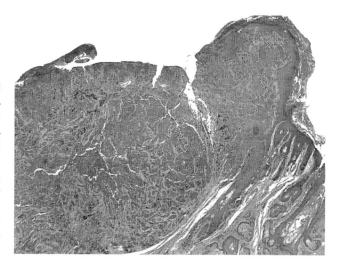

FIGURE 24
Combined melanoma and squamous cell carcinoma: scanning magnification discloses a neoplasm with attributes suggesting both melanocytic and squamous lines of differentiation. An invasive melanoma of the lentigo maligna type (Breslow thickness: 3.39 mm, mitotic rate: 11 per mm², ulceration: present) is intimately admixed with a basaloid squamous cell carcinoma.

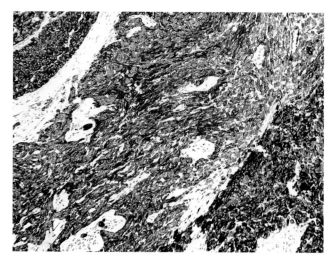

FIGURE 25
Combined melanoma and squamous cell carcinoma: expression of HMB45 in many of the same tumor cells. The same microscopic field (not shown) has demonstrated expression of cytokeratin 5/6 suggesting biphenotypic differentiation.

Differential Diagnosis

The fundamental task for the histopathologist is to verify the benign or malignant nature of the tumor and if conventional melanoma is clearly present or not. One must attempt to assign a given neoplasm into one of the categories outlined above, i.e., as a collision tumor; a tumor colonized by either benign dendritic melanocytes or melanoma cells; a combined tumor comprised of two distinct malignant cellular populations, closely intermingled but without evident biphenotypic differentiation in individual tumor cells; and finally a tumor with biphenotypic differentiation which can only be confirmed by immunohistochemistry, electron microscopy, or other advanced technique.

Prognosis

Because so few cases have been reported, because of the difficulty of classifying precisely many of these neoplasms, because of the difficulty of knowing their biological nature, and finally because of the difficulty of measuring Breslow thickness for many such lesions, there are no robust data available about the general category of composite melanomas. Nonetheless, one would presume that the major prognostic indicators for cutaneous melanoma including Breslow thickness, mitotic rate, ulceration, and stage would be applicable to these neoplasms exhibiting true biologic melanoma. Thus standardized microstaging and reporting of melanoma should be applied to composite melanomas in general.

Management

If true biologic melanoma is confirmed to be present, the same management strategy as for all conventional melanomas should be applicable.

■ REFERENCES

1. Melanocytic tumors. In: LeBoit P, Burg G, Weedon D, Sarasin A, eds. *World Health Organization Classification of Tumours: Pathology and Genetics of Skin Tumours.* Lyon: IARC, 2006.
2. Curtin JA, Fridlyand J, Kageshita T, et al. Distinct sets of genetic alterations in melanoma. *N Engl J Med.* 2005;353(20):2135–2147.
3. Bruijn JA, Salasche S, Sober AJ, Mihm MC, Barnhill RL. Desmoplastic melanoma: clinicopathologic aspects of six cases. *Dermatology (Basel).* 1992;185(1):3–8.
4. Carlson JA, Dickersin GR, Sober AJ, Barnhill RL. Desmoplastic neurotropic malignant melanoma: a clinicopathologic analysis of 28 cases. *Cancer.* 1994;75:478–494.
5. Tsao H, Sober AJ, Barnhill RL. Desmoplastic neurotropic melanoma. *Sem Cutan Med Surg.* 1997;16:131–136.
6. Lens MB, Newton-Bishop JA, Boon AP. Desmoplastic malignant melanoma: a systematic review. *Br J Dermatol.* 2005; 152:673–678.
7. Cummins DL, Esche C, Barrett TL, et al. Lymph node biopsy results for desmoplastic malignant melanoma. *Cutis.* 2007;79:390–394.
8. Posther KE, Selim MA, Mosca PJ, et al. Histopathologic characteristics, recurrence patterns, and survival of 129 patients with desmoplastic melanoma. *Ann Surg Oncol.* 2006;13:728–739.
9. Quinn MJ, Crotty KA, Thompson JF, et al. Desmoplastic and desmoplastic neurotropic melanoma: experience with 280 patients. *Cancer.* 1998;83:1128–1135.
10. Skelton HG, Smith KJ, Laskin WB, et al. Desmoplastic malignant melanoma. *J Am Acad Dermatol.* 1995;32:717–725.
11. Livestro DP, Muzikansky A, Kaine EM, et al. Biology of desmoplastic melanoma: a case-control comparison with other melanomas. *J Clin Oncol.* 2005;23:6739–6746.
12. Hawkins WG, Busam KJ, Ben-Porat L, et al. Desmoplastic melanoma: a pathologically and clinically distinct form of cutaneous melanoma. *Ann Surg Oncol.* 2005;12:207–213.

13. Barnhill R. Malignant melanoma. In: Barnhill R, Piepkorn M, Busam KJ, eds. *Pathology of Melanocytic Nevi and Malignant Melanoma.* 2nd ed. New York: Springer Verlag, 2004:303–311.

14. Winnepenninckx V, De Vos R., Stas M, et al. New phenotypical and ultrastructural findings in spindle cell (desmoplastic/neurotropic) melanoma. *Appl Immunohistochem Mol Morphol.* 2003;11:319–325.

15. Nonaka D, Chiriboga L, Rubin BP. Sox10: a pan-schwannian and melanocytic marker. *Am J Surg Pathol.* 2008;32(9):1291–1298.

16. Penneys NS. Excision of melanoma after initial biopsy. An immunohistochemical study. *J Am Acad Dermatol.* 1985;13:995–998.

17. Chorny JA, Barr RJ. S100-positive spindle cells in scars: a diagnostic pitfall in the re-excision of desmoplastic melanoma. *Am J Dermatopathol.* 2002;24:309–312.

18. Robson A, Allen P, Hollowood K. S100 expression in cutaneous scars: a potential diagnostic pitfall in the diagnosis of desmoplastic melanoma. *Histopathology.* 2001;38:135–140.

19. Schmoeckel C, Castro CE, Braun-Falco O. Nevoid malignant melanoma. *Arch Dermatol Res.* 1985;277(5):362–369.

20. Wong TY, Duncan LM, Mihm MC Jr. Melanoma mimicking dermal and Spitz's nevus ("nevoid" melanoma). *Semin Surg Oncol.* 1993;9:188–193.

21. Wong TY, Suster S, Duncan LM, Mihm MC Jr. Nevoid melanoma: a clinicopathological study of seven cases of malignant melanoma mimicking spindle and epithelioid cell nevus and verrucous dermal nevus. *Hum Pathol.* 1995;26(2):171–179.

22. McNutt NS, Urmacher C, Hakimian J, Hoss DM, Lugo J. Nevoid malignant melanoma: morphologic patterns and immunohistochemical reactivity. *J Cutan Pathol.* 1995;22(6):502–517.

23. McNutt NS. "Triggered trap": nevoid malignant melanoma. *Semin Diagn Pathol.* 1998;15(3):203–209.

24. Zembowicz A, McCusker M, Chiarelli C, Dei Tos AP, Granter SR, Calonje E, et al. Morphological analysis of nevoid melanoma: a study of 20 cases with a review of the literature. *Am J Dermatopathol.* 2001; 23(3):167–175.

25. Spitz S. Melanomas of childhood. *Am J Pathol.* 1948;24(3):591–609.

26. Echevarria R, Ackerman LV. Spindle and epitheloid cell nevi in the adult. Clinicopathologic report of 26 cases. *Cancer.* 1967;20(2):175–189.

27. Reed RJ, Ichinose H, Clark WH Jr, Mihm MC Jr. Common and uncommon melanocytic nevi and borderline melanomas. *Semin Oncol.* 1975;2(2):119–147.

28. Weedon D, Little JH. Spindle and epithelioid cell nevi in children and adults. A review of 211 cases of the Spitz nevus. *Cancer.* 1977;40(1):217–225.

29. Paniago-Pereira C, Maize JC, Ackerman AB. Nevus of large spindle and/or epithelioid cells (Spitz's nevus). *Arch Dermatol.* 1978;114(12):1811–1823.

30. Requena C, Requena L, Kutzner H, Sánchez Yus E. Spitz nevus: a clinicopathological study of 349 cases. *Am J Dermatopathol.* 2009; 31(2):107–116.

31. Crotty KA, Scolyer RA, Li L, Palmer AA, Wang L, McCarthy SW. Spitz naevus versus spitzoid melanoma: when and how can they be distinguished? *Pathology.* 2002;34(1):6–12.

32. Barnhill RL. The spitzoid lesion: rethinking Spitz tumors, atypical variants, 'spitzoid melanoma' and risk assessment. *Mod Pathol.* 2006;19(suppl 2):S21–33.

33. Da Forno PD, Fletcher A, Pringle JH, Saldanha GS. Understanding spitzoid tumours: new insights from molecular pathology. *Br J Dermatol.* 2008;158(1):4–14.

34. Sepehr A, Chao E, Trefrey B, Blackford A, Duncan LM, Flotte TJ, et al. Long-term outcome of Spitz-type melanocytic tumors. *Arch Dermatol.* 2011;147(10):1173–1179.

35. Cerrato F, Wallins JS, Webb ML, McCarty ER, Schmidt BA, Labow BI. Outcomes in pediatric atypical Spitz tumors treated without sentinel lymph node biopsy. *Pediatr Dermatol.* 2012;29(4):448–453.

36. Vollmer RT. Use of Bayes rule and MIB-1 proliferation index to discriminate Spitz nevus from malignant melanoma. *Am J Clin Pathol.* 2004;122(4):499–505.

37. Kapur P, Selim MA, Roy LC, Yegappan M, Weinberg AG, Hoang MP. Spitz nevi and atypical Spitz nevi/tumors: a histologic and immunohistochemical analysis. *Mod Pathol.* 2005;18:197–204.

38. Kanter-Lewensohn L, Hedblad MA, Wejde J, et al. Immunohistochemical markers for

distinguishing Spitz nevi from malignant melanomas. *Mod Pathol.* 1997;10:917–920.

39. Bastian BC, Wesselmann U, Pinkel D, LeBoit PE. Molecular cytogenetic analysis of Spitz nevi shows clear differences to melanoma. *J Invest Dermatol.* 1999; 113(6):1065–1069.

40. Bastian BC, LeBoit PE, Pinkel D. Mutations and copy number increase of HRAS in Spitz nevi with distinctive histopathological features. *Am J Pathol.* 2000;157(3):967–972.

41. Raskin L, Ludgate M, Iyer RK, Ackley TE, Bradford CR, Johnson TM, et al. Copy number variations and clinical outcome in atypical Spitz tumors. *Am J Surg Pathol.* 2011; 35(2):243–252.

42. Gerami P, Li G, Pouryazdanparast P, et al. A highly specific and discriminatory FISH assay for distinguishing between benign and malignant melanocytic neoplasms. *Am J Surg Pathol.* 2012;36(6):808–817.

43. Gaiser T, Kutzner H, Palmedo G, et al. Classifying ambiguous melanocytic lesions with FISH and correlation with clinical long-term follow up. *Mod Pathol.* 2010;23(3):413–419.

44. Gerami P, Jewell SS, Morrison LE, et al. Fluorescence in situ hybridization (FISH) as an ancillary diagnostic tool in the diagnosis of melanoma. *Am J Surg Pathol.* 2009;33(8):1146–1156.

45. Gammon B, Beilfuss B, Guitart J, Gerami P. Enhanced detection of spitzoid melanomas using fluorescence in situ hybridization with 9p21 as an adjunctive probe. *Am J Surg Pathol.* 2012;36(1):81–88.

46. Gerami P, Scolyer RA, Xu X, et al. Risk Assessment for atypical spitzoid melanocytic neoplasms using FISH to identify chromosomal copy number aberrations. *Am J Surg Pathol.* 2012;in press.

47. Kerl K, Palmedo G, Wiesner T, Mentzel T, Rütten A, Schärer L, et al. A proposal for improving multicolor FISH sensitivity in the diagnosis of malignant melanoma using new combined criteria. *Am J Dermatopathol.* 2012;34(6):580–585.

48. George E, Polissar NL, Wick M. Immunohistochemical evaluation of p16INK4A, E-cadherin, and cyclin D1: expression in melanoma and Spitz tumors. *Am J Clin Pathol.* 2010;133:370–379.

49. Healy E, Belgaid C, Takata M, et al. Allelotypes of primary cutaneous melanoma and benign melanocytic nevi. *Cancer Res.* 1996;56:589–593.

50. Bogdan I, Burg G, Boni R. Spitz nevi display allelic deletions. *Arch Dermatol.* 2001;137:1417–1420.

51. Gill M, Cohen J, Renwick N, et al. Genetic similarities between Spitz nevus and spitzoid melanoma in children. *Cancer.* 2004; 101:2636–2640.

52. Barnhill RL, Flotte TJ, Fleischli M, Perez-Atayde A. Cutaneous melanoma and atypical Spitz tumors in childhood. *Cancer.* 1995;76(10):1833–1845.

53. Barnhill RL, Argenyi ZB, From L, Glass LF, Maize JC, Mihm MC Jr, et al. Atypical Spitz nevi/tumors: lack of consensus for diagnosis, discrimination from melanoma, and prediction of outcome. *Hum Pathol.* 1999; 30(5):513–520.

54. Lohmann CM, Coit DG, Brady MS, Berwick M, Busam KJ. Sentinel lymph node biopsy in patients with diagnostically controversial spitzoid melanocytic tumors. *Am J Surg Pathol.* 2002;26(1):47–55.

55. Busam KJ, Pulitzer M. Sentinel lymph node biopsy for patients with diagnostically controversial spitzoid melanocytic tumors? *Adv Anat Pathol.* 2008;15(5):253–262.

56. Murali R, Sharma RN, Thompson JF, Stretch JR, Lee CS, McCarthy SW, et al. Sentinel lymph node biopsy in histologically ambiguous melanocytic tumors with spitzoid features (so-called atypical spitzoid tumors). *Ann Surg Oncol.* 2008;15(1):302–309.

57. Ludgate MW, Fullen DR, Lee J, Lowe L, Bradford C, Geiger J, et al. The atypical Spitz tumor of uncertain biologic potential: a series of 67 patients from a single institution. *Cancer.* 2009;115(3):631–641.

58. Barnhill RL, Lugassy C. Angiotropic malignant melanoma and extravascular migratory metastasis: description of 36 cases with emphasis on a new mechanism of tumour spread. *Pathology.* 2004;36:485–490.

59. Lugassy C, Barnhill RL. Angiotropic malignant melanoma and extravascular migratory metastasis: a review. *Adv Anat Pathol.* 2007;14(3):195–201.

60. Lugassy C, Eyden BP, Christensen L, Escande JP: Angio-tumoral complex in human malignant melanoma characterised by free laminin: ultrastructural and immuno-histochemical observations. *J Submicrosc Cytol Pathol.* 1997; 29:19–28.

61. Lugassy C, Dickersin GR, Christensen L, et al. Ultrastructural and immunohistochemical

studies of the periendothelial matrix in malignant melanoma: evidence for an amorphous matrix containing laminin. *J Cutan Pathol.* 1999;26:78–83.

62. Lugassy C, Shahsafaei A, Bonitz P, Busam KJ, Barnhill RL. Tumor microvessels in melanoma express the beta-2 chain of laminin. Implications for melanoma metastasis. *J Cutan Pathol.* 1999;26:222–226.

63. Barnhill R, Dy K, Lugassy C. Angiotropism in cutaneous melanoma: a prognostic factor strongly predicting risk for metastasis. *J Invest Dermatol.* 2002;119:705–706.

64. Van Es SL, Colman M, Thompson JF, McCarthy SW, Scolyer RA. Angiotropism is an independent predictor of local recurrence and in-transit metastasis in primary cutaneous melanoma. *Am J Surg Pathol.* 2008;32(9):1396–403.

65. Lugassy C, Vernon SE, Busam, K, Engbring, JA, Welch, DR, Poulos, EG, et al. Angiotropism of human melanoma: studies involving in transit and other cutaneous metastases and the chicken chorioallantoic membrane: implications for extravascular melanoma invasion and metastasis. *Am J Dermatopathol.* 2006;28:187–193.

66. Lugassy C, Haroun RI, Brem H, et al. Pericytic-like angiotropism of glioma and melanoma cells. *Am J Dermatopathol.* 2002;24:473–478.

67. Lugassy C, Kleinman HK, Fernandez PM, et al. Human melanoma cell migration along capillary-like structures in vitro: a new dynamic model for studying extravascular migratory metastasis. *J Invest Dermatol.* 2002; 119:703–704.

68. Lugassy C, Kleinman HK, Vernon SE, Welch DR, Barnhill RL. C16 laminin peptide increases angiotropic extravascular migration of human melanoma cells in a shell-less chick cam assay. *Br J Dermatol.* 2007;157(4):780–782.

69. Lugassy C, Lazar V, Dessen P, van den Oord JJ, Winnepenninckx V, Spatz A, et al. Gene expression profiling of human angiotropic primary melanoma: selection of 15 differentially expressed genes potentially involved in extravascular migratory metastasis. *Eur J Cancer.* 2011;47:1267–1275.

70. Wilmott J, Haydu L, Bagot M, Zhang Y, Jakrot V, McCarthy S, et al. Angiotropism is an independent predictor of microscopic satellites in primary cutaneous melanoma. *Histopathology.* 2012;epub ahead of print. doi: 10.1111/j.1365–2559.

71. Allen AC: A reorientation on the histogenesis and clinical significance of cutaneous nevi and melanomas. *Cancer.* 1949;2:28–56.

72. Temple-Camp CRE, Saxe N, King H. Benign and malignant cellular blue nevus. A clinicopathological study of 30 cases. *Am J Dermatopathol.* 1988;10:289–296.

73. Goldenhersh MA, Savin RC, Barnhill RL, Stenn KS. Malignant blue nevus. *J Am Acad Dermatol.* 1988;19:712–722.

74. Connelly J, Smith JL Jr. Malignant blue nevus. *Cancer.* 1991;67:2653–2657.

75. Granter SR, McKee PH, Calonje E, Mihm MC, Busan K. Melanoma associated with blue nevus and melanoma mimicking cellular blue nevus: a clinicopathologic study of 10 cases on the spectrum of so-called "malignant blue nevus." *Am J Surg Pathol.* 2001;25:316–323.

76. Rodriguez HA, Ackerman LV. Cellular blue nevus. Clinicopathologic study of forty-five cases. *Cancer.* 1968;21:393–405.

77. Tran TA, Carlson JA, Basaca B, Mihm MC Jr. Cellular blue nevus with atypia (atypical cellular blue nevus): a clinicopathologic study of nine cases. *J Cutan Pathol.* 1998;25:252–258.

78. Barnhill R. Malignant melanoma. In: Barnhill R, Piepkorn M, Busam KJ, eds. *Pathology of Melanocytic Nevi and Malignant Melanoma.* 2nd ed. New York: Springer Verlag, 2004:322–328.

79. Maize JC Jr, McCalmont TH, Carlson JA, Busam KJ, Kutzner H, Bastian BC. Genomic analysis of blue nevi and related dermal melanocytic proliferations. *Am J Surg Pathol.* 2005;29(9):1214–1220.

80. Barnhill RL, Argenyi Z, Berwick M, Duray PH, Erickson L, Guitart J, et al. Atypical cellular blue nevi (cellular blue nevi with atypical features): lack of consensus for diagnosis and distinction from cellular blue nevi and malignant melanoma ("malignant blue nevus"). *Am J Surg Pathol.* 2008;32(1):36–44.

81. Martin RC, Murali R, Scolyer RA, Fitzgerald P, Colman MH, Thompson JF. So-called "malignant blue nevus": a clinicopathologic study of 23 patients. *Cancer.* 2009; 115(13):2949–2955.

82. Van Raamsdonk CD, Bezrookove V, Green G, Bauer J, Gaugler L, O'Brien JM, et al. Frequent somatic mutations of GNAQ in uveal melanoma and blue naevi. *Nature.* 2009; 457(7229):599–602.

83. Gammon B, Beilfuss B, Guitart J, Busam KJ, Gerami P. Fluorescence in situ hybridization for distinguishing cellular blue nevi from blue nevus-like melanoma. *J Cutan Pathol.* 2011;38(4):335–341.

84. Hantschke M, Mentzel T, Rütten A, Palmedo G, Calonje E, Lazar AJ, et al. Cutaneous clear cell sarcoma: a clinicopathologic, immunohistochemical, and molecular analysis of 12 cases emphasizing its distinction from dermal melanoma. *Am J Surg Pathol.* 2010;34(2):216–222.

85. Novick M, Gard DA, Hardy SB, Spira M. Burn scar carcinoma: a review and analysis of 46 cases. *J Trauma.* 1977;17(10):809–817.

86. Rosen LB, Williams WD, Benson J, Rywlin AM. A malignant neoplasm with features of both squamous cell carcinoma and malignant melanoma. *Am J Dermatopathol.* 1984;6(suppl):213–219.

87. Erickson LA, Myers JL, Mihm MC, Markovic SN, Pittelkow MR. Malignant basomelanocytic tumor manifesting as metastatic melanoma. *Am J Surg Pathol.* 2004;28(10):1393–1396.

88. Rodriguez J, Nonaka D, Kuhn E, Reichel M, Rosai J. Combined high-grade basal cell carcinoma and malignant melanoma of the skin ("malignant basomelanocytic tumor"): report of two cases and review of the literature. *Am J Dermatopathol.* 2005;27(4):314–318.

89. Satter EK, Metcalf J, Lountzis N, Elston DM. Tumors composed of malignant epithelial and melanocytic populations: a case series and review of the literature. *J Cutan Pathol.* 2009;36(2):211–219.

90. Scruggs JM, Rensvold EA, Parekh PK, Butler DF. Cutaneous collision cancers: a report of two squamomelanocytic malignancies and review of the literature. *Dermatol Surg.* 2011;37(11):1679–1683.

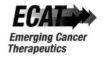

Controversies in the Management of the Regional Node Basin in Cutaneous Melanoma

Ioannis Hatzaras and Julie R. Lange*

Johns Hopkins Medicine, Department of Surgery, Division of Surgical Oncology, Baltimore, MD

■ ABSTRACT

In patients with primary cutaneous melanoma, the regional lymph nodes have always been important for staging and treatment. Many advances have been made in our assessment and management of the regional nodes, and yet, many controversies and challenges remain. The regional lymph node status is an important prognostic factor for patients with newly diagnosed cutaneous melanoma. There is great variation in the prognosis of patients with lymph node metastasis. This chapter will discuss the indications for lymph node basin assessment and the related prognostic implications of node-positive disease. Controversies in management of the lymph node basin will be discussed in the setting of the following challenging scenarios: (a) sentinel lymph node biopsy in thin (<1 mm) melanoma, thick melanoma, in-transit metastasis, or recurrent lesions; (b) lymph node assessment using ultrasound technology; (c) completion lymphadenectomy in a positive sentinel lymph node biopsy; and (d) indications for radiation treatment in the clinically positive lymph node basin.

Keywords: melanoma, lymph node metastasis, lymphadenectomy, controversies

*Corresponding author, Associate Professor of Surgery, Oncology, and Dermatology, Department of Surgery, 600 North Wolfe Street, Carnegie 681, Baltimore, MD

E-mail address:jlange@jhmi.edu

Emerging Cancer Therapeutics 3:3 (2012) 461–470.
© 2012 Demos Medical Publishing LLC. All rights reserved.
DOI: 10.5003/2151–4194.3.3.461

■ INTRODUCTION

The incidence of cutaneous melanoma has steadily been rising. Melanoma is increasing in men more rapidly than any other malignancy, and in women more rapidly than any other malignancy, except for lung cancer (1). There is an estimated 1 million melanoma survivors living in the United States, and an estimated 76,250 individuals will be diagnosed in 2012 (2). For patients with cutaneous melanoma, the regional node basin has long been a major focus of concern. Several controversies remain with regard to the management of the regional node basin. In this chapter, we review the selection of patients for sentinel node biopsy, whether ultrasound (US) can replace sentinel node biopsy in some patients, the growing controversy with regard to completion dissection for patients with nodal micrometastases, and the use of radiation therapy to the regional basin in selected patients.

■ THE IMPORTANCE OF THE REGIONAL NODES

Melanoma has long been viewed as a surgical disease, where extirpation of the primary tumor offers good local control of the disease (3). Cutaneous melanoma generally metastasizes by the lymphatic route in a predictable and orderly fashion (4). In patients with primary cutaneous melanoma, the status of the regional nodes is the most important prognostic factor. The American Joint Committee on Cancer (AJCC) melanoma database analysis of more than 17,600 patients showed that the presence of any regional nodal metastases is associated with poorer survival (5). Management of the primary tumor and the lymphatic basin has evolved, and several advancements have been made; yet, many areas of controversy remain (6).

Before the development of sentinel lymph node biopsy (SLNB), some experts recommended that patients with melanomas between 1 and 4 mm in thickness and a clinically negative regional node basin should undergo elective lymph node dissection. Approximately 20% of such patients undergoing elective dissection had a positive lymph node and, thus, were the only patients likely to benefit from the dissection. The majority of patients had pathologically negative nodes but lived with the morbidity of complete node dissection. In 1992, Morton and colleagues described the sentinel lymph node (SLN) technique for patients with cutaneous melanoma as a method of determining the status of the clinically negative regional node basin without an elective dissection (7). Numerous studies have since documented the great prognostic significance of the sentinel node status, and the sentinel node biopsy has been widely adopted as a staging procedure (4,5,8–11).

The Multicenter Selective Lymphadenectomy Trial (MLST-1) (10), a large international study, randomized intermediate thickness melanoma patients to wide local excision with SLNB versus wide local excision with an observational approach to the regional nodes. The trial demonstrated that evaluation of the regional lymphatic basin provides important prognostic information, and in fact, the SLN status was the most important predictor of survival by multivariate analysis. The patients who were randomized to the observation arm of the study had frequent assessment of their lymphatic basins; in patients with recurrence in the regional basin, subsequent lymph node dissections revealed, on the average, more involved lymph nodes than the lymphadenectomy specimens from patients in the sentinel node arm of the study (3.3 metastatic nodes vs. 1.4). Moreover, in the observation arm, approximately the same percentage of participants had a regional recurrence as had positive sentinel nodes in the sentinel node arm. Although MSLT I did not find any difference in the overall survival in the two arms, the sentinel node arm had significantly better disease-free survival.

There is great variation in the prognosis of patients with regional lymph node metastasis, with several variables identified with prognostic importance. The most important characteristic is the number of affected nodes, with substantially worsening prognosis with the increasing number of positive nodes. Also of substantial importance is whether the positive nodes are clinically apparent or microscopically involved, such as those found by sentinel node biopsy, with significantly better outcomes for patients with microscopic disease compared with macroscopic (palpable) disease (5). Any amount of metastatic disease in the regional lymph nodes is a poor prognostic sign associated with a drop in survival in both short- and long-term follow-up (5,12–17). Survival curves for patients with positive nodes slope steeply downward in the first 2 to 3 years after diagnosis but thereafter bend toward nearly a plateau once the patient is past 10 years after diagnosis. The node-positive population of melanoma patients is a high-risk group, but a substantial minority of patients will be alive at 10 and more years after diagnosis. Management of the regional node basin currently remains a critically important part of melanoma surgical care.

■ SELECTION OF PATIENTS FOR SENTINEL NODE BIOPSY

To assess which patients should have SLNB as part of their initial management, the benefits of the technique for an individual should be considered. For patients with a new diagnosis of invasive cutaneous melanoma and a clinically negative regional node basin, SLNB is a staging tool that allows us to better understand an individual's future risk of recurrence and assists with clinical decision making. A node-positive patient is at increased risk of recurrence both in the regional node basin and at distant sites. Node-positive patients are generally recommended to have a completion dissection of the affected basin and are considered for systemic adjuvant therapies.

The thickness, or the T stage, of the primary tumor is closely associated with the risk of a positive node. In the group of patients with lesions <1mm, the overall chance that they harbor a positive SLN is 5% or less; in patients with lesions between 1 and 2 mm, it is about 10%; for lesions that are 2 to 4 mm, the chance is approximately 25%; and melanomas that are thicker than 4 mm have greater than 40% chance of having a positive SLN (18–20). Sentinel node staging is appropriate for patients for whom the information about node status would be useful in clinical decision making and for patients who may consider enrollment in clinical trials.

Current Guidelines for the Use of Sentinel Node Biopsy

Guidelines for the use of SLNB have been developed by oncology organizations in the USA, Australia, and Europe. There is a general agreement that SLNB should be offered to appropriate patients with newly diagnosed invasive cutaneous melanoma. In the United States, the most widely used guidelines are from the National Comprehensive Cancer Network (NCCN). The NCCN endorses SLNB for patients with melanoma >1 mm in thickness with a clinically negative node basin. SLNB should be done either before or with the wide excision, because the accuracy of the procedure in patients who have had a wide excision is uncertain. Sentinel nodes should pathologically be evaluated with multiple step sections and immunohistochemistry. Patients found to have a histologically positive node should receive a recommendation for completion node dissection or consideration for enrollment of clinical trials of dissection versus observation.

Clinicians should be aware that the accuracy of SLNB after prior wide excision may be decreased. Some reports have described results of SLNB in patients who had previous wide local excision (21–23). It is sometimes possible to identify positive nodes in patients who have had a prior wide excision, although the accuracy of the technique in patients who have undergone complex reconstruction of the primary excision site is unknown. As such, wide excision before planned SLNB should be discouraged. Patients can, however, be considered for the SLNB on an individual basis if they present after initial wide excision, taking into account the patient's risk of nodal metastases, the importance of the staging for that patient, and the extent of tissue disruption by the wide excision. Simultaneous SLNB with wide local excision is preferred whenever possible (21,22).

Controversies in the Use of Sentinel Lymph Node Biopsy

Thin Melanoma

Most newly diagnosed cases of invasive melanoma are <1 mm. Patients with in situ melanoma or thin melanoma (<1 mm) with no adverse features are not candidates for SLNB. Thin melanoma,

in general, is associated with good prognosis, and most cases are well managed with a simple wide local excision alone. Of these patients overall, a small minority (<5%) will have regional nodal metastases, and therefore, SLNB is not appropriate for most patients with thin melanoma. However, there is growing recognition that there is a subgroup of patients with thin melanoma who are node positive and growing endorsement for consideration of SLNB for patients with thin melanoma with adverse features that indicate a somewhat higher risk of nodal metastases.

Several retrospective series of sentinel node biopsy in patients with thin melanoma have identified risk factors that are associated with positive sentinel nodes. Thickness of 0.76 to 1.0 mm, elevated mitotic rate, and ulceration were identified as factors most strongly associated with positive sentinel nodes in patients with thin melanoma. Weaker factors that were cited include Clark's level IV/V and young age; these factors are of unknown significance and are generally not used to support a decision for SLNB. Currently, the NCCN endorses consideration of SLNB in patients who have thin melanoma with a thickness of 0.76 to 1.0 mm, histologic ulceration, or an elevated mitotic rate (>1/mm2) (24–29).

Thick Melanoma

Most studies of SLNB have included either mostly or exclusively patients with intermediate thickness melanoma. Patients with thick (>4 mm) melanoma are at high risk of recurrence, and the value of SLNB in this population has been questioned. However, several retrospective series have demonstrated that SLN status is a strong independent predictor of outcome, even in patients with thick melanoma (5,8,30,31). Thus, in these high-risk patients, SLNB, at the very least, provides prognostic information that can be useful in clinical decision making. It is reasonable to offer SLNB to help define the extent of disease and appropriately stratify for participation in clinical trials of adjuvant therapy.

In-transit or Locally Recurrent Melanoma

Two scenarios in which the value of SLNB remains controversial is a patient with a transit lesion and a patient with a local recurrence. About 5%–10% of melanoma patients develop in-transit recurrence. In-transit lesions themselves define a patient having stage III disease and are associated with high regional and distant recurrence rates. Therefore, in this population, the information from a sentinel node biopsy may not provide useful prognostic information. Although patients with in-transit disease have a high probability of occult nodal involvement, the effect of SLNB on clinical decisions and on outcome remains uncertain (11,32).

Locally recurrent disease encompasses two distinct entities: true local scar recurrence after inadequate initial excision, which most likely represents persistent local disease, and local recurrence after adequate initial excision, which likely represents dermal lymphatic disease appearing in proximity to the wide excision scar (11). The available data are sparse on the appropriate management of these conditions, but established guidelines recommend reexcision to appropriate margins with SLNB in the first scenario and metastatic workup, followed by surgical excision in the second scenario. SLNB is of uncertain benefit and should be considered on a case-by-case basis (11,33).

■ ULTRASOUND AS AN ALTERNATIVE TO SENTINEL NODE BIOPSY

Most sentinel nodes are histologically negative. SLNB seems to confer no overall survival advantage, and there is a financial cost associated with the application of the technique, with overall charges ranging from $10,000 to $15,000 in the U.S. These increased costs have also been noted in European and Australian literature (34). An effective alternative to SLNB could potentially have significant savings in cost and, perhaps, morbidity. Preoperative US has recently been proposed as such a technology that might serve these functions.

Voit and colleagues (34) assessed 400 consecutive patients who underwent preoperative lymphoscintigraphy for melanoma in preparation for SLNB and also underwent a US examination of the regional node basin. When the US examination showed a suspicious or malignant pattern, patients were further assessed with fine-needle aspiration cytology (FNAC) before the SN procedure. US-guided FNAC identified 51 (65%) of 79 SN metastases. Specificity was 99% (317 of 321), with a positive predictive value of 93% and a negative predictive value of 92%. The SN-positive identification rate by US-guided FNAC increased from 40% in stage pT1a/b disease to 79% in stage pT4a/b disease. The authors concluded that 65% of the patients with positive SLN could have been spared a SLNB and been given a complete regional node dissection from the outset.

The promising results from Dr. Voit's group have not yet been replicated elsewhere. A study from the Melanoma Institute of Australia concluded that targeted US examination of the regional node basin can detect metastatic melanoma deposits with a sensitivity of only approximately 24% (35). A follow-up analysis from the Sydney group concluded that US technology is not yet an appropriate substitute for SLNB (36). At present, the existing evidence shows that US is not ready for widespread use to replace sentinel node biopsy. However, further investigation of the technique is warranted.

■ COMPLETION NODE DISSECTION FOR A POSITIVE SENTINEL NODE

Goals and Current Guidelines

Patients with a positive SLN should be recommended for a complete lymph node dissection of the involved nodal basin (11). The goals of dissection in this population are staging, regional control, and, possibly, survival benefit. Patients with a larger number of positive regional nodes have worse prognosis; this information may be valuable to both the patient and their providers. Regional control after completion dissection for a positive sentinel node is excellent, with most series reporting 0% to 2% regional basin recurrence rates. In the past, it was assumed that dissection of positive regional nodes would improve melanoma-specific survival, but this traditional goal is now challenged. In the era of sentinel node biopsies, most patients with positive nodes have microscopic nodal deposits, and the benefits of completion dissection have been called into question.

Among patients who had a completion dissection for a positive sentinel node, published studies have revealed positive nonsentinel nodes in approximately 15% to 20% of these complete lymph node dissection specimens (9,37). Therefore, most patients undergoing completion dissection have no further disease identified in their dissection specimen. These patients do run a risk of complications

related to the dissection, including a risk of lymphedema after axillary or inguinal dissection. The rate of complications after inguinal lymph node dissection can be higher than after axillary or modified radical neck dissection. Complete lymph node dissection at any site is associated with a higher rate of complications when there are clinically evident lymph nodes compared with patients who are having a lymphadenectomy after a positive SLNB (38,39).

To address the uncertain benefit of completion node dissection for patients with a positive sentinel node, the MLST II was designed. The MLST II study is a large ongoing multi-institutional randomized trial for patients with a positive SLNB (40). Such patients are randomized 1:1 to either standard completion node dissection versus no further surgery with US surveillance. Recruitment for the study has progressed well and is ongoing. The primary objective of the study is to determine whether completion node dissection is associated with better melanoma-specific survival compared to observation with US surveillance. Secondary goals are to evaluate disease-free survival, rate of lymph node basin recurrence in the observation arm, and quality of life. This study should yield important information on the question of whether complete lymph node dissection has a true benefit in patients with a positive sentinel node.

A multicenter dataset from the Netherlands (41) reported that patients with micrometastases less than 0.1 mm have the same prognosis as SN negative patients do and might be spared a completion lymph node dissection (CLND). The European Organization for Research and Treatment of Cancer (EORTC) has designed the MINITUB study as an observational cohort study for patients with minimal tumor burden in their sentinel node who have chosen to forgo a completion dissection. The primary objective is to define the time to recurrence in this cohort. Other centers have reported that minimal disease in the sentinel node is associated with poorer survival compared with node-negative patients (42,43). Until further trial information is available, completion dissection for positive sentinel nodes is considered the standard of care. The uncertainty with regard to the benefit of completion dissection is a substantial problem in clinical decision making for melanoma patients, and trial participation is particularly encouraged.

■ RADIATION THERAPY FOR THE REGIONAL NODE BASIN

Today, most patients undergoing completion dissection are patients with a positive sentinel node, and most of these are at very low risk of subsequent in-basin recurrence. However there are still patients who require node dissection for palpable nodal disease, either at the time of original diagnosis or as a regional recurrence. Several factors can be identified as associated with in-basin recurrence after complete node dissection, including having more than three positive nodes, nodal deposit of greater than 3 cm, extracapsular extension, and regional recurrence after prior dissection. Series reported from the M. D. Anderson Cancer Center have demonstrated that postdissection node basin adjuvant irradiation can safely and effectively be delivered in high-risk patients (44,45).

A retrospective study of patients with clinically advanced melanoma having lymphadenectomy with or without adjuvant radiation therapy showed significantly improved regional control associated with the addition of radiation therapy after dissection. However, patients receiving radiation were also more likely to have lymphedema, particularly after radiation to the inguinal node basin (44). A multicenter international randomized clinical trial of radiation versus observation after nodal dissection for high-risk regional disease showed a significantly decreased risk of lymph node basin recurrence in the group randomized to radiation therapy, although it failed to show a benefit in terms of the overall survival (46). On the basis of these data, adjuvant radiation therapy to the nodal bed after dissection should be considered for patients with high-risk nodal disease: multiple positive nodes, enlarged nodes, or extracapsular extension. Radiation therapy should judiciously be offered for inguinal disease, because chronic lymphedema can be exacerbated by adjuvant radiation therapy at that site.

■ SUMMARY

The incidence of cutaneous melanoma is high. Patients with lesions thicker than 1 mm and a clinically negative regional node basin should be offered SLNB. Select patients with lesions thinner than 1 mm with adverse features such as ulceration or a high mitotic rate should also be offered SLNB. At this point, US evaluation of the regional basin cannot replace sentinel node biopsy. If an SLNB is positive for melanoma, the patient should be recommended to have completion lymph node dissection or participation in MSLT II. Radiation therapy to the dissected lymph node basin improves regional control for patients with several positive regional node, large nodal tumor deposits, or extranodal extension.

■ REFERENCES

1. Jemal A, Siegel R, Xu J, Ward E. Cancer statistics, 2010. *CA Cancer J Clin.* 2010;60(5):277–300.
2. Siegel R, Desantis C, Virgo K, et al. Cancer treatment and survivorship statistics, 2012. *CA Cancer J Clin.* 2012; 62(4):220–241.
3. Ewing J. The problems of melanoma. *BMJ.* 1930;2(3646):852–856.
4. Mansfield PF, Lee JE, Balch CM. Cutaneous melanoma: current practice and surgical controversies. *Curr Probl Surg.* 1994;31(4):253–374.
5. Balch CM, Soong SJ, Gershenwald JE, et al. Prognostic factors analysis of 17,600 melanoma patients: validation of the American Joint Committee on Cancer melanoma staging system. *J Clin Oncol.* 2001; 19(16):3622–3634.
6. Balch CM, Soong SJ, Atkins MB, et al. An evidence-based staging system for cutaneous melanoma. *CA Cancer J Clin.* 2004;54(3):131–149.
7. Morton DL, Wen DR, Wong JH, et al. Technical details of intraoperative lymphatic mapping for early stage melanoma. *Arch Surg.* 1992; 127(4):392–399.
8. Gershenwald JE, Mansfield PF, Lee JE, Ross MI. Role for lymphatic mapping and sentinel lymph node biopsy in patients with thick (> or = 4 mm) primary melanoma. *Ann Surg Oncol.* 2000;7(2):160–165.
9. Lee JH, Essner R, Torisu-Itakura H, Wanek L, Wang H, Morton DL. Factors predictive of tumor-positive nonsentinel lymph nodes after tumor-positive sentinel lymph node dissection for melanoma. *J Clin Oncol.* 2004;22(18):3677–3684.
10. Morton DL, Thompson JF, Cochran AJ, et al. Sentinel-node biopsy or nodal observation in melanoma. *New Engl J Med.* 2006;355(13):1307–1317.
11. Coit DG, Andtbacka R, Bichakjian CK, et al. Melanoma. *JNCCN.* 2009;7(3):250–275.
12. Morton DL, Wanek L, Nizze JA, Elashoff RM, Wong JH. Improved long-term survival after lymphadenectomy of melanoma metastatic to regional nodes: analysis of prognostic factors in 1134 patients from the John Wayne Cancer Clinic. *Ann Surg.* 1991;214(4):491–499; discussion 499–501.
13. Kadison AS, Morton DL. Immunotherapy of malignant melanoma. *Surg Clin North Am.* 2003;83(2):343–370.
14. Kirkwood JM, Strawderman MH, Ernstoff MS, Smith TJ, Borden EC, Blum RH. Interferon alfa-2b adjuvant therapy of high-risk resected cutaneous melanoma: the Eastern Cooperative Oncology Group Trial EST 1684. *J Clin Oncol.* 1996;14(1):7–17.
15. Karakousis CP, Velez A, Driscoll DL, Takita H. Metastasectomy in malignant melanoma. *Surgery.* 1994;115(3):295–302.
16. Lee ML, Tomsu K, Von Eschen KB. Duration of survival for disseminated malignant melanoma: results of a meta-analysis. *Melanoma Res.* 2000;10(1):81–92.
17. Leong SP. Selective sentinel lymphadenectomy for malignant melanoma. *Surg Clin North Am.* 2003;83(1):157–185, vii.
18. Gershenwald JE, Thompson W, Mansfield PF, et al. Multi-institutional melanoma lymphatic mapping experience: the prognostic value of sentinel lymph node status in 612 stage I or II melanoma patients. *J Clin Oncol.* 1999;17(3):976–983.
19. Sondak VK, Taylor JM, Sabel MS, et al. Mitotic rate and younger age are predictors of sentinel lymph node positivity: lessons learned from the generation of a probabilistic model. *Ann Surg Oncol.* 2004;11(3):247–258.
20. Andtbacka RH, Gershenwald JE. Role of sentinel lymph node biopsy in patients with thin melanoma. *JNCCN.* 2009;7(3):308–317.
21. Ariyan S, Ali-Salaam P, Cheng DW, Truini C. Reliability of lymphatic mapping after wide local excision of cutaneous melanoma. *Ann Surg Oncol.* 2007;14(8):2377–2383.
22. Gannon CJ, Rousseau DL, Jr., Ross MI, et al. Accuracy of lymphatic mapping and sentinel lymph node biopsy after previous wide local excision in patients with primary melanoma. *Cancer.* 2006;107(11):2647–2652.
23. Karakousis CP, Grigoropoulos P. Sentinel node biopsy before and after wide excision of the primary melanoma. *Ann Surg Oncol.* 1999;6(8):785–789.
24. Wong SL, Brady MS, Busam KJ, Coit DG. Results of sentinel lymph node biopsy in patients with thin melanoma. *Ann Surg Oncol.* 2006;13(3):302–309.
25. Kesmodel SB, Karakousis GC, Botbyl JD, et al. Mitotic rate as a predictor of sentinel lymph

node positivity in patients with thin melanomas. *Ann Surg Oncol.* 2005;12(6):449–458.

26. Ranieri JM, Wagner JD, Wenck S, Johnson CS, Coleman JJ, 3rd. The prognostic importance of sentinel lymph node biopsy in thin melanoma. *Ann Surg Oncol.* 2006;13(7):927–932.

27. Puleo CA, Messina JL, Riker AI, et al. Sentinel node biopsy for thin melanomas: which patients should be considered? *Cancer Control.* 2005; 12(4):230–235.

28. Wright BE, Scheri RP, Ye X, et al. Importance of sentinel lymph node biopsy in patients with thin melanoma. *Arch Surg.* 2008;143(9):892–899; discussion 899–900.

29. Murali R, Haydu LE, Quinn MJ, et al. Sentinel lymph node biopsy in patients with thin primary cutaneous melanoma. *Ann Surg.* 2012;255(1):128–133.

30. Ferrone CR, Panageas KS, Busam K, Brady MS, Coit DG. Multivariate prognostic model for patients with thick cutaneous melanoma: importance of sentinel lymph node status. *Ann Surg Oncol.* 2002;9(7):637–645.

31. Gutzmer R, Satzger I, Thoms KM, et al. Sentinel lymph node status is the most important prognostic factor for thick (> or = 4 mm) melanomas. *J Dtsch Dermatol Ges.* 2008;6(3):198–203.

32. Yao KA, Hsueh EC, Essner R, Foshag LJ, Wanek LA, Morton DL. Is sentinel lymph node mapping indicated for isolated local and in-transit recurrent melanoma? *Ann Surg.* 2003;238(5):743–747.

33. Wolf IH, Richtig E, Kopera D, Kerl H. Locoregional cutaneous metastases of malignant melanoma and their management. *Dermatol Surg.* 2004;30(2 Pt 2):244–247.

34. Voit CA, van Akkooi AC, Schafer-Hesterberg G, et al. Rotterdam Criteria for sentinel node (SN) tumor burden and the accuracy of ultrasound (US)-guided fine-needle aspiration cytology (FNAC): can US-guided FNAC replace SN staging in patients with melanoma? *J Clin Oncol.* 2009;27(30):4994–5000.

35. Starritt EC, Uren RF, Scolyer RA, Quinn MJ, Thompson JF. Ultrasound examination of sentinel nodes in the initial assessment of patients with primary cutaneous melanoma. *Ann Surg Oncol.* 2005;12(1):18–23.

36. Sanki A, Uren RF, Moncrieff M, et al. Targeted high-resolution ultrasound is not an effective substitute for sentinel lymph node biopsy in patients with primary cutaneous melanoma. *J Clin Oncol.* 2009;27(33):5614–5619.

37. Cascinelli N, Bombardieri E, Bufalino R, et al. Sentinel and nonsentinel node status in stage IB and II melanoma patients: two-step prognostic indicators of survival. *J Clin Oncol.* 2006; 24(27):4464–4471.

38. Pawlik TM, Ross MI, Johnson MM, et al. Predictors and natural history of in-transit melanoma after sentinel lymphadenectomy. *Ann Surg Oncol.* 2005;12(8):587–596.

39. Sabel MS, Griffith KA, Arora A, et al. Inguinal node dissection for melanoma in the era of sentinel lymph node biopsy. *Surgery.* 2007;141(6):728–735.

40. Morton DL. Overview and update of the phase III Multicenter Selective Lymphadenectomy Trials (MSLT-I and MSLT-II) in melanoma. *Clin Exp Metastas.* [Published online ahead of print, 2012].

41. van der Ploeg AP, van Akkooi AC, Rutkowski P, et al. Prognosis in patients with sentinel node-positive melanoma is accurately defined by the combined Rotterdam tumor load and Dewar topography criteria. *J Clin Oncol.* 2011;29(16):2206–2214.

42. Murali R, Scolyer RA, Thompson JF. Can we better identify thin cutaneous melanomas that are likely to metastasize and cause death? *Ann Surg Oncol.* 2012;19(11):3310–3312.

43. Morton DL, Scheri RP, Balch CM. Can completion lymph node dissection be avoided for a positive sentinel node in melanoma? *Ann Surg Oncol.* 2007; 14(9):2437–2439.

44. Agrawal S, Kane JM, 3rd, Guadagnolo BA, Kraybill WG, Ballo MT. The benefits of adjuvant radiation therapy after therapeutic lymphadenectomy for clinically advanced, high-risk, lymph node-metastatic melanoma. *Cancer.* 2009; 115(24):5836–5844.

45. Ballo MT, Bonnen MD, Garden AS, et al. Adjuvant irradiation for cervical lymph node metastases from melanoma. *Cancer.* 2003;97(7):1789–1796.

46. Burmeister BH, Henderson MA, Ainslie J, et al. Adjuvant radiotherapy versus observation alone for patients at risk of lymph-node field relapse after therapeutic lymphadenectomy for melanoma: a randomised trial. *Lancet Oncol.* 2012;13(6):589–597.

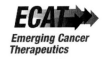

Adjuvant Therapy for Melanoma

Tara C. Gangadhar* and Lynn M. Schuchter

Abramson Cancer Center of the University of Pennsylvania, Philadephia, PA

■ ABSTRACT

Surgical resection is the standard of care for early stage melanoma. Recurrence rates after surgical resection of advanced stage II and stage III melanoma remain high. High-dose interferon is the only approved agent for adjuvant therapy in melanoma and results in an improved relapse-free survival; however, there is no definite overall survival benefit. This chapter reviews the data in support of the use of high-dose interferon for the adjuvant treatment of melanoma as well as new approaches and current adjuvant therapy clinical trials.

Keywords: interferon, immune therapy, chemotherapy, clinical trials, melanoma

*Corresponding author, Abramson Cancer Center of the University of Pennsylvania, Philadelphia, PA
  E-mail address: Tara.Gangadhar@uphs.upenn.edu

Emerging Cancer Therapeutics 3:3 (2012) 471–484.
DOI: 10.5003/2151-4194.3.3.471

demosmedpub.com/ecat

■ INTRODUCTION

The primary treatment for most patients with early stage melanoma is surgical resection. The most recent version of the American Joint Committee on Cancer (AJCC) melanoma staging guidelines has made it possible for clinicians to more accurately predict recurrence rates and to identify the patients at highest risk for disease recurrence and death because of metastatic melanoma. Postoperative adjuvant therapy can be considered for patients at high risk for recurrent melanoma. Incorporated into the staging system of the AJCC are the most important determinants of prognosis: tumor thickness, mitotic rate, ulceration, and the extent of regional nodal involvement. Patients with stage IIC disease (T4b melanoma > 4 mm thick and with ulceration), for example, have 5 and 10 year survival rates of 53% and 39%, respectively. Patients with stage III disease have 10 year survival rates as low as 33%, and 5 year survival rates of 78%, 59%, and 40%, respectively, for patients with stages IIIA, IIIB, and IIIC disease (1). Given this high risk of recurrence and death because of melanoma for patients who initially present with locally or regionally advanced disease, the availability of effective adjuvant therapy would greatly improve survival rates in melanoma patients who have undergone complete resection of their disease.

Adjuvant therapy of melanoma has been under investigation since the 1980s, with a number of approaches tested in an effort to reduce recurrence rates in high-risk patient subsets. The intent of this chapter is to summarize the recent updates and emerging new adjuvant therapy approaches for patients with high-risk melanoma, which is generally defined as melanomas that are either more than 4 mm thick or are node positive (stage III)

disease. Because high-dose interferon (HD IFN) remains the only United States Food and Drug Administration (FDA)-approved adjuvant therapy for melanoma, the main focus will be on the role of adjuvant HD IFN.

■ EARLY ADJUVANT THERAPY STUDIES

Over the last 40 years, more than 100 randomized adjuvant clinical trials have investigated numerous therapies, including cytotoxic chemotherapy and non-specific immunostimulants such as the bacillus Calmette–Guérin (BCG) vaccine, corynbacterium parvum, or levamisole, but none has shown any survival benefit in the adjuvant setting. Trials of dacarbazine (DTIC) either alone (2) or in combination regimens (3) did not result in any survival benefit. Neither the biologic agents BCG vaccine (either alone or in combination with DTIC) (4) and interferon (IFN)-gamma (5) improve survival in high-risk postoperative patients, nor did high-dose chemotherapy with autologous bone marrow support (6) or hormonal therapy with megestrol (7).

■ ADJUVANT THERAPY WITH HIGH-DOSE INTERFERON

Biology of Immune Therapy With Interferon

IFNs were initially discovered in 1957 and constitute a family of proteins that are capable of inducing antiviral effects (8). Further characterization of human IFNs in the late 1970s led to the identification of 2 antigenic species of IFN, with leukocyte derived IFN (mainly IFN-b) being distinct from fibroblast-derived IFN (mainly IFN-a) (9). Ultimately, several IFN species had been cloned by the early 1980s, marking the inception of their clinical therapeutic use and followed by the development of industrial-scale production through recombinant DNA techniques in bacteria, purification, or monoclonal immunosorbent antibody (10). Type 1 IFNs, which include both IFN-a species and IFN-b, are a very heterogeneous subfamily and affect their actions through IFN receptors with signaling classically mediated through the Janus kinase/signal transducers and activators of transcription (JAK-STAT) pathway proteins (11), although many additional signaling pathways have been described (12). There is evidence to suggest that IFN also upregulates STAT1, a tumor suppressor, downregulates STAT3, which may play a role in tumor progression, and modulates chemokine receptor expression (11). Downstream signaling results in the expression of several genes with diverse biological functions, including genes that are involved in the regulation of apoptosis (13), p53, and cell-cycle inhibitors while also affecting immune modulation to promote a host response against melanoma (14).

Review of Adjuvant Interferon Clinical Studies

On the basis of potent immunologic effects of IFN and its modest activity in patients with metastatic melanoma, a series of studies with IFN have been conducted in the postoperative adjuvant setting. These studies have explored a variety of doses, schedules, durations, and varying formulations of IFN with an optimal approach not firmly established. On the basis of early results from the Eastern Cooperative Oncology Group (ECOG) trial E1684, high-dose IFN alfa-2b was approved in 1996 by the FDA for the adjuvant treatment of melanoma patients with a high

risk of recurrence after complete surgical resection. In that study, 280 patients with thick primary melanoma, Stage IIB (more than 4 mm thick), and node-negative disease or with node-positive Stage III melanoma were randomly assigned to receive either high-dose IFN for 1 year or to be observed with no therapy. An intensive dose was deliberately chosen to deliver IFN at the maximally tolerated dose to achieve peak drug levels. The patients were treated with IFN alfa-2b, 20 million units per square meter per day, intravenously given 5 times per week for a 4 week induction phase, followed by 10 million units per square meter per day give by subcutaneous injection 3 times per week for a 48 week maintenance phase. For patients who were randomized to the IFN arm, there was a 9 month prolongation in the median relapse free survival (RFS; 1.7 years vs. 1.0 years; $p = 0.002$), and there was a 1 year prolongation in the median OS (3.8 years vs. 2.8 years; $p = 0.02$), with an absolute increase of 9% in survival at 5 years (46% vs. 37%) (15). This trial was the first study of adjuvant therapy in which an improvement in OS was demonstrated, and based on these results, the high-dose IFN treatment regimen was FDA approved for patients with stage III and high-risk stage II melanoma. It should be noted, however, that, in updated results and subsequent analysis with a median follow-up of 12.6 years, although the RFS benefit was maintained, the improvement in the overall survival was no longer statistically significant (16). The diminished survival benefit after longer follow-up led many physicians and patients to question whether high-dose IFN was worth the benefit, given the substantial side effects associated with treatment.

The interpretation of the role of high-dose adjuvant IFN therapy has further been complicated by results of subsequent studies, which were designed to evaluate the optimal dose and duration of IFN treatment. In particular, 2 subsequent large randomized ECOG studies were conducted after the initial E1684 study, including E1690 and E1694. ECOG protocol 1690, involved a 3-way randomization with patients receiving high-dose IFN alfa-2b, low-dose IFN alfa-2b (3 million units/day SC 3 times a week for 2 years), or no therapy for patients with thick primary melanomas > 4mm thick or node-positive disease. The lower dose given for a longer duration was included because of the significant toxicity observed with the 52 week regimen tested in the E1684 study and emerging studies suggesting a benefit for low-dose IFN regimens. The study enrolled 642 patients. At a median follow-up of 4.3 years, high-dose IFN alfa-2b led to a reduction in the risk of recurrence compared with no treatment (HR = 1.28; p = 0.025). However, neither the high- nor the lower-dose regimen improved the OS compared with observation (17). It should be noted that the median survival for patients in the observation arm was 6 years, which was much better than that in the previous E1684 study. It is possible that the OS benefit initially seen in the E1684 study was not observed in the E1690 study, because lymphadenectomies were not required for clinical stage II disease on the E1690 study. Because of the commercial availability of IFN alfa-2b beginning in 1996, several of the patients randomized to observation arm went on to receive adjuvant IFN therapy at the time of regional nodal relapse and resection, which had not been available to patients randomized to observation on E1684, making the E1690 OS data more difficult to interpret.

In ECOG protocol E1694, 880 high-risk patients were randomized to high-dose IFN alfa-2b for 52 weeks or a GM2-ganglioside vaccine (GMK) for 96 weeks. The GMK vaccine consisted of purified ganglioside GM2 coupled to keyhole limpet hemocyanin (KLH). An external data safety and monitoring committee unblinded the study at a median follow-up of 1.3 years after an interim analysis identified a superior RFS and OS for high-dose IFN alfa-2b. The estimated RFS (62% vs. 49%; HR = 1.47; p = 0.0015) and OS (78% vs. 73%; HR = 1.52; p = 0.009) rates at 2 years for the patients receiving high-dose IFN alfa-2b were superior to those for the vaccine (18). However, it is not possible to assess whether high-dose IFN in this study was superior to observation, because the study did not include an observation arm. Similarly, it is not possible to assess whether the vaccine would have been inferior or equivalent to observation.

A pooled analysis of ECOG trials upheld the finding of prolonged RFS, but not OS, in patients treated with high-dose IFN alfa-2b versus observation on a 2-sided univariate log-rank analysis of E1684 and E1690 pooled data (16).

Other Interferon Alfa-2b Schedules

Given the high toxicity observed in the initial E1684 study, several studies addressed the question of whether alternate dosing schedules of high-dose IFN alfa-2b might offer a DFS or OS benefit with less toxicity. Trials of very-low-dose, low-dose, or intermediate-dose IFN alfa-2b given for time periods ranging from 6 months to 2 years were all ineffective in improving OS (19–25). It should be noted that a trial that compared the 4 week induction high-dose IFN alfa-2b alone versus the standard 52 week regimen did not improve the OS (26). In addition, a 3-arm randomized study of intermediate-dose IFN compared observation versus 4 weeks of induction with a flat dose of IFN alfa-2b 10 million units subcutaneously 5 days per week followed by 12 months of maintenance therapy (IFN alfa-2b 10 million units flat dose subcutaneously 3 days per week) versus 1 month of induction and 24 months of maintenance. At a median follow-up time of 72.4 months, intermediate-dose IFN alfa-2b did not improve the overall survival. IFN alfa-2b with 1 year of maintenance therapy improved the RFS, but the RFS benefit was not seen for the 2 year maintenance therapy arm compared with observation (27). Another EORTC protocol (18991) that tested an extended course of pegylated IFN alfa-2b for 5 years versus observation in 1256 stage III melanoma patients demonstrated improved relapse-free survival, but not improved overall survival (28). This regimen of pegylated IFN is now used by some clinicians as a reasonable alternative to the standard high-dose IFN formulation. Although the toxicity profile is similar to standard high-dose IFN, the absence of daily intravenous dosing for the induction period and weekly dosing makes the pegylated long-acting formulation appealing to some patients. The dose used in the trial was 6 mcg per kg by subcutaneous injection weekly for an 8 week induction period, followed by 3 mcg per kg weekly for an intended duration of 5 years. It should be noted that a DFS benefit was observed, although 31% of the patients discontinued therapy because of toxicity; the intended treatment duration, however, was 5 years. One caveat to the use of this regimen is that, although an OS benefit had initially been observed with the standard 52 week HD IFN regimen, no such OS benefit has ever been observed with the pegylated IFN formulation.

Interferon Studies Meta-Analyses

Several meta-analyses of adjuvant IFN studies and systematic reviews have been conducted. The first included 12 trials of high-, intermediate-, and low-dose IFN alfa-2a and IFN alfa-2b and indicated a clear improvement in the RFS versus control (HR = 0.83; 95% CI 0.77–0.90) and some improvement in the overall survival (HR=0.93; 95% CI 0.85–1.02; p = 0.1) (29). A follow-up meta-analysis, which also included EORTC 18991 with PegIFN 2b, indicated statistically significant improvements in both DFS (HR for recurrence = 0.82 95% CI 0.77–.87; p < 0.001) and OS (HR for death = 0.89; 95% CI 0.83–0.96; p = 0.002) (30). Petrella et al. have recently conducted an updated meta-analysis and systematic review and essentially confirmed the conclusions of prior reviews with a significant DFS benefit for high-dose IFN or pegylated IFN treatment. The available evidence shows that adjuvant IFN may have a small long-term survival advantage; however, it has been shown to consistently improve the RFS or DFS. Important new results from this analysis showed a DFS benefit for pegylated IFN compared with observation (31).

Adverse Events and Supportive Care During High-Dose Interferon Therapy

High-dose IFN alfa-2b is associated with a number of toxicities, which necessitate dose reductions and delays in a majority of patients (32). Given that a shorter treatment course has not been as effective as the standard 52 week regimen and dose-related responses have been observed for IFN, understanding the common reasons for dose reduction and discontinuation are essential. Familiarity with the common toxicities allows clinicians to provide the level of supportive care needed to optimize efficacy by increasing the chance of completing the full course of adjuvant therapy at the highest dose tolerated. Effective communication with the patient and their support network is also an important part of the supportive care; patients who have thorough understanding of the high probability of toxicity and the possibility of dose interruption may be less likely to become discouraged during therapy. The adverse events associated with IFN are, for the most part, reversible with dose interruption.

Almost all patients experience constitutional symptoms, including fatigue, fevers, chills, headaches, and myalgia, which can be severe in many patients. Nausea and vomiting also occur in a majority of patients. These "flu-like" symptoms acutely occur, with the highest severity after the initial treatment with high-dose IFN, last 4 to 8 hours, and are related to the release of cytokines in response to exogenous IFN. Tolerance develops, and these symptoms decrease with subsequent treatments but may reoccur after dose interruptions. These symptoms can be managed with prophylactic acetaminophen or nonsteroidal anti-inflammatory drugs at the time of administration during early treatment cycles and as needed. Antiemetics can be used as needed, and adequate fluid intake should be encouraged to avoid dehydration.

The most common side effect resulting in treatment discontinuation is fatigue, which occurs, to some extent, in almost 100% of the treated patients and can be severe in about 25% of the patients, leading to disruption of daily activity and function. Unlike the other constitutional and flu-like symptoms, which decrease with time, fatigue can worsen with increasing duration of therapy. Fatigue may be multifactorial, and thyroid function, mood, and nutritional status can also be assessed when evaluation fatigue. Dose reductions or discontinuation should be considered when the quality of life or the ability to carry on daily activity and function is impaired.

Mood disorders are associated with high-dose IFN and most commonly consist of depressive symptoms, which can range from mild changes to severe clinical depression, although severe symptoms, suicidal ideation, and suicide attempts are rare. Some symptoms of depression can occur in up to 40% of the treated patients and may be related to effects of IFN on the hypothalamic–pituitary–adrenal axis and cytokine effects on neurotransmitters. Other neuropsychiatric adverse events include anxiety and impaired cognitive function; patients and family members should be aware of a wide range of possible symptoms and know to immediately report any changes in mood, behavior, or cognition. Clinicians should have a careful discussion of these risks with all patients, in particular, patients with a prior history of psychiatric symptoms, when discussing the risks versus the potential benefit of treatment with adjuvant IFN therapy. Patients who do develop mood symptoms should be followed very closely, with medical intervention or psychiatric referral if clinically indicated and dose interruption or discontinuation when needed.

Myelosuppression also occurs in almost all patients and consists predominantly of neutropenia. Elevations in transaminases (AST and ALT) occur in about 2/3 of all patients and can be severe in up to 1/3 of the patients. Therefore, patients require frequent blood draws during treatment with HDI, including weekly blood counts and blood chemistry during the initial 4 week induction phase, followed by monthly lab evaluations during the maintenance phase. Other lab evaluations, such as thyroid-stimulating hormone, may be checked periodically or as clinically indicated in the setting of fatigue or depression. The purpose of the routine labs evaluations is primarily to detect either neutropenia or an elevated AST/ALT, both of which are common, so that appropriate dose interruptions or modifications can be made as needed to maintain safety and increase the chance of completing the full treatment course. A 33% dose reduction from the starting dose is recommended for a granulocyte count of less than 500 per cubic millimeter or AST/ALT greater than 5 times the upper limit of normal, with interruption of therapy until resolution to grade 1 or normal before resuming treatment at the reduced dose. A 66% reduction from the starting dose is recommended for a second occurrence, with treatment discontinuation for a third occurrence of either neutropenia or elevated AST/ALT as previously defined. Therapy may also be interrupted or reduced for severe constitutional or mood adverse events if maximal supportive care is ineffective in reducing symptoms or based on clinical judgment and discussion with the patient. The dose reduction recommendations previously outlined apply to both the induction- and the maintenance-phase dosing. Patients who require dose reductions during the induction phase may initiate the maintenance phase at full dose, with subsequent dose reductions following the same recommendations when indicated for neutropenia or elevated AST/ALT or other severe adverse events. Approximately 1/3 of the patients will require dose reductions or delays in the induction phase, with some patients requiring discontinuation. Approximately 1/3 of the patients initiating the maintenance phase of treatment will also require dose reductions or delays.

Other symptoms include anorexia, which occurs, to some extent, in a majority of patients, and weight loss, which can be multifactorial; a patient's weight should periodically be measured on high-dose IFN. Less common toxicities include dermatologic reactions such as alopecia, increased triglycerides, and thyroid dysfunction.

Patient Selection for Adjuvant Therapy

After complete resection of stage III melanoma, clinicians may consider following a patient with close observation, treating with adjuvant high-dose IFN for 1 year, or offering a patient the opportunity to participate in a clinical trial.

Many patients are not candidates for high-dose IFN alfa-2b, because the risk of toxicity may outweigh any potential benefit because of their age or comorbid conditions. The high toxicity associated with HDI and the lack of a definite OS benefit make close observation without adjuvant therapy an equally reasonable alternative to IFN for many patients. When discussing these options with patients, clinicians must present the high risk of toxicity and the potential benefit of therapy.

Although preliminary data have suggested subsets of patients who may be more likely to benefit from adjuvant therapy, including the development of autoimmunity, the presence of an ulcerated primary tumor, and tumor signatures associated with response (33,34), no data support the clinical use of any definitive predictive marker in deciding which patients are more likely to benefit from adjuvant therapy. Manifestations of autoimmunity, including thyroid dysfunction, vitiligo, and the development of autoantibodes, occur in approximately15%–20% of patients who are treated with IFN. As aforementioned, there are conflicting results with regard to the prognostic or predictive role of development of autoimmunity. Because autoimmunity may not be observed until months after initiation of therapy, there is no way, at present, of prospectively identifying patients who are most likely to derive benefit from IFN.

Last, the decision to treat either the primary tumor resection site or the regional nodal basin with adjuvant radiation therapy can be considered in selected patient situations. Surgical excision with a wide excision margin remains the standard initial treatment for the primary tumor and results in a very low local recurrence rate. However, in cases in which tumor location and anatomic considerations do not permit an adequate wide resection margin, radiation therapy to the primary resection site can be considered in the case of close or positive margins. Although studies have demonstrated that multiple involved nodes (>3), large nodes (>3cm), or extracapsular extension may confer a higher risk of regional nodal recurrence, which can be reduced with adjuvant radiation therapy, randomized studies have not demonstrated any overall survival benefit for adjuvant radiation therapy after standard lymph node dissection. In the absence of any overall survival benefit, individual patient clinical considerations, including the risks of morbidity and risks of local–regional and distant metastatic disease, must carefully be considered before recommending adjuvant radiation therapy (35).

Vaccine Therapy in Adjuvant Therapy

A number of melanoma vaccine strategies have been pursued over the last 40 years. In general, 2 approaches are under clinical investigation: whole-cell vaccine (autologous or allogeneic) and peptide-based, or defined, antigens. Peptides have been selected from 2 classes: melanocyte differentiation antigens and cancer testes antigens. The most widely studied peptides are derived from glycoprotein (gp) 100, tyrosinase, melan-A, and NY-ESO-1 and melanoma antigen encoding gene (MAGE) proteins. However, despite the active development of several vaccine based therapies in melanoma, no vaccine therapy has been effective in the adjuvant setting when tested in a randomized clinical trial. Morton and colleagues conducted phase III adjuvant therapy study of CancerVax (CancerVax Corporation), an allogeneic whole-cell vaccine composed of 3 highly antigenic, irradiated melanoma cell lines based on a retrospective study that suggested benefit of Canvaxin for patients with resected stage III melanoma. In the randomized clinical trial for patients with restected stage III or stage IV melanoma, patients were randomized to Canvaxin with BCG versus BCG alone. There was no improvement in the RFS or OS. The study was stopped early after an interim analysis suggested a low likelihood of a survival benefit (36).

Additional phase III adjuvant vaccine trials have been completed, including a vaccinia melanoma oncolysate vaccine (37), a vaccinia viral lysate of melanoma Melacine (Corixa Corp., Seattle, WA) (38), a cell-lysate vaccine (39), and the GM2-ganglioside vaccine examined in the E1694 study, none of which were effective. EORTC 18961, a randomized postoperative adjuvant clinical trial for patients with stage II melanoma, tested the ganglioside GM2-KLH21 vaccine compared with observation. Preliminary results showed that the vaccine was ineffective and could possibly be detrimental, although more mature follow-up data have suggested no differences in any outcome of the trial (40). Currently, the largest ongoing adjuvant vaccine study is a randomized controlled phase III study of the MAGE-A3 vaccine compared with placebo (GSK "DERMA" study). The MAGE-A3 protein is expressed on 70% of melanomas; therefore, this vaccine may be suitable for many patients. The primary end point of the study is DFS with a total accrual goal of 1,349 patients. Results from this trial are pending.

Granulocyte-Macrophage Colony-Stimulating Factor in Adjuvant Therapy

Granulocyte-macrophage colony-stimulating factor (GM-CSF) is approved for the treatment of bone marrow transplant graft delay or failure and for supporting neutrophil recovery after induction chemotherapy for acute myelogenous leukemia. The drug also promotes melanoma antigen presentation through activation of macrophages, monocytes, and dendritic cells. A randomized placebo-controlled phase III study GM-CSF was conducted in patients with resected high-risk stage III and IV melanoma (protocol E4697). Although adjuvant GM-CSF did improve DFS, there was no improvement in the OS (41). The drug is commercially available, but it is not approved for any indication in melanoma.

Adjuvant Biochemotherapy

Biochemotherapy, the combination of immunotherapy and chemotherapy, has been studied in patients with metastatic melanoma and in the adjuvant setting. Most studies have combined IFN and IL-2 and various chemotherapy regimens. The Southwest Oncology Group (SWOG) trial S0008 conducted a randomized clinical trial comparing 3 cycles of biochemotherapy (BCT) with 1 year of high-dose IFN alfa-2b in high-risk patients with high-risk stage III disease (N1a disease was not included). Biochemotherapy as used in the study consisted of dacarbazine 800 mg/m^2 day 1, cisplatin 20 mg/m^2/ days 1 to 4, vinblastine 1.2 mg/m^2 days 1 to 4, IL-2 9 MIU/m^2/day continuous IV days 1 to 4, IFN 5 MU/m^2/day SC days 1 to 4, 8,10,12, and G-CSF 5 mcg/kg/day SC days 7 to 16. BCT cycles were given every 21 days for 3 cycles (9 weeks total). At a median follow-up of 6 years, BCT improved the RFS compared with 1 year of high-dose IFN, 47% versus 39% (HR 0.77; $p = 0.02$; 95% CI 0.58–0.98), although there was no improvement in the OS with a 5 year survival of 56% for both arms (HR 1.02; 95% CI 0.76–1.37) (42). Biochemotherapy is associated with significant toxicity, including myelosuppression, GI side effects, hypotension, and skin rash. On the basis of these new results, it may be reasonable to consider biochemotherapy in a highly selected patient population in hospitals with an experience in the administration of this complex treatment regimen.

New Approaches in Adjuvant Therapy

The recent FDA approvals of vemurafenib, a BRAF-targeted therapy, and ipilimumab, an anti-CTLA-4 monoclonal antibody, has led to the evaluation of these newer agents in the adjuvant setting for high-risk patients with melanoma (Table 1).

Two CTLA-4 blocking antibodies have been evaluated in patients with melanoma, ipilimumab (developed by Medarex/Bristol Myers Squibb), and tremelimumab (developed by Pfizer/Medimmune), the former FDA-approved for stage IV and unrestectable stage III melanoma. With the success of ipilumumab in the metastatic setting, trials that evaluate ipilumumab in the adjuvant setting have already begun. EORTC 18071 is an adjuvant study of ipilimumab compared with placebo for patients with stage III cutaneous melanoma. Accrual is complete, and results are expected in 2013 or 2014. ECOG protocol E1609 compares high-dose IFN with ipilimumab, with a primary end point of RFS and a target accrual of 1500 patients. In this chapter, 2 different doses of ipilimumab are studied, as well as the role of maintenance therapy. Given the high

TABLE 1 Ongoing Adjuvant Therapy Trials

Study sponsor	Agents	Patient population	Primary end point	Accrual goal	Study status
EORTC 18071 BMS	Ipilimumab vs. placebo	High-risk stage III cutaneous melanoma	RFS	950	Accrual completed
EORTC 18081 BMS	Peg-IFN (2 years) vs. observation	Ulcerated primary cutaneous melanoma T(2–4) bN0M0	RFS	1200	Start date 2012
DERMA GSK	MAGE-A3 vaccine vs. placebo	Stage III cutaneous melanoma with macroscopic involvement	DFS	1349	Accrual completed
ECOG 1609	Ipilimumab vs. HD IFN	High-risk stage III cutaneous melanoma	RFS	1500	Open to accrual
Genentech/ Roche	Vemurafenib (1 year) vs. placebo	Stage IIC and III cutaneous melanoma	DFS	725	Open to accrual
GSK	Dabrafenib and trametinib vs. placebo	Stage III cutaneous melanoma	RFS	852	Start date 2012

TABLE 2 Adjuvant Therapy Recommendations

Patients with high-risk melanoma should be encouraged to participate in clinical trials.

High-dose IFN therapy for 1 year is a reasonable therapy to offer patients with high-risk melanoma to increase DFS.

Pegylated IFN for 1 year is a reasonable alternative to high-dose IFN.

There is insufficient evidence to recommend 1 month of IFN.

cost and toxicities of ipilimumab, clinically relevant biomarkers or predicators of response are desperately needed to identify which patients are most likely to derive benefit from therapy. Ongoing studies are exploring these critical questions.

Adjuvant studies with BRAF inhibitors are just beginning. A study in patients with high-risk BRAF mutated melanoma, including patients with resected stage IIC disease will compare vemurafenib with placebo for 1 year. Last, a trial of the novel BRAF inhibitor dabrafenib in combination with the MEK inhibitor trametinib will be compared with placebo in an adjuvant therapy trial of 852 patients. Another question that remains is whether immune therapy in combination with targeted therapy can improve outcomes when used in the adjuvant setting.

SUMMARY AND FUTURE DIRECTIONS

During the last 30 years, numerous agents have been evaluated in a series of randomized and nonrandomized adjuvant therapy trials in melanoma. Many of these studies suffered from serious methodological problems such as inadequate statistical power, the use of inappropriate controls, and the lack of stratification for known prognostic factors. However, the major obstacle to the success of adjuvant therapy has been a lack of active agents. One important message, overall, is that there are now more effective treatments for advanced melanoma, including molecularly targeted therapies and new immunotherapy strategies. Active drugs targeting BRAF, KIT, and the anti-CTLA4 antibody ipilimumab have shown an overall survival advantage for patients with metastatic disease. Clinical trials with these agents are now underway in the adjuvant setting. Two important questions arise. First, what is the appropriate control arm for these studies? Many of the new adjuvant studies have observation as the control arm which is entirely appropriate given the small overall benefit of IFN and side effect profile of IFN. The second question is: What is the correct end point for adjuvant melanoma studies; in other words, how should success be measured? The RFS or DFS has been the primary end point for most adjuvant melanoma trials; however, many believe that prolongation

of the overall survival is the most appropriate end point. With the development of more successful treatment options for metastatic disease, which can prolong survival after relapse, this end point needs to be reconsidered, and RFS should strongly be considered as an appropriate end point for phase III randomized adjuvant studies.

IFN is an appropriate option for some patients with melanoma. IFN consistently improves RFS by approximately 20% to 30% and may have a modest effect on the overall survival in meta-analysis in the range of approximately 3% to 10%. The optimal schedule and dose for IFN is still not defined. High-dose IFN, as approved by the FDA, is a reasonable regimen for surgically resected stage IIB,C and III patients, with pegylated IFN being a more convenient alternative option, FDA approved for stage III patients.

The optimal care for a patient with high-risk melanoma requires the integration of the existing evidence and should be individualized based on an estimate of the patient's risk of relapse and other comorbid decisions, the judgment of experienced clinicians, and the informed input from our patients. More and more, appropriate patient care will require earlier somatic molecular profiling and new techniques to allow for testing on smaller amounts of tumor tissue. Continued participation by physicians and our patients in well-designed clinical trials remains a priority and will facilitate the continued progress in the treatment of melanoma.

REFERENCES

1. Balch CM, Gershenwald JE, Soong SJ, et al. Final version of 2009 AJCC melanoma staging and classification. *J Clin Oncol.* 2009;27(36):6199–6206.
2. Hill GJ 2nd, Moss SE, Golomb FM, et al. DTIC and combination therapy for melanoma:

III. DTIC (NSC 45388) Surgical Adjuvant Study COG PROTOCOL 7040. *Cancer.* 1981;47(11):2556–2562.

3. Tranum BL, Dixon D, Quagliana J, et al. Lack of benefit of adjunctive chemotherapy in stage I malignant melanoma: a Southwest Oncology Group Study. *Cancer Treat Rep.* 1987; 71(6):643–644.

4. Veronesi U, Adamus J, Aubert C, et al. A randomized trial of adjuvant chemotherapy and immunotherapy in cutaneous melanoma. *N Engl J Med.* 1982;307(15):913–916.

5. Meyskens FL Jr, Kopecky K, Samson M, et al. Recombinant human interferon gamma: adverse effects in high-risk stage I and II cutaneous malignant melanoma. *J Natl Cancer Inst.* 1990;82(12):1071.

6. Meisenberg BR, Ross M, Vredenburgh JJ, et al. Randomized trial of high-dose chemotherapy with autologous bone marrow support as adjuvant therapy for high-risk, multi-node-positive malignant melanoma. *J Natl Cancer Inst.* 1993;85(13):1080–1085.

7. Markovic S, Suman VJ, Dalton RJ, et al. Randomized, placebo-controlled, phase III surgical adjuvant clinical trial of megestrol acetate (Megace) in selected patients with malignant melanoma. *Am J Clin Oncol.* 2002;25(6):552–556.

8. Borden EC, Sen GC, Uze G, et al. Interferons at age 50: past, current and future impact on biomedicine. *Nat Rev Drug Discov.* 2007;6(12):975–990.

9. Havell EA, Berman B, Ogburn CA, Berg K, Paucker K, Vilcek J. Two antigenically distinct species of human interferon. *Proc Natl Acad Sci USA.* 1975;72(6):2185–2187.

10. Kirkwood JM, Ernstoff MS. Interferons in the treatment of human cancer. *J Clin Oncol.* 1984;2(4):336–352.

11. Ascierto PA, Gogas HJ, Grob JJ, et al. Adjuvant interferon alfa in malignant melanoma: An interdisciplinary and multinational expert review. *Crit Rev Oncol Hematol.* 2012; Aug 5 [Epub ahead of print].

12. Platanias LC. Mechanisms of type-I- and type-II-interferon-mediated signalling. *Nat Rev Immunol.* 2005;5(5): 375–386.

13. Der SD, Zhou A, Williams BR, Silverman RH. Identification of genes differentially regulated by interferon alpha, beta, or gamma using oligonucleotide arrays. *Proc Natl Acad Sci USA.* 1998;95(26):15623–15628.

14. Moschos S, Kirkwood JM. Present role and future potential of type I interferons in adjuvant therapy of high-risk operable melanoma. *Cytokine Growth Factor Rev.* 2007; 18(5–6):451–458.

15. Kirkwood JM, Strawderman MH, Ernstoff MS, Smith TJ, Borden EC, Blum RH. Interferon alfa-2b adjuvant therapy of high-risk resected cutaneous melanoma: the Eastern Cooperative Oncology Group Trial EST 1684. *J Clin Oncol.* 1996;14(1):7–17.

16. Kirkwood JM, Manola J, Ibrahim J, Sondak V, Ernstoff MS, Rao U; Eastern Cooperative Oncology Group. A pooled analysis of eastern cooperative oncology group and intergroup trials of adjuvant high-dose interferon for melanoma. *Clin Cancer Res.* 2004;10(5):1670–1677.

17. Kirkwood JM, Ibrahim JG, Sondak VK, et al. High- and low-dose interferon alfa-2b in high-risk melanoma: first analysis of intergroup trial E1690/S9111/C9190. *J Clin Oncol.* 2000; 18(12):2444–2458.

18. Kirkwood JM, Ibrahim JG, Sosman JA, et al. High-dose interferon alfa-2b significantly prolongs relapse-free and overall survival compared with the GM2-KLH/QS-21 vaccine in patients with resected stage IIB-III melanoma: results of intergroup trial E1694/S9512/C509801. *J Clin Oncol.* 2001;19(9):2370–2380.

19. Kleeberg UR, Suciu S, Bröcker EB, et al.; EORTC Melanoma Group in cooperation with the German Cancer Society (DKG). Final results of the EORTC 18871/DKG 80–1 randomised phase III trial. rIFN-alpha2b versus rIFN-gamma versus ISCADOR M versus observation after surgery in melanoma patients with either high-risk primary (thickness >3 mm) or regional lymph node metastasis. *Eur J Cancer.* 2004;40(3):390–402.

20. Cameron DA, Cornbleet MC, Mackie RM, et al.; Scottish Melanoma Group. Adjuvant interferon alpha 2b in high risk melanoma - the Scottish study. *Br J Cancer.* 2001;84(9):1146–1149.

21. Pehamberger H, Soyer HP, Steiner A, et al. Adjuvant interferon alfa-2a treatment in resected primary stage II cutaneous melanoma. Austrian Malignant Melanoma Cooperative Group. *J Clin Oncol.* 1998;16(4):1425–1429.

22. Grob JJ, Dreno B, de la Salmonière P, et al. Randomised trial of interferon alpha-2a as adjuvant therapy in resected primary

melanoma thicker than 1.5 mm without clinically detectable node metastases. French Cooperative Group on Melanoma. *Lancet.* 1998;351(9120):1905–1910.

23. Hancock BW, Wheatley K, Harris S, et al. Adjuvant interferon in high-risk melanoma: the AIM HIGH Study–United Kingdom Coordinating Committee on Cancer Research randomized study of adjuvant low-dose extended-duration interferon Alfa-2a in high-risk resected malignant melanoma. *J Clin Oncol.* 2004;22(1):53–61.

24. Cascinelli N, Belli F, MacKie RM, Santinami M, Bufalino R, Morabito A. Effect of long-term adjuvant therapy with interferon alpha-2a in patients with regional node metastases from cutaneous melanoma: a randomised trial. *Lancet.* 2001; 358(9285):866–869.

25. Eggermont AM, Suciu S, MacKie R, et al.; EORTC Melanoma Group. Post-surgery adjuvant therapy with intermediate doses of interferon alfa 2b versus observation in patients with stage IIb/III melanoma (EORTC 18952): randomised controlled trial. *Lancet.* 2005;366(9492):1189–1196.

26. Pectasides D, Dafni U, Bafaloukos D, et al. Randomized phase III study of 1 month versus 1 year of adjuvant high-dose interferon alfa-2b in patients with resected high-risk melanoma. *J Clin Oncol.* 2009;27(6):939–944.

27. Hansson J, Aamdal S, Bastholt L, et al.; Nordic Melanoma Cooperative Group. Two different durations of adjuvant therapy with intermediate-dose interferon alfa-2b in patients with high-risk melanoma (Nordic IFN trial): a randomised phase 3 trial. *Lancet Oncol.* 2011;12(2):144–152.

28. Eggermont AM, Suciu S, Santinami M, et al.; EORTC Melanoma Group. Adjuvant therapy with pegylated interferon alfa-2b versus observation alone in resected stage III melanoma: final results of EORTC 18991, a randomised phase III trial. *Lancet.* 2008;372(9633):117–126.

29. Wheatley K, Ives N, Hancock B, Gore M, Eggermont A, Suciu S. Does adjuvant interferon-alpha for high-risk melanoma provide a worthwhile benefit? A meta-analysis of the randomised trials. *Cancer Treat Rev.* 2003;29(4):241–252.

30. Mocellin S, Pasquali S, Rossi CR, Nitti D. Interferon alpha adjuvant therapy in patients with high-risk melanoma: a systematic review and meta-analysis. *J Natl Cancer Inst.* 2010;102(7):493–501.

31. Petrella T, Verma S, Spithoff K, Quirt I, McCready D; Melanoma Disease Site Group. Adjuvant interferon therapy for patients at high risk for recurrent melanoma: an updated systematic review and practice guideline. *Clin Oncol (R Coll Radiol).* 2012; 24(6):413–423.

32. Kirkwood JM, Bender C, Agarwala S, et al. Mechanisms and management of toxicities associated with high-dose interferon alfa-2b therapy. *J Clin Oncol.* 2002;20(17):3703–3718.

33. Gogas H, Ioannovich J, Dafni U, et al. Prognostic significance of autoimmunity during treatment of melanoma with interferon. *N Engl J Med.* 2006;354(7):709–718.

34. Eggermont AM, Suciu S, Testori A, et al. Ulceration and stage are predictive of interferon efficacy in melanoma: results of the phase III adjuvant trials EORTC 18952 and EORTC 18991. *Eur J Cancer.* 2012;48(2):218–225.

35. Gonzalez RJ, Kudchadkar R, Rao NG, Sondak VK. Adjuvant Immunotherapy and Radiation in the Management of High-risk Resected Melanoma. *Ochsner J.* 2010;10(2):108–116.

36. Morton DL, Mozzillo N, Thompson JF, et al. An international, randomized, phase III trial of bacillus Calmette–Guerin (BCG) plus allogeneic melanoma vaccine (MCV) or placebo after complete resection of melanoma metastatic to regional or distant sites. *JCO.* 2007;25(18S):Abstract 8508.

37. Wallack MK, Sivanandham M, Balch CM, et al. Surgical adjuvant active specific immunotherapy for patients with stage III melanoma: the final analysis of data from a phase III, randomized, double-blind, multicenter vaccinia melanoma oncolysate trial. *J Am Coll Surg.* 1998;187(1):69–77; discussion 77.

38. Hersey P, Coates AS, McCarthy WH, et al. Adjuvant immunotherapy of patients with high-risk melanoma using vaccinia viral lysates of melanoma: results of a randomized trial. *J Clin Oncol.* 2002;20(20):4181–4190.

39. Sondak VK, Liu PY, Tuthill RJ, et al. Adjuvant immunotherapy of resected, intermediate-thickness, node-negative melanoma with an allogeneic tumor vaccine: overall results of a randomized trial of the Southwest Oncology Group. *J Clin Oncol.* 2002;20(8): 2058–2066.

40. Eggermont AM, Suciu S, Ruka W, et al. EORTC 18961: Post-operative adjuvant

ganglioside GM2-KLH21 vaccination treatment vs observation in stage II (T3-T4N0M0) melanoma: 2nd interim analysis led to an early disclosure of the results. *J Clin Oncol.* 2008;26: Abstract 9004.

41. Lawson DH, Lee SJ, Tarhini AA, et al. E4697: Phase III cooperative group study of yeast-derived granulocyte macrophage colony-stimulating factor (GM-CSF) versus placebo as adjuvant treatment of patients with completely resected stage III-IV melanoma. *J Clin Oncol.* 2010;28:15s (Supplement; Abstract 8504).

42. Flaherty LE, Moon J, Atkins MB, et al. Phase III trial of high-dose interferon alpha-2b versus cisplatin, vinblastine, DTIC plus IL-2 and interferon in patients with high-risk melanoma (SWOG S0008): an intergroup study of CALGB, COG, ECOG, and SWOG. *JCO.* 2012;30 (Supplement; Abstract 8504).

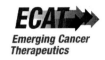

Emerging Cancer
Therapeutics

RAF Kinase Inhibitor Therapy in Melanoma

James J. Harding and Paul B. Chapman*

*Melanoma and Sarcoma Division, Department of Medicine,
Memorial Sloan-Kettering Cancer Center, New York, NY*

■ ABSTRACT

It is now clear that the majority (and perhaps all) of melanomas are driven by extracellular signal-regulated kinase (ERK) signaling because of abnormal activation of the mitogen-activated protein kinase (MAPK) cascade. In most cases, this is a result of an activating mutation in v-Raf murine sarcoma viral oncogene homolog B1 (*BRAF*). This observation has led to the development of the RAF kinase inhibitors vemurafenib and dabrafenib. These agents are associated with response rates ≥50%, improved progression-free survival compared with dacarbazine chemotherapy, and, in the case of vemurafenib, improved overall survival. As a result, vemurafenib has been approved for use by both the Food and Drug Administration (FDA) and European Medicines Agency (EMA) in patients with BRAF^{V600E} metastatic melanoma. Dabrafenib is likely to be approved in the near future. Here, we review the role of *BRAF* mutations in melanoma and the mechanism of action of the 2 RAF kinase inhibitors. We summarize the pivotal clinical studies of vemurafenib and dabrafenib and discuss the toxicities of these 2 drugs. Because the median progression-free survival in patients treated with the RAF inhibitors is ≤7 months, it is clear that melanomas rapidly develop resistance. We describe what is known so far about the mechanisms of resistance and speculate as to how this might be overcome.

Keywords: melanoma, BRAF, vemurafenib, dabrafenib, ERK signaling

*Corresponding author, Melanoma and Sarcoma Division, Department of Medicine, Memorial Sloan-Kettering Cancer Center, New York, NY
   E-mail address: chapmanp@mskcc.org

Emerging Cancer Therapeutics 3:3 (2012) 485–500.
DOI: 10.5003/2151–4194.3.3.485

■ INTRODUCTION

Metastatic melanoma has historically been relatively refractory to cytotoxic chemotherapy, immunotherapy, and radiotherapy (1). Despite decades of intense scientific research, the only treatments for advanced melanoma approved by the Food and Drug Administration (FDA) before 2010 were high-dose interleukin-2 and dacarbazine. These agents are each associated with an objective response of 10% to 20% but have never been subjected to randomized trials to see if they improve the median overall survival of melanoma patients. Most investigators in the field feel they would fail such a test. As such, the expected median overall survival for patients with metastatic melanoma was less than 1 year before 2010 (2).

A major breakthrough in melanoma biology occurred in 2002, when Davies and colleagues showed that approximately 60% of melanomas harbor activating mutations in the gene encoding BRAF kinase (3). In the next 8 years, preclinical investigations demonstrated the importance of the BRAF^{V600E} mutation for the survival of melanomas with this mutation. Inhibitors of RAF kinase were developed and exhibited unprecedented antitumor activity in both preclinical models and a number of clinical trials (Table 1). Vemurafenib, the first RAF kinase inhibitor to reach the clinic, was shown to improve the overall survival in patients with BRAF-mutated metastatic melanoma (4). This agent was approved by the FDA for use in 2011 and approved by the European Medicines Agency (EMA) the following year. In this chapter, we will describe the normal function of the MAPK pathway, the scientific basis for targeting mutant BRAF kinase, the pivotal clinical trials demonstrating the efficacy of RAF kinase inhibitors in BRAF-mutant melanoma, the unique toxicities observed with this class of compound, the mechanisms of resistance to these agents, and how rational drug combinations may augment the efficacy of RAF kinase inhibitors.

■ THE MITOGEN-ACTIVATED PROTEIN KINASE PATHWAY

Signal transduction involves a series of enzymatic reactions that transmit an extracellular signal to the nucleus, ultimately leading to the transcription of a set of genes that control and coordinate a number of diverse cellular processes such as cellular proliferation, reproduction, differentiation, migration, and apoptosis. Several signal transduction cascades have been identified; the best characterized is the classic mitogen-activated protein kinase pathway (Figure 1) (5,6). External growth factors engage the appropriate receptor tyrosine kinase (RTK) embedded in the phospholipid bilayer at the cell surface. Ligand binding leads to activation of the RTK, followed by transphosphorylation of the cytoplasmic components of the receptor. The phosphorylated cytoplasmic tail recruits a variety of accessory and regulatory molecules, which leads to activation of the rat sarcoma (RAS) kinases (HRAS, KRAS, and NRAS) (7). RAS subsequently activates the RAF kinases, of which there are 3 isoforms: ARAF, BRAF, and CRAF (8). RAF kinase activation is a complex molecular event that is not fully understood at present. It is clear that activated RAS recruits RAF to the cell membrane. RAS subsequently induces conformational changes in the RAF protein, leading to RAF dimerization, phosphorylation, and kinase activation. These dimers, which can form as homodimers or heterodimers, have the ability to phosphorylate and activate MAPK/ERK kinase (MEK). Subsequently,

TABLE 1 RAF kinase inhibitors in Braf-mutated, unresectable locally advanced or metastatic melanoma.

Study	Citation	Agent	N	ORR	Median PFS (months)	Median OS (months)	12-month Survival
BRIM-1	(33)	Vemurafenib	32	56%* (18/32)	7	NR	NR
BRIM-2	(35)	Vemurafenib	132	53% (70/132)	6.8	15.9	58%
BRIM-3	(4, 37)	Vemurafenib	337	57% (192/337)	6.9	13.6	56%
BREAK-1	(39)	Dabrafenib	36	69% (25/36)	5.5	NR	NR
BREAK-2	(40)	Dabrafenib	76	59%† (45/76)	6.8	NR	NR
BREAK-3	(42)	Dabrafenib	187	50% (93/187)	5.1	NR	NR

The results of the major clinical trials of the RAF kinase inhibitors are summarized here. All patients initially received vemurafenib at 960 mg PO BID or dabrafenib 150 mg PO BID. Dose escalation cohorts, expansion cohorts that included patients with brain metastases, and BREAK-MB are not listed here and are discussed in the text.

Abbreviations/Footnotes: overall response rate (ORR), progression-free survival (PFS), overall survival (OS), not reported (NR), * At the time of publication of BRIM-1, the unconfirmed response rate was reported as 81% (26/36). The updated confirmed RECIST response rate is reported here; †BREAK-2, the phase II trial of patients with metastatic BRAF-mutated melanoma enrolled patients with both V600E and V600K mutations, the results listed here are only for those with a V600E mutation.

phosphorylated MEK (p-MEK) activates ERK-1 and ERK-2. Phosphorylation of ERK by MEK leads to the modification of a number of substrates (i.e. Cyclin D, Myc, and Elk) that, in turn, regulate protein synthesis, transcription, and entrance into the cell cycle. In addition, several negative feedback mechanisms that modulate the activity of the signaling cascade have been identified. One important negative feedback loop involves sprouty proteins, which are activated by ERK phosphorylation. SPRY feed back and inhibit RAS activation, which leads to decreased RAF dimerization and downregulation of

the pathway. This downregulation of RAF dimerization may be important for the specificity of these RAF inhibitors (discussed as follows).

■ THE BRAF[V600E] MUTATION IN MELANOMA

Since the original report by Davies et al. (3), several investigators have confirmed that mutations in *BRAF* are present in 40% to 60% of all melanomas (9–12). The majority of the mutations occur at codon 600 on exon 15 of the *BRAF* gene. The

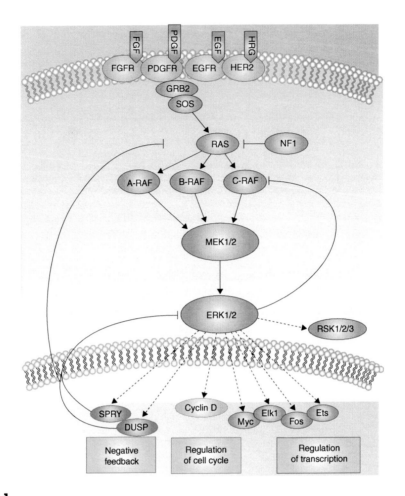

FIGURE 1

Mitogen-activated protein kinase (MAPK) pathway. The MAPK pathway can be activated in mela-nomas by mutations in RAS or BRAF. The presence of such mutations increases ERK signaling output in the absence of normal external stimuli. Inappropriate ERK activation leads to the transcription of a number of target genes that promote melanoma survival and growth.

Reprinted with permission from the American Association for Cancer Research (5).

most common mutation at this position is a missence mutation that results in the substitution of glutamic acid for valine (i.e., BRAF^{V600E}). Other less frequently observed variants are V600K, V600R, and V600D (11,13). *BRAF* mutations cor-relate with several factors specific to both the patient and the antecedent primary melanoma, including patient age, histo-pathologic subtype, and tumor location (10,13). For example, such mutations are infrequent in melanomas from mucosal, acral, and chronically sun-damaged sites. Data from a number of independent groups indicate that *BRAF* mutations are present in 9% to 17% of mucosal melanomas, 0% to 20% of acral mela-nomas, and 10% to 20% of melanomas arising from chronically sun-damaged skin (9–12). In contrast, 50% to 60% of primary nodular or superficial spreading melanomas originating in nonchronically sun-damaged skin harbor mutations in *BRAF* (9–11). *BRAF* mutations have not been reported in patients with uveal melanomas (14). With the exception of uveal melanomas, all patients with metastatic melanoma should undergo routine molecular diagnostic testing for mutations in *BRAF*.

Acquisition of the BRAF^{V600E} mutation serves to destabilize the inactive conformation of the kinase that promotes an active conformation of the molecule (15). In contrast with wild-type BRAF kinase, mutant BRAF kinase requires neither RAS for its activation nor dimerization to activate MEK (16). BRAF-mutant melanoma cells are clearly dependent on ERK signaling for their survival. Several groups have demonstrated that interruption of the MAPK pathway in BRAF^{V600E} mutant melanoma cell lines and mouse models, either by RNA interference or by inhibition of RAF and MEK, results in the suppression of ERK activity, followed by rapid cell cycle arrest, decreased cellular proliferation, and apoptosis (16,17). These data predict that blocking BRAF^{V600E} would have profound inhibitory effects in patients with BRAF^{V600E}-mutated melanoma.

However, BRAF^{V600E} is commonly found in benign human nevi, consistent with the observation that introduction of the BRAF^{V600E} mutation into normal cells induces senescence (18). In mouse models, conditional expression of BRAF^{V600E} leads only to melanocytic hyperplasia; an additional genetic mutation is required for development of frankly invasive melanoma (19). These data indicate that the BRAF^{V600E} mutation is a necessary initial step in developing melanoma but it is not sufficient. This initially led to skepticism that inhibiting BRAF^{V600E} in melanoma might not be effective because melanomas might no longer be dependent on the BRAF^{V600E} mutation. As shown in the following text, this is not the case.

■ PRECLINICAL DEVELOPMENT OF RAF KINASE INHIBITORS

Given the dependence of BRAF-mutated melanomas on the MAPK pathway, investigators evaluated a number of kinase inhibitors to determine the utility and feasibility of targeting BRAF^{V600E} kinase. Sorafenib (Nexavar, BAY-43–9006) was the first widely available molecule that had demonstrable inhibitory activity in vitro (20). Initial studies of sorafenib in cell culture and xenograft models demonstrated promising activity against melanoma (21,22). In retrospect, several preclinical observations would explain the failure of sorafenib in the clinic. In biochemical assays, sorafenib exhibited greater inhibitory effects on wild-type CRAF (CRAF^{WT}) and wild-type BRAF (BRAF^{WT}) kinase. The antitumor effects of sorafenib were also observed in both BRAF mutant and wild-type cell lines, suggesting that sorafenib was not specific for melanoma driven by BRAF^{V600E} kinase (23).

Second-generation BRAF kinase inhibitors have greater potency for mutant BRAF^{V600E} kinase. Vemurafenib (Zelboraf, or PLX4032), and its analog PLX4720 profoundly reduce BRAF^{V600E} kinase activity in vitro and in vivo (16,24–26). In biochemical assays, vemurafenib preferential inhibits BRAF^{V600E} and CRAF^{WT} at 31 and 48 nM, respectively. It inhibits BRAF^{WT} at 100 nM (24). Thus, vemurafenib is not specific for BRAF^{V600E} but can inhibit all isoforms of the RAF kinases (27).

Why does vemurafenib only inhibit BRAF mutant cells, although vemurafenib can inhibit all isoforms of RAF kinase? The basis for this functional specificity is that tumors driven by an activating BRAF mutation are "wired" slightly differently. In BRAF^{WT} cells, upstream RAS activation results in dimerization of RAF kinases; both homodimers and heterodimers probably form. This leads to downstream activation of MEK and, then, ERK. If vemurafenib (or other RAF kinase inhibitors) is added to these cells, the drug binds and inhibits 1 member of the RAF dimer but transactivates the partner RAF kinase, leading to enhanced ERK signaling (27). Thus, vemurafenib does not inhibit these cells but, in fact, results in increased proliferation. In tumor cells containing a BRAF^{V600E} mutation, ERK signaling is already increased, which, through feedback inhibition, decreases RAS activation. This inhibits RAF dimer formation, and as a result, ERK signaling in these cells is largely driven by BRAF^{V600E} monomers. When vemurafenib is added, these monomers are inhibited, turning off the pathway.

This model predicts that only tumors with a BRAF^{V600E} mutation will be sensitive to vemurafenib. It also predicts that these tumors might become resistant to vemurafenib through any mechanism that encourages RAF dimer formation, such as RAS activation.

■ CLINICAL DEVELOPMENT OF RAF KINASE INHIBITORS

Sorafenib

Sorafenib is currently licensed by the FDA for the treatment of renal cell carcinoma and hepatocellular carcinoma. It is also used off-label to treat gastrointestinal stromal tumors, angiosarcomas, and thyroid carcinomas. Multiple clinical trials examining both sorafenib monotherapy and combination therapy failed to demonstrate the antitumor activity of this agent in melanoma (28–32). The preclinical activity of sorafenib indicates low potency as a RAF inhibitor, and its antitumor activity seems to be a result of its ability to inhibit vascular endothelial growth factor

receptor-2/3 (VEGFR-2/3). As such, it is not considered a RAF inhibitor.

Vemurafenib

The phase I (BRAF inhibitor in melanoma [BRIM]-1) clinical study of vemurafenib in BRAF-mutated solid tumor patients established the maximum tolerated oral dose to be 960 mg twice a day (33). Rash and arthralgias were the major dose-limiting toxicities; other adverse events included fatigue, photosensitivity, pruritus, palmar–plantar dysesthesias, and cutaneous proliferations such as keratoacanthomas and squamous-cell carcinomas. Consistent with the preclinical model, antitumor activity was observed only in tumors with a BRAF^{V600E} mutation and not in melanomas expressing wild-type BRAF. The clinical efficacy of vemurafenib at the maximum tolerated dose was quite impressive. By day 15 of treatment, tumor uptake of glucose was dramatically reduced in virtually all patients, as assessed by FDG-positron emission tomography (34). Pharmacodynamic analysis in paired tumor biopsies, before treatment and at day 15 of vemurafenib, also confirmed the rapid suppression of ERK signaling and early reduction in tumor cell viability. Antitumor responses were seen in most patients, and 56% had a confirmed partial or complete response by *response evaluation criteria in solid tumors* (RECIST). Two of these patients had a complete response. In the majority of cases, significant tumor shrinkage was observed within 2 months of treatment.

Given the early signal of efficacy in phase I, vemurafenib was moved rapidly through clinical development. In fact, the phase II (BRIM-2, for previously-treated patients) and phase III (BRIM-3, for previously untreated patients) trials of vemurafenib in melanoma were opened almost simultaneously (4,35). Both trials were restricted to melanoma patients with BRAF^{V600}-mutated melanomas. The results of the phase II trial confirmed the efficacy of the agent (35). The overall objective response rate was 53% (8 CRs and 62 PRs). It is also important to note that, retrospectively, 10 of 132 patients were found to have had a BRAF^{V600K} mutation; 4 of these patients achieved a partial response. This indicates that vemurafenib is also effective for melanomas that harbor a BRAF^{V600K} mutation. Although the majority of responses occurred rapidly, the durability of the response was limited. The median progression-free survival was 6.8 months. This indicates that resistance to BRAF kinase inhibition occurs rapidly. Nevertheless, patients on the phase II trial seemed to do favorable compared with historic controls with a 1-year overall survival rate of 58% and median overall survival of 15.9 months.

The activity of vemurafenib is not restricted to a particular metastatic site or substage of metastatic disease. Responses were documented in metastases within the subcutis, lymph nodes, lungs, bones, viscera, and brain (33,35,36). Limited data are available with regard to the efficacy of vemurafenib as a treatment for brain metastases because the phase I, II, and III trials of vemurafenib excluded patients with active brain metastases. A multicenter phase II trial (NCT01378975) investigating the effects of vemurafenib in BRAF-mutated melanoma with brain metastases is ongoing.

The pivotal, multicenter, randomized phase III trial comparing vemurafenib to dacarbazine for patients with BRAF-mutant, surgically unresectable stage IIIC, or IV melanoma established vemurafenib as a new standard of care in melanoma (4). In this study, 675 treatment-naïve melanoma patients were randomly assigned (1:1) to receive vemurafenib at a dose of 960 mg twice daily or dacarbazine at a dose of 1000 mg/m^2

intravenously every 3 weeks. Participants were further stratified based on the American Joint Committee on Cancer (AJCC) stage (i.e., unresectable IIIC, M1a, M1b, and M1c), serum lactate dehydrogenase (LDH), Eastern Cooperative Oncology Group (ECOG) performance status, and geographic region. The coprimary end points of the trial were progression-free and overall survival. Secondary end points included the determination of response rate, response duration, and safety. Cross-over was initially not allowed; however, once the predetermined end points were met at interim analysis, the data and safety-monitoring board recommend that patients in the dacarbazine group be allowed to cross over to vemurafenib.

At the first interim analysis, the median follow-up time was 3.8 and 2.3 months for patients in the vemurafenib and dacarbazine arm, respectively. The overall response rate in 439 evaluable patients was consistent with prior reports—48% of patients in the vemurafenib arm achieved a confirmed RECIST response. This was in comparison with an overall response rate of 5% in the dacarbazine group. Similar to BRIM-2, a small proportion of patients on BRIM-3 were found, retrospectively, to have had a BRAF^{V600K} mutation, and these tumors seemed to show the same response rate as BRAF^{V600E}-mutated melanomas. The estimated median progression-free survival was superior in the vemurafenib arm: 1.6 months for dacarbazine and 5.3 months for vemurafenib. This corresponded to a hazard ratio of 0.26, representing a relative reduction in the risk of death or progression of 74% in favor of vemurafenib. It is important to note that the hazard ratio for death in the vemurafenib arm was 0.37, which translates to a 63% relative reduction in the risk of death in favor of vemurafenib.

Updated results from BRIM-3 were recently presented at the American Society of Clinical Oncology (ASCO) Annual Meeting in 2012 (37). The median follow-up for analysis was 12.5 months for patients in the vemurafenib group and 9.5 months for those in the dacarbazine arm. With longer follow-up, all patients were evaluable for objective response. The confirmed objective response rate to vemurafenib was 57%. Similar to the initial analysis, vemurafenib significantly improved progression-free survival in comparison with dacarbazine. The median progression-free survival was 1.6 months for dacarbazine and 6.9 months for vemurafenib. This benefit was observed in all prespecified patient subgroups. Adequate follow-up was also available to estimate the overall median survival for both study arms. Censoring patients who crossed over to vemurafenib, the estimated median overall survival for dacarbazine was 9.7 months versus 13.6 months for vemurafenib. This corresponds to a hazard ratio of 0.70, which ultimately translates to a 30% relative reduction in the risk of death in favor of vemurafenib. On subset analysis, the survival benefit was primarily seen in patients with M1c disease. An ad hoc analysis showed that patients with stage IIIC, IVM1a, or IVM1b who progressed after receiving dacarbazine were the most likely cohort to receive ipilimumab, an immunotherapy that is known to improve the overall survival in patients with melanoma (38). This may partly explain the lack of an overall survival benefit seen in this group. However, it may be that vemurafenib's greatest effect is in patients with the shortest expected survival.

It is also unclear if a subset of patients treated with vemurafenib will attain long-term disease control. That is, is there a tail of the curve? At the time of publication of the phase II trial, 11% of patients had ongoing responses exceeding 1 year. Two patients have continued therapy for at least 18 months, suggesting that durable disease control is possible, albeit infrequent. Long-term follow-up of BRIM-3 will add more data about long-term benefits of vemurafenib. What seems to be clear so far is that, if vemurafenib therapy is discontinued in responding patients, the melanoma will almost invariably recur. This seems to be true, even in patients who have had a complete response. It thus seems that, even in the setting of an apparent complete response, BRAF^{V600E} melanoma cells persist and are capable of growth once vemurafenib is withdrawn. Patients must indefinitely remain on vemurafenib.

Dabrafenib

Dabrafenib, a second, ATP-competitive, RAF inhibitor has been developed. The multicenter phase I/II dabrafenib in patients with metastatic solid tumors did not identify the maximum tolerated dose, despite several dose escalations (39). Dose-limiting toxicities and common adverse events included pyrexia, syncope, fatigue, and cutaneous squamous-cell carcinomas (cuSCCs). Dabrafenib at 150 mg twice a day was ultimately selected as the recommended phase II dose. This schedule was comparable in antitumor activity, pharmacokinetic properties, and pharmacodynamic effect to higher doses. Similar to vemurafenib, dabrafenib exhibits substantial antitumor activity for BRAF^{V600E} and BRAF^{V600K} mutant melanomas but is not effective in melanomas expressing BRAF^{WT} kinase. Twenty-five of the 36 (69%) BRAF-mutant metastatic melanoma patients who were treated with the recommend phase II achieved an unconfirmed partial or complete response. The median duration of response was 6.2 months; the median progression-free survival was 5.5 months. The trial also assessed the efficacy of dabrafenib in patients with active brain metastases. Nine of the 10 patients with brain metastases, ranging from 3 to 15 mm, had disease shrinkage, 4 of whom had a complete response.

Two phase II studies of dabrafenib have confirmed its antitumor activity in melanoma. BREAK-2, a single-arm phase II of dabrafenib in BRAF-mutated melanoma without intracranial metastasis, demonstrated that 59% of the patients with a BRAF^{V600E} mutation attain a RECIST response (40). A multicenter phase II trial (BREAK-MB) evaluated the efficacy of dabrafenib in patients with metastatic melanoma harboring a BRAF^{V600E} or BRAF^{V600K} melanoma and active asymptomatic intracranial metastases (41). Patients were enrolled into 2 separate cohorts: either no prior intracranial therapy or prior intracranial therapy. Objective response rates were equivalent between both cohorts: 31% for the group without prior brain therapy and 39% for patients who had prior intracranial therapy. Responses in brain metastases were generally concordant with responses in other metastatic sites. It is important to note that the proportion of patients with disease control (CR +PR +SD) exceeded 80%. The median progression-free survival was approximately 16 weeks. Sites of progression were equally distributed among intracranial sites only, extracranial sites only, or both intracranial and extracranial sites. These results are in stark contrast with historical experiences with systemic chemotherapy or whole brain radiation therapy, in which only anecdotal responses were seen.

In a multicenter, open-label, randomized phase III clinical trial (BREAK-3) in patients with unresectable stage IIIC or IV BRAF-mutated melanoma, dabrafenib was found to improve progression-free survival compared with dacarbazine (42). In this study, 250 patients were randomized (3:1) to oral dabrafenib 150 mg twice a day or dacarbazine 100 mg/m^2 intravenously. Eligible patients could have received prior immunotherapy with interleukin-2 but no other systemic therapy. Patients were stratified according to AJCC stage (IIIC, M1a, M1b, and M1c). Cross-over from dacarbazine to dabrafenib was allowed at progression. The primary end point of the trial was progression-free survival. The overall response rate for dabrafenib was 50% (6 CR, 87 PR). The trial met its primary end point, demonstrating a significant improvement in the progression-free survival in favor of dabrafenib. The median progression-free survival was 5.1 months for dabrafenib compared with 2.7 months with dacarbazine with a hazard ratio for progression of 0.30. There were too few events to make any conclusions about the overall survival, which was not a primary end point of the trial.

■ ADVERSE EVENTS ASSOCIATED WITH RAF INHIBITORS

The RAF kinase inhibitors are quite tolerable and have a unique spectrum of manageable drug-related toxicities. Dose reductions are required for 38% of patients receiving vemurafenib and for 28% of patients receiving dabrafenib (4,42). Drug discontinuation as a result of intolerable toxicity is rare and occurs in less than 10% of the patients. Dermatologic manifestations are the most common adverse events and include rash, pruritus, hyperkeratosis, actinic keratosis, palmar–plantar erythrodysesthesia, alopecia, photosensitivity, keratoacanthomas, and cuSCCs. Arthralgias, fatigue, pyrexia, and gastrointestinal toxicities are also frequently observed side effects of the RAF kinase inhibitors. The development of new primary melanomas has been reported in patients undergoing treatment with vemurafenib and dabrafenib (42–45).

Although there are clearly class effects of the RAF inhibitors, subtle differences in the toxicity profile of both vemurafenib and dabrafenib are certainly notable. Arthralgias and photosensitivity seem to be more prevalent with vemurafenib, whereas clinically significant pyrexia seems more prominent with dabrafenib. Keratoacanthomas and cuSCCs developed in 6% of the patients treated with dabrafenib (42) and 18% of the patients treated with vemurafenib (4). The induction of cutaneous proliferations and premalignant lesions is a unique adverse event that characterizes the RAF kinase inhibitors. In general, these lesions develop with a median onset of approximately 10 weeks, do not result in treatment discontinuation, and are easily treated with complete local resection (33). The cuSCCs examined have been low-grade, well-differentiated neoplasia that do not locally recur or metastasize (39). The paradoxical activation of wild-type BRAF kinase by the selective BRAF kinase inhibitors is thought to be responsible for the development of these lesions (44).

■ MECHANISMS OF RESISTANCE TO RAF INHIBITORS

Intrinsic Resistance

Three to 14% of melanoma patients have primary progressive disease, despite treatment with a RAF inhibitor (4,35,42). This indicates that a small subset of BRAF-mutated melanomas is intrinsically resistant to inhibitors of BRAF kinase (25). The basis for this de novo resistance is not known but may involve mutations in other signaling

pathways or tumor suppressor genes. To this end, concomitant mutational inactivation of phosphatase and tensin homolog (PTEN) and retinoblastoma protein (RB1) has been observed in BRAF-mutated cell lines, and these comutations render these cell lines resistant to BRAF kinase inhibition (46,47). The analysis of tumor samples from patients receiving dabrafenib and vemurafenib are consistent with these preclinical findings (47,48). Patients with co-occurring PTEN mutations or low levels of PTEN expression exhibited lower response rates to dabrafenib or vemurafenib, respectively, compared with patients with BRAF-mutated melanoma with normal PTEN function and expression. These data suggest that simultaneous inhibition of both MAPK and phosphatidylinositol 3-kinase/AKT (PI3K-AKT) pathways could further improve response rates and circumvent some mechanisms of intrinsic resistance. This approach is currently being explored in a phase I/II trial of vemurafenib and BKM120, a PI3K inhibitor, in patients with BRAF-mutated melanoma (NCT01512251).

Acquired Resistance

The trials from both RAF inhibitors vemurafenib and dabrafenib indicate that half of the tumors acquire resistance to these drugs within 7 months and, ultimately, at least 80% of tumors develop resistance. These observations underscore the importance of understanding the mechanisms of resistance. In studying the resistant tumors and cell lines, 2 observations have generally held true. First, melanomas develop resistance by reactivating ERK signaling. Second, this reactivation is not a result of a new gatekeeper mutation in BRAF. That is, the inhibitors can still bind to the kinase domain of the BRAF^{V600E} protein. So far, acquired resistance has not been observed as a result of activation of bypass pathways such as the PI3K/AKT pathway, although this is still a possibility.

Several mechanisms of acquired resistance and reactivation of ERK signaling have been described, although not all have yet to be confirmed by investigators at more than 1 institution to occur in actual human tumors. Most of these mechanisms of resistance reestablish the ability of RAF kinases to dimerize. Some resistant tumors have been found to have acquired an activating mutation in *NRAS*, which can not only drive cell proliferation but also enhance RAF dimerization, leading to resistance (49,50). Another mechanism is that a splicing event of the mutated *BRAF* mRNA can occur, leading to a truncated BRAF^{V600E} kinase that eliminates the RAS-binding domain. This allows the truncated BRAF^{V600E} to dimerize with unmutated forms of RAF, leading to increased ERK signaling in the presence of vemurafenib (49). There have been reports of activation of receptor tyrosine kinases such as the platelet-derived growth factor (50) or insulin-like growth factor (51) receptor, which would be expected to enhance RAF dimerization. It seems that some melanomas may become resistant to BRAF inhibition through activation of hepatocyte growth factor receptor (HGFR or MET), which has been reported to be expressed on approximately 1/3 of metastatic melanomas (52). Stroma express hepatocyte growth factor, the ligand for MET, leading to RAS activation and resistance to BRAF inhibitors (53). Activation of any of these RTKs would lead to RAS activation, which enhances RAF dimerization, leading to vemurafenib resistance.

Another mechanism of resistance that was predicted from preclinical experiments is amplification of the mutated BRAF allele leading to overexpression of the activated kinase, overwhelming the ability of the inhibitors to block proliferation (54).

This has now been observed in resistant tumors from patients treated with vemurafenib (55).

Additional resistance mechanisms that result in direct activation of MEK either through expression of mitogen-activated protein kinase 8 (MAP3K or COT) (56), which activates MEK, or development of an activating mutation in MEK1 (57) have been proposed. It is not yet clear how common these occur in tumors that acquire resistance to RAF inhibitors.

These data suggest that, in the setting of acquired resistance, it will be necessary to block the MAPK pathway downstream of RAF. With this in mind, combination trials of RAF inhibitors plus MEK inhibitors are ongoing. In patients who develop resistance as a result of activation of MET, adding a MET inhibitor or a monoclonal antibody to block activation of MET would be a rational approach. In tumors that amplify the mutated BRAF allele, withdrawal of BRAF inhibitor would be predicted to result in the loss of amplification and reestablishment of sensitivity (58). It is possible that treating patients with these combinations as initial therapy will delay or prevent the development of resistance. There is also speculation that treating patients with discontinuous schedules of BRAF inhibitor could delay resistance (58).

■ CONCLUDING REMARKS AND FUTURE DIRECTIONS

The activity of the RAF kinase inhibitors vemurafenib and dabrafenib in the treatment of metastatic melanoma has changed the treatment paradigm for metastatic melanoma. It is now required that tumors be genotyped to determine if they carry the BRAF^{V600E} mutation. This should be part of routine pathological evaluation of metastatic melanoma.

Nevertheless, several important clinical questions remain; we point out 3 in particular. First, treatment with single-agent RAF inhibitors routinely leads to short median time to progression. In half of the patients treated, the tumors become resistant to RAF inhibition within 7 months. As discussed in this chapter, several mechanisms of resistance have been described, and additional mechanisms will likely be discovered. This information will inform us as to how to overcome or prevent resistance. Second, among responding patients, very few complete responses have been observed, and even in these cases, discontinuation of drug generally results in rapid regrowth of the tumor. This indicates that a small subset of BRAF^{V600E}-mutated melanoma cells can remain senescent but viable in the presence of RAF inhibitors. This has meant that responding patients must indefinitely remain on RAF inhibitors. Third, there is a wide range of sensitivity to RAF inhibitors among BRAF^{V600E}-mutated melanomas, ranging from dramatic responses to minimal responses and complete resistance. It seems clear that other genetic changes in these tumors have a major effect on the degree of sensitivity, and much needs to be learned about this.

Investigators are now actively exploring ways of preventing or overcoming resistance to RAF inhibitors. Because all the resistance mechanisms identified so far involve reactivation of MEK, it seems logical to combine a MEK inhibitor with a RAF inhibitor. The hypothesis would be that the combination might improve responses and could delay (or prevent) resistance. An added benefit might be that a MEK inhibitor should minimize the paradoxical ERK activation in wild-type BRAF cells thereby reducing the occurrence of keratoacanthomas and secondary malignancies such as cutaneous squamous cell carcinomas. Preliminary results from an ongoing phase I/II of dabrafenib combined with trametinib, an oral MEK inhibitor, in patients with BRAF-mutant solid tumors were recently reported at ASCO 2012 (59). Forty-three of the 77 (57%) treatment-naïve metastatic melanoma patients who were treated with varying doses of the combination had a confirmed overall response. Although this response rate was not different than that seen with RAF inhibitor alone, the median duration of response was 11.3 months. In contrast, the median duration of response to BRAF inhibitor monotherapy is only 5 to 7 months. Two phase III trials will formally investigate the combination of dabrafenib and trametinib in comparison with either vemurafenib (NCT01597908) or dabrafenib (NCT01584648) in patients BRAF-mutated melanoma.

There is also intense interest in combining RAF inhibition with immunotherapy. Ipilimumab, an anti-cytotoxic T-lymphocyte associated antigen-4 (CTLA-4) monoclonal antibody, has been FDA approved because of its ability to induce durable responses and improve overall survival compared with dacarbazine. Combining ipilimumab with the RAF inhibitor vemurafenib is very appealing, and a phase I trial is currently under way. In the absence of data combining these 2 drugs, there is interest in learning how to sequence the drugs. We have reported on the occurrence of vemurafenib drug hypersensitivity reactions, particularly within 1 month after ipilimumab therapy (60). Other groups have retrospectively evaluated the outcomes of patients who were treated with ipilimumab followed by vemurafenib, and vice versa (61). The small sample size in these reports makes it difficult to definitively recommend a particular treatment sequence. A randomized trial is currently being planned by cooperative groups and will hopefully answer this important question.

We have finally entered the age of targeted therapy directed by the genotype of the melanoma. Much is still unknown to us, but it is clear that, if we identify the driving mutation of the patient's melanoma and we treat with a drug that blocks that activated protein, dramatic tumor shrinkage is seen, which can improve the patient's survival. We can now build on this understanding, with the hope that survival will further be improved.

■ REFERENCES

1. Yang AS, Chapman PB. The history and future of chemotherapy for melanoma. *Hematol Oncol Clin North Am*. 2009;23(3):583–97, x.

2. Balch CM, Gershenwald JE, Soong SJ, et al. Final version of 2009 AJCC melanoma staging and classification. *J Clin Oncol*. 2009; 27(36):6199–6206.

3. Davies H, Bignell GR, Cox C, et al. Mutations of the BRAF gene in human cancer. *Nature*. 2002; 417(6892):949–954.

4. Chapman PB, Hauschild A, Robert C, et al.; BRIM-3 Study Group. Improved survival with vemurafenib in melanoma with BRAF V600E mutation. *N Engl J Med*. 2011; 364(26):2507–2516.

5. Pratilas CA, Solit DB. Targeting the mitogen-activated protein kinase pathway: physiological feedback and drug response. *Clin Cancer Res*. 2010;16(13):3329–3334.

6. Chang L, Karin M. Mammalian MAP kinase signalling cascades. *Nature*. 2001; 410(6824):37–40.

7. McCormick F. Signal transduction. How receptors turn Ras on. *Nature*. 1993;363 (6424):15–16.

8. Wellbrock C, Karasarides M, Marais R. The RAF proteins take centre stage. *Nat Rev Mol Cell Biol*. 2004;5(11):875–885.

9. Curtin JA, Fridlyand J, Kageshita T, et al. Distinct sets of genetic alterations in melanoma. *N Engl J Med*. 2005;353(20):2135–2147.

10. Long GV, Menzies AM, Nagrial AM, et al. Prognostic and clinicopathologic associations of oncogenic BRAF in metastatic melanoma. *J Clin Oncol*. 2011;29(10):1239–1246.

11. Menzies AM, Haydu LE, Visintin L, et al. Distinguishing Clinicopathologic Features of Patients with V600E and V600K BRAF-mutant Metastatic Melanoma. *Clin Cancer Res*. 2012.

12. Carvajal RD, Antonescu CR, Wolchok JD, et al. KIT as a therapeutic target in metastatic melanoma. *JAMA*. 2011;305(22):2327–2334.

13. Jakob JA, Bassett RL, Jr., Ng CS, et al. NRAS mutation status is an independent prognostic factor in metastatic melanoma. *Cancer*. 2011.

14. Van Raamsdonk CD, Bezrookove V, Green G, et al. Frequent somatic mutations of GNAQ in uveal melanoma and blue naevi. *Nature*. 2009;457(7229):599–U108.

15. Wan PT, Garnett MJ, Roe SM, et al.; Cancer Genome Project. Mechanism of activation of the RAF-ERK signaling pathway by oncogenic mutations of B-RAF. *Cell*. 2004; 116(6):855–867.

16. Joseph EW, Pratilas CA, Poulikakos PI, et al. The RAF inhibitor PLX4032 inhibits ERK signaling and tumor cell proliferation in a V600E BRAF-selective manner. *Proc Natl Acad Sci USA*. 2010;107(33):14903–14908.

17. Hoeflich KP, Gray DC, Eby MT, et al. Oncogenic BRAF is required for tumor growth and maintenance in melanoma models. *Cancer Res*. 2006;66(2):999–1006.

18. Michaloglou C, Vredeveld LC, Soengas MS, et al. BRAFE600-associated senescence-like cell cycle arrest of human naevi. *Nature*. 2005;436(7051):720–724.

19. Dankort D, Curley DP, Cartlidge RA, et al. Braf(V600E) cooperates with Pten loss to induce metastatic melanoma. *Nat Genet*. 2009;41(5):544–552.

20. Mangana J, Levesque MP, Karpova MB, Dummer R. Sorafenib in melanoma. *Expert Opin Investig Drugs*. 2012;21(4):557–568.

21. Karasarides M, Chiloeches A, Hayward R, et al. B-RAF is a therapeutic target in melanoma. *Oncogene*. 2004;23(37):6292–6298.

22. Panka DJ, Wang W, Atkins MB, Mier JW. The Raf inhibitor BAY 43–9006 (Sorafenib) induces caspase-independent apoptosis in melanoma cells. *Cancer Res*. 2006;66(3):1611–1619.

23. Wilhelm SM, Carter C, Tang L, et al. BAY 43–9006 exhibits broad spectrum oral antitumor activity and targets the RAF/MEK/ERK pathway and receptor

tyrosine kinases involved in tumor progression and angiogenesis. *Cancer Res.* 2004; 64(19):7099–7109.

24. Bollag G, Hirth P, Tsai J, et al. Clinical efficacy of a RAF inhibitor needs broad target blockade in BRAF-mutant melanoma. *Nature.* 2010;467(7315):596–599.

25. Søndergaard JN, Nazarian R, Wang Q, et al. Differential sensitivity of melanoma cell lines with BRAFV600E mutation to the specific Raf inhibitor PLX4032. *J Transl Med.* 2010;8:39.

26. Tsai J, Lee JT, Wang W, et al. Discovery of a selective inhibitor of oncogenic B-Raf kinase with potent antimelanoma activity. *Proc Natl Acad Sci USA.* 2008;105(8):3041–3046.

27. Poulikakos PI, Zhang C, Bollag G, Shokat KM, Rosen N. RAF inhibitors transactivate RAF dimers and ERK signalling in cells with wild-type BRAF. *Nature.* 2010;464(7287):427–430.

28. Eisen T, Ahmad T, Flaherty KT, et al. Sorafenib in advanced melanoma: a Phase II randomised discontinuation trial analysis. *Br J Cancer.* 2006;95(5):581–586.

29. Margolin KA, Moon J, Flaherty LE, et al. Randomized phase II trial of sorafenib with temsirolimus or tipifarnib in untreated metastatic melanoma (S0438). *Clin Cancer Res.* 2012;18(4):1129–1137.

30. McDermott DF, Sosman JA, Gonzalez R, et al. Double-blind randomized phase II study of the combination of sorafenib and dacarbazine in patients with advanced melanoma: a report from the 11715 Study Group. *J Clin Oncol.* 2008;26(13):2178–2185.

31. Hauschild A, Agarwala SS, Trefzer U, et al. Results of a phase III, randomized, placebo-controlled study of sorafenib in combination with carboplatin and paclitaxel as second-line treatment in patients with unresectable stage III or stage IV melanoma. *J Clin Oncol.* 2009;27(17):2823–2830.

32. Flaherty KT. Where does the combination of sorafenib and interferon in renal cell carcinoma stand? *Cancer.* 2010;116(1):4–7.

33. Flaherty KT, Puzanov I, Kim KB, et al. Inhibition of mutated, activated BRAF in metastatic melanoma. *N Engl J Med.* 2010;363(9):809–819.

34. McArthur GA, Puzanov I, Amaravadi R, et al. Marked, homogeneous, and early [18F] fluorodeoxyglucose-positron emission tomography responses to vemurafenib in BRAF-mutant advanced melanoma. *J Clin Oncol.* 2012; 30(14):1628–1634.

35. Sosman JA, Kim KB, Schuchter L, et al. Survival in BRAF V600-mutant advanced melanoma treated with vemurafenib. *N Engl J Med.* 2012;366(8):707–714.

36. Rochet NM, Kottschade LA, Markovic SN. Vemurafenib for melanoma metastases to the brain. *N Engl J Med.* 2011;365(25):2439–2441.

37. Chapman PB, Hauschild A, Robert C, et al. Updated overall survival results for BRIM-3, a phase III randomized, open-label, multicenter trial comparing BRAF inhibitor vemurafenib with dacarbazine in previously untreated patients with BRAFV600E-mutated melanoma. Paper presented at the American Society of Clinical Oncology (ASCO) Annual Meeting: Collaborating to Conquer Cancer; 2012; Chicago, IL.

38. Hodi FS, O'Day SJ, McDermott DF, et al. Improved survival with ipilimumab in patients with metastatic melanoma. *N Engl J Med.* 2010; 363(8):711–723.

39. Falchook GS, Long GV, Kurzrock R, et al. Dabrafenib in patients with melanoma, untreated brain metastases, and other solid tumours: a phase 1 dose-escalation trial. *Lancet.* 2012;379(9829):1893–1901.

40. Trefzer U, Minor D, Ribas A. BREAK-2: a Phase IIA trial of the selective BRAF kinase inhibitor GSK2118436 in patients with BRAF mutation-positive (V600E/K) metastatic melanoma. *Pigment Cell Melanoma Res.* 2011;24:1020.

41. Kirkwood J, Long GV, Trefzer U, et al. BREAK-MB: A phase II study assessing overall intracranial response rate to dabrafenib in patients with BRAF V600E/k mutation-positive melanoma with brain metastases Paper presented at the American Society of Clinical Oncology (ASCO) Annual Meeting: Collaborating to Conquer Cancer; 2012; Chicago, IL.

42. Hauschild A, Grob JJ, Demidov LV, et al. Dabrafenib in BRAF-mutated metastatic melanoma: a multicentre, open-label, phase 3 randomised controlled trial. *Lancet.* 2012.

43. Zimmer L, Hillen U, Livingstone E, et al. Atypical Melanocytic Proliferations and New Primary Melanomas in Patients With Advanced Melanoma Undergoing Selective BRAF Inhibition. *J Clin Oncol.* 2012.

44. Su F, Viros A, Milagre C, et al. RAS mutations in cutaneous squamous-cell carcinomas in patients treated with BRAF inhibitors. *N Engl J Med.* 2012;366(3):207–215.

45. Dalle S, Poulalhon N, Thomas L. Vemurafenib in melanoma with BRAF V600E mutation. *N Engl J Med.*.2011;365(15):1448–1449; author reply 1450.

46. Xing F, Persaud Y, Pratilas CA, et al Concurrent loss of the PTEN and RB1 tumor suppressors attenuates RAF dependence in melanomas harboring (V600E)BRAF. *Oncogene.* 2012; 31(4):446–457.

47. Nathanson KL, Martin A, Letrero R, et al. Tumor genetic analyses of patients with metastatic melanoma treated with the BRAF inhibitor GSK2118436 (GSK436). Paper presented at the American Society of Clinical Oncology (ASCO) Annual Meeting: Patients, Pathways, Progress; 3–7, 2011; Chicago, IL.

48. Sosman JA, Pavlick AC, Schuchter L, et al. Analysis of molecular mechanisms of response and resistance to vemurafenib in BRAFV600E melanoma. Presented at the American Society of Clinical Oncology (ASCO) Annual Meeting: Collaborating to Conquer Cancer; 2012; Chicago, IL.

49. Poulikakos PI, Persaud Y, Janakiraman M, et al. RAF inhibitor resistance is mediated by dimerization of aberrantly spliced BRAF(V600E). *Nature.* 2011;480(7377): 387–390.

50. Nazarian R, Shi H, Wang Q, et al. Melanomas acquire resistance to B-RAF(V600E) inhibition by RTK or N-RAS upregulation. *Nature.* 2010;468(7326):973–977.

51. Villanueva J, Vultur A, Lee JT, et al. Acquired resistance to BRAF inhibitors mediated by a RAF kinase switch in melanoma can be overcome by cotargeting MEK and IGF-1R/PI3K. *Cancer Cell.* 2010;18(6):683–695.

52. Natali PG, Nicotra MR, Di Renzo MF, et al. Expression of the c-Met/HGF receptor in human melanocytic neoplasms: demonstration of the relationship to malignant melanoma tumour progression. *Br J Cancer.* 1993;68(4):746–750.

53. Straussman R, Morikawa T, Shee K, et al. Tumour micro-environment elicits innate resistance to RAF inhibitors through HGF secretion. *Nature.* Jul 4 2012.

54. Corcoran RB, Dias-Santagata D, Bergethon K, Iafrate AJ, Settleman J, Engelman JA. BRAF gene amplification can promote acquired resistance to MEK inhibitors in cancer cells harboring the BRAF V600E mutation. *Sci Signal.* 2010;3(149):ra84.

55. Shi H, Moriceau G, Kong X, et al. Melanoma whole-exome sequencing identifies (V600E) B-RAF amplification-mediated acquired B-RAF inhibitor resistance. *Nat Commun.* 2012;3:724.

56. Johannessen CM, Boehm JS, Kim SY, et al. COT drives resistance to RAF inhibition through MAP kinase pathway reactivation. *Nature.* 2010;468(7326):968–972.

57. Emery CM, Vijayendran KG, Zipser MC, et al. MEK1 mutations confer resistance to MEK and B-RAF inhibition. *Proc Natl Acad Sci USA.* 2009;106(48):20411–20416.

58. Neyns B, Seghers AC, Wilgenhof S, Lebbe C. Successful rechallenge in two patients with BRAF-V600-mutant melanoma who experienced previous progression during treatment with a selective BRAF inhibitor. *Melanoma Res.* 2012.

59. Weber JS, Flaherty KT, Infante JR, et al. Updated safety and efficacy results from a phase I/II study of the oral BRAF inhibitor dabrafenib (GSK2118436) combined with the oral MEK 1/2 inhibitor trametinib (GSK1120212) in patients with BRAFi-naive metastatic melanoma. Presented at the American Society of Clinical Oncology (ASCO) Annual Meeting: Collaborating to Conquer Cancer; 2012; Chicago, IL.

60. Harding JJ, Pulitzer M, Chapman PB. Vemurafenib sensitivity skin reaction after ipilimumab. *N Engl J Med.* 2012; 366(9):866–868.

61. Ascierto PA, Simeone E, Giannarelli D, Grimaldi AM, Romano A, Mozzillo N. Sequencing of BRAF inhibitors and ipilimumab in patients with metastatic melanoma: a possible algorithm for clinical use. *J Transl Med.* 2012;10:107.

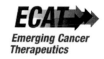

Emerging Targets for Melanoma Therapy Besides BRAF

Young Kwang Chae, Sapna P. Patel, and Kevin B. Kim*

Department of Melanoma Medical Oncology, The University of Texas MD Anderson Cancer Center, Houston, TX

■ ABSTRACT

The discovery of a high incidence of *BRAF* mutations and the successful development of selective BRAF inhibitors have paved the way for a field of targeted therapy for melanoma. However, most patients who are treated with a BRAF inhibitor ultimately require other systemic therapies, because their melanomas develop resistance to a BRAF inhibitor. In addition, approximately 50% of patients with metastatic melanoma do not have a *BRAF* mutation in their tumor and, therefore, do not benefit from BRAF inhibitors. Several targeted therapies for melanoma have emerged as our understanding of various biomarkers has rapidly advanced through preclinical and clinical studies in which biomarker evaluation has heavily been emphasized. These molecular targets include antiangiogenic proteins, mutated *KIT*, AKT/mammalian target of rapamycin kinases, cyclin-dependent kinases, and unique molecular aberrations found in uveal melanoma, such as *GNAQ*, *GNA11*, and *BAP1*.

Keywords: non-BRAF melanoma, MEK, KIT, ocular melanoma

*Corresponding author, Department of Melanoma Medical
Oncology, Unit 430, The University of Texas MD Anderson
Cancer Center, 1515 Holcombe Boulevard, Houston, TX
  E-mail address: kkim@mdanderson.org

Emerging Cancer Therapeutics 3:3 (2012) 501–516.
DOI: 10.5003/2151–4194.3.3.501
demosmedpub.com/ecat

■ INTRODUCTION

Treatment of advanced melanoma was challenging for many years until the recent success of novel molecular targeted therapy using selective v-raf murine sarcoma viral oncogene homologe B1 (BRAF) inhibitors and immune checkpoint inhibitors such as anti-cytotoxic T-lymphocyte antigen 4 (CTLA4) antibodies. However, BRAF inhibitors work only in melanomas that carry a *BRAF* mutation, and more than half of melanomas do not harbor an oncogenic *BRAF* mutation. Moreover, most patients with *BRAF*-mutant melanoma treated with a selective BRAF inhibitor have disease progression within 1 year of treatment despite a significant initial tumor regression (1,2). In addition, a majority of patients who are treated with ipilimumab, the CTLA4-blocking antibody that represents the most advanced of the current generation of molecularly targeted immunotherapies, are not cured and need other systemic therapies.

Further improvements in molecular-targeted therapy are thus clearly needed and also highly desirable, because this approach allows for the selection of appropriate patients with clinically relevant molecular targets for certain drugs and is less likely than chemotherapeutic agents to cause lethal toxic effects such as severe myelosuppression. One of the first targeted drugs that were tested for advanced melanoma in a clinical setting was oblimersen, an antisense oligonucleotide that targets the mRNA of Bcl-2 which is an antiapoptotic protein. Despite encouraging preclinical and early phase clinical study data (3,4), a large phase III study did not show an overall survival (OS) benefit of oblimersen over dacarbazine (5). That study did not enroll patients on the basis of a molecular biomarker profile such as tumoral Bcl-2 expression; therefore, it is impossible to determine whether the lack of survival benefit with oblimersen was a resulta of insufficient inhibition of the target (Bcl-2) or because of the lack of patient selection according to the presence of the target biomarker. This experience underscores the importance of identifying robust molecular targets for therapy and selecting appropriate patients with predictive biomarkers.

Several molecular targets for melanoma therapy have garnered interest, including molecules involved in signal transduction pathways and tumor environment factors such as those that promote angiogenesis. Different subsets of melanoma, such as mucosal melanoma, acral lentiginous melanoma or uveal melanoma, have a biology and clinical course different from those of cutaneous melanomas and thus have a distinct set of biomarkers. Understanding the clinical relevance of these biomarkers in the context of each type of melanomas cannot be overemphasized in the attempt to advance the field of targeted therapy. In this chapter, we discuss a number of molecular targets for melanoma therapy, including antiogenic proteins, KIT kinase, AKT/mammalian target of rapamycin (mTOR), and cyclin-dependent kinase 4 (CDK4). In addition, we review the potential targets of uveal melanoma, which has unique clinical features.

■ ANGIOGENIC TARGETS

Angiogenesis, a dynamic process where new blood vessels are formed through a remodeling of the existing vasculature, is essential for tumor growth and metastasis (6). New vasculatures that are formed within or adjacent to enlarging tumor lesions express various molecules that are potential therapeutic targets (7). The induction of angiogenesis was first reported when human melanoma cells were transplanted into hamsters (8). However, the prognostic importance of angiogenesis in melanoma remains controversial. Although some researchers found an inverse relationship between tumor microvasculature and the survival outcomes of patients with melanoma, these findings were not validated in subsequent studies (9,10). Several important angiogenic factors are involved in melanoma progression, but no single predominant protein has been shown to be responsible for neovasculature formation and tumor progression in melanoma.

Vascular Endothelial Growth Factors and Their Receptors

Neovascularization in melanoma is accomplished through a hypoxia-driven mechanism that is stimulated by several growth factors such as vascular endothelial growth factor (VEGF) (6). VEGF consists of 5 glycoproteins: VEGF-A, VEGF-B, VEGF-V, VEGF-D, and placental growth factor (PIGF). Serum levels of VEGF-A, commonly known as VEGF, have been reported to be strongly associated with melanoma progression and poorer survival outcomes (9). VEGF ligands bind to the extracellular domains of structurally similar tyrosine receptor kinases, vascular endothelial growth factor receptor (VEGFR)-1, VEGFR-2, and VEGFR-3. VEGFR-1 and VEGFR-2 are primarily expressed on the surface of blood endothelial cells, whereas VEGFR-3 is primarily expressed on lymphatic endothelial cells. Both ligands and receptors have been identified as potential targets of antiangiogenic therapy for melanoma.

Preclinical studies have shown that VEGF inhibition through either RNA interference or a neutralizing antibody led to reduced growth and metastatic potential in various xenograft models, including those of melanoma. Consistent with the promising preclinical data, bevacizumab, a humanized monoclonal immunoglobulin G antibody against VEGF, has been shown to have antiangiogenic activity and to yield clinical benefits in the treatment of metastatic non–small cell lung, colorectal, and renal cell cancer and glioblastoma, thus leading to this agent's approval by the U.S. Food and Drug Administration (FDA).

In a randomized phase II trial of patients with metastatic melanoma treated with bevacizumab alone or in combination with low-dose interferon (IFN)-alpha-2b, bevacizumab monotherapy resulted in a median progression-free survival (PFS) duration of 3 months and a median OS duration of 8.5 months, and low-dose IFN-alpha-2b did not augment its activity, thereby suggesting that bevacizumab yields a modest clinical benefit as a single agent (11). Bevacizumab has also been investigated in combination with other chemotherapeutic agents such as temozolomide (12), paclitaxel (13), and both carboplatin and paclitaxel (14) on the basis of its additive clinical benefit when administered with cytotoxic agents in the treatment of colon cancer and non–small cell lung cancer. In a phase II trial of a combination of bevacizumab and temozolomide in treatment-naive patients with metastatic melanoma, the response rate was 16% among 62 patients (12). The median progression-free survival (PFS) and OS durations were 4.2 and 9.6 months, respectively. Despite the small number of patients in each subset, the OS duration was greater in patients with wild-type *BRAF* melanoma than in those with *V600E BRAF*-mutated melanoma (12.0 versus 9.2 months; *P* = 0.014). In a phase II trial of bevacizumab with dacarbazine and daily low-dose IFN-alpha-2a as first-line treatment for metastatic melanoma, the response rate was 23%, and the median PFS duration was 2.3 months in

26 patients; however, in the responders, the median PFS duration was 8.1 months (15). Nonetheless, the regimen was associated with remarkable vascular toxicity. In a phase II trial of a combination of bevacizumab and everolimus in patients who had received up to 2 prior systemic regimens, the response rate was 12%, and the median PFS duration was 4 months (16).

To better elucidate the clinical benefit of adding bevacizumab to cytotoxic chemotherapeutic agents, a large placebo-controlled, randomized phase II study was conducted in patients with previously untreated advanced melanoma (17). A total of 214 patients were randomly assigned to receive either a combination of carboplatin, paclitaxel, and bevacizumab (CPB) or a combination of carboplatin, paclitaxel, and placebo (CP) in a 2:1 ratio; the median PFS duration was 5.6 months and 4.2 months, respectively, and the median OS was 12.3 months and 9.2 months, respectively, but the differences were not statistically significant. It is interesting to note that the difference in

OS was more pronounced in patients with high serum lactate dehydrogenase levels and stage IV-M1c melanoma. Taken together, these data from clinical trials with bevacizumab have shown a modest benefit in the setting of metastatic melanoma. Because angiogenesis plays a role in metastasis, it could also be an attractive target for adjuvant therapy in patients with resected melanoma. In fact, a phase III trial comparing bevacizumab and observation in patients with fully resected high-risk cutaneous melanoma is ongoing (18). Initial safety data have indicated that bevacizumab after surgery is well tolerated.

Another VEGF ligand inhibitor, VEGF-Trap, also known as aflibercept, is designed to bind to VEGF-A, VEGF-B, and Aflibercept acts as a high-affinity soluble decoy VEGFR and thereby inhibits angiogenesis. A multicenter phase II study in chemo-naive patients with inoperable stage III or IV cutaneous or uveal melanoma was conducted to evaluate the efficacy of aflibercept (19). Of 40 patients, 3 (8%) had a partial response, and 20 (50%) had a PFS duration of 4 months or longer. The median OS duration in this trial was 16.3 months. Currently, a randomized phase II study of interleukin-2 with or without aflibercept is under way to evaluate the clinical benefit of VEGF-Trap.

In addition to the drugs targeting VEGF, tyrosine kinase inhibitors (TKIs) that target VEGFR are currently being investigated in metastatic melanoma. Among them, sorafenib is the most extensively studied drug that was initially developed as a (both CRAF and BRAF) inhibitor. It inhibits multiple targets, including VEGFR-2, VEGFR-3, platelet-derived growth factor receptor (PDGFR)-beta, Flt-3, and KIT, and it was shown to block both tumor cell proliferation and angiogenesis (20). As a single agent, sorafenib, however, did not render a significant benefit in a randomized phase II study of metastatic melanoma (21). In previous phase I and II clinical trials of therapy for advanced melanoma, sorafenib had promising clinical activity when combined with various chemotherapeutic agents, including dacarbazine (22) and temozolomide (23). In a phase I/II study of a combination of carboplatin, paclitaxel, and sorafenib, the response rate was 26%, and 74% of the patients did not have disease progression at the first staging evaluation at 6 weeks (24). However, in large randomized phase III studies of the addition of sorafenib to carboplatin and paclitaxel, the response rates, PFS durations, and OS durations were similar between the sorafenib-containing arm and the placebo-containing chemotherapy arm in both the first- (25) and second-line (26) settings.

Sorafenib was also investigated in combination with other targeted agents such as temsirolimus or tipifarnib, but the clinical benefits of these combinations were only modest (27).

Axitinib is another small-molecule tyrosine kinase inhibitor (TKI) that inhibits multiple targets, including VEGFR-1, VEGFR-2, VEGFR-3, PDGFR, and KIT, and it was approved by the U.S. Food and Drug Administration (FDA) as second-line treatment for metastatic renal cell carcinoma (28). In a multicenter phase II study of axitinib in 32 patients with metastatic melanoma, the objective response rate was 19%, and the median PFS and response durations were 3.9 and 5.9 months, respectively (29). Axitinib selectively decreased plasma concentrations of soluble VEGFR-2 and VEGFR-3. Further evaluation of axitinib alone or in combination with conventional chemotherapy is ongoing. In an interim analysis of a single-arm phase II trial assessing another VEGFR TKI, pazopanib, in combination with paclitaxel as first-line treatment for unresectable stage III and IV melanoma, yielded a 48% overall response rate. Disease control (objective response and disease stabilization as the best response) was observed in 80% of the patients (30). Further clinical development of pazopanib in combination with cytotoxic drug(s) is under way.

Fibroblast Growth Factors and Their Receptors

Deregulation of fibroblast growth factors (FGFs), their receptors (FGFRs) and downstream signaling components have been associated with autocrine stimulation of melanoma growth (31). Inhibition of the FGF pathway leads to tumor cell apoptosis and growth retardation (32). In addition, resistance to VEGF blockade in antiangiogenic

therapy may partially be contributed by other proangiogenic factors, such as FGFs, that restimulate tumor angiogenesis (33). Dovitinib (TKI258) is an orally available inhibitor of basic FGF (bFGF), VEGF, and PDGRF that suppresses both tumor proliferation and angiogenesis. In a phase I/II study of dovitinib in patients with advanced melanoma that was resistant or refractory to standard therapies or for whom no standard therapy was available, no confirmed response was observed, and stable disease as the best tumor response was observed in 12 of the 47 patients, thereby suggesting only limited efficacy (34). Although administration of dovitinib did not result in significant tumor regression, dovitinib induced a decrease in tumor blood flow and vascular permeability in a dose-dependent manner, as demonstrated by dynamic contrast-enhanced magnetic resonance imaging and also a decrease in FGFR phosphorylation within the tumor lesions.

Another agent, lenvatinib (E7080), an inhibitor of VEGFR, PDGFR, and bFGF, has been investigated in clinical trials of patients with various tumor types, including melanoma. Two phase I studies of lenvatinib revealed that 2 of the 14 patients with metastatic melanoma had a confirmed clinical response, and 5 patients had tumor reductions of 20% to 85% (35). A median PFS duration of 7 months in the patients with metastatic melanoma was encouraging. A phase II study of lenvatinib for melanoma is under way to evaluate its clinical activity in 2 cohorts: patients with wild-type BRAF melanoma and patients with *BRAF*-mutated melanoma who previously received a BRAF inhibitor.

Integrin

Adhesion molecules, in particular integrins, which modulate the extracellular matrix, are key players in tumor cell migration and angiogenesis (36). The αvβ3 and αvβ5 integrins that are expressed on the surface of endothelial cells promote invasion and neovascularization (37). Cilengitide (EMD121974) is a cyclic pentapeptide that is an antagonist of both the $αvβ_3$ and $αvβ_5$ integrins. In a preclinical study, cilengitide and temozolomide exerted synergistic antiproliferative effects against melanoma and endothelial cells and retarded the growth of melanoma in vivo (38). In a recent randomized phase II study in patients with metastatic melanoma, treatment with cilengitide was well tolerated; however, although tumoral $αvβ_3$ expression was lower after 1 week of treatment, the clinical efficacy of cilengitide at either 500 or 2,000 mg twice weekly was minimal (39). Similarly, vitaxin (a humanized version of a monoclonal antibody against the $αvβ_3$ integrin) and volociximab (a high-affinity chimeric immunoglobulin G_4 monoclonal antibody against the $α_5β_1$ integrin) had negligible clinical activity as a single agent in phase II clinical trials (40,41).

KIT Kinase

KIT (CD117) is a receptor tyrosine kinase that binds to the stem cell factor (SCF), and its signaling induced by KIT mutations or SCF binding is crucial for the survival, migration, and proliferation of melanocyte precursors (42–44). Immunohistochemical analysis has shown that KIT is overexpressed in 74% to 96% of melanomas (45,46). However, the role of the KIT signaling pathway in the proliferation and survival of melanoma cells is less clear than its role in the survival, migration, and proliferation of melanocyte precursors, because KIT expression is downregulated as melanomas progress to more advanced stages, and transient expression of KIT inhibits melanoma cell proliferation and metastasis (45–47).

In in vivo experiments, imatinib, a KIT inhibitor, did not significantly inhibit the growth of melanoma lesions established in the subcutaneous tissue of athymic nude mice (48). It is not surprising that 3 phase II studies showed that imatinib had minimal clinical efficacy in patients with metastatic melanoma who were selected, regardless of their KIT expression or mutation status (49–51). In these 3 studies, only 1 of the 63 patients who received 400 mg of imatinib twice a day had a durable objective response, which lasted more than 12 months (51). It is interesting to note that this patient's tumor had a high intensity of KIT expression and high percentage of cells expressing KIT, but without a KIT mutation (51).

However, clinical interest in KIT inhibitors was renewed when Curtin and colleagues demonstrated the presence of KIT aberrations in subtypes of melanoma (52). Of the 102 primary melanomas that they analyzed using comparative genomic hybridization assays and mutation analysis, 36% of acral lentiginous melanomas, 39% of mucosal melanomas, and 28% of melanomas arising from chronically sun-damaged skin had KIT mutations or increases in the KIT gene copy number. In contrast, BRAF mutations were less common than were KIT aberrations in these types of melanomas. In another study of 189 samples, Beadling and colleagues found KIT mutations in 23% of acral melanomas, 16% of mucosal melanomas, and 8% of conjunctival melanomas (53).

Most of the KIT mutations found in melanoma occur in either the juxtamembrane or the kinase domain, suggesting a functional significance of these aberrations in melanoma progression and the sensitivity of these melanoma lesions to imatinib (52,54). These mutated KIT proteins activate both the mitogen-activated protein kinase (MAPK) and the PI3K/AKT pathways, thereby resulting in melanoma cell proliferation, invasion, and metastasis. The KIT mutations in melanomas are usually the substitution of a single amino acid in exons 11, 13, and 17, whereas the most common KIT mutations in gastrointestinal stromal tumors are deletions or insertions primarily in exon 11, suggesting a possibility that the sensitivity of KIT-mutated cells to KIT inhibitors may be different between these 2 malignancies.

Imatinib was investigated in several phase II trials of patients with metastatic acral lentiginous melanoma, mucosal melanoma, or melanoma occurring in the chronic sun-damaged skin. Hodi and colleagues reported that 5 of the 10 patients with KIT-mutant melanoma had a clinical response, whereas none of the 10 patients with KIT amplification but not a KIT mutation responded (55). In a phase II study conducted in China, 10 (23%) of the 43 patients with metastatic melanoma harboring a KIT mutation or amplification achieved a partial response to imatinib administered at 400 to 800 mg per day (56). In this study, 9 of the 10 responders had a KIT mutation in exon 11 or 13, and despite the small number of patients, the median PFS and OS durations were significantly longer in the responders than in the nonresponders.

In another phase II study of imatinib in patients with advanced melanoma harboring KIT mutation or amplification, treated with imatinib at 400 mg twice daily, 4 of the 25 patients (16%) achieved an objective response that lasted for more than 1 year (57). It is interesting to note that the response rate was 40% in cases with mutations that affected recurrent hotspots or with a ratio of mutant to wild-type alleles of more than 1, thereby suggesting that a more refined selection of

KIT mutations could lead to the identification of better predictive biomarkers for imatinib response. Several clinical studies are currently under way to evaluate the clinical benefit of other KIT inhibitors such as dasatinib and nilotinib in patients with acral lentiginous, mucosal, or KIT-mutant melanoma.

AKT and Mammalian Target of Rapamycin

In melanoma, the PI3K (phosphatidylinositol-3 kinase)/AKT (also known as protein kinase B) signaling pathways are known to constitutively be activated through various mechanisms (58). In particular, deregulated AKT3, 1 of the 3 isoforms of AKT, promotes the development of malignant melanoma (59). Phosphatase and tensin homologue (PTEN) is an important tumor suppressor gene that inhibits cell growth by increasing cells' susceptibility to apoptotic processes through suppression of the AKT pathway (60). In melanoma cells, targeted reduction of AKT3 activity or overexpression of active PTEN protein stimulates apoptosis, thereby suggesting that both AKT and PTEN are potential targets for melanoma treatment (59). Targeted delivery of PTEN to melanoma cells could be an effective strategy for treating melanoma and may theoretically be achieved using liposome-based PTEN expression vectors conjugated with specific antibodies that can recognize melanoma cells. However, successfully delivering genes to tumor cells in humans still remains challenging because of the lack of efficient carriers for gene delivery.

AKT, which is activated in approximately 2/3 of melanomas (61), has been pursued as an ideal target for melanoma treatment. Isoselenocyanates are compounds that are synthesized by combining selenium (62) and isothiocyanates (63), both of which have been shown to down-regulate AKT activity. In a preclinical model, 2 isoselenocyanates, ISC-4 and ISC-6, decreased melanoma by inhibiting AKT and thereby increasing apoptosis by 3-fold (64). BI-69A11, another AKT inhibitor, has also shown antitumor activity in melanoma in vitro and in vivo by suppressing both the AKT and nuclear factor kappa-B pathways (65). Several selective AKT inhibitors, such as perifosine (66), MK-2206 (67), and GSK-2141795 (68), have been evaluated in patients with metastatic solid tumors in a phase I study setting, which included only a small number of patients with metastatic melanoma. To date, no AKT inhibitors have been shown to have substantial clinical activity in metastatic melanoma, thus indicating that inhibiting the AKT pathway alone is not sufficient to promote tumor regression.

AKT inhibitors are likely to be more useful when they are combined with drugs that target other clinically relevant signaling pathways. The PTEN/AKT pathway may affect the resistance of melanoma cells to inhibitors of the MAPK pathway (69). In vitro studies showed that BRAF or MEK inhibitors induced apoptosis in *BRAF*-mutant cell lines with normal PTEN expression, but they induced only cell-cycle arrest and minimal apoptosis in BRAF-mutant PTEN-null cell lines (70). The role of *PTEN* aberration in the resistance to BRAF inhibitors was also suggested in a phase I study of dabrafenib (GSK2118436), a selective RAF inhibitor (71), which showed a strong trend of association between PTEN deletions or mutations in pretreatment tumor specimens and shorter PFS. Accordingly, AKT inhibition has been implicated in overcoming the resistance of melanoma cells to BRAF or MEK inhibitors in melanoma cell lines

(72). A phase II study of a combination of selumetinib (AZD6244), a selective MEK inhibitor, and MK-2206, a selective AKT inhibitor, in patients with metastatic BRAF-mutant melanoma who had disease progression while being treated with a BRAF inhibitor, is ongoing to determine whether dual targeting of the MAPK and AKT pathways can sufficiently suppress the growth of such tumors.

One of the major direct effectors of AKT are the mammalian target of rapamycin (mTOR) and its downstream effector ribosomal protein S6 kinase, 70-KD, which are involved in cell-cycle progression, apoptosis regulation, and angiogenesis (73). Small-molecule drugs that inhibit the activation of mTOR have been evaluated in patients with metastatic melanoma, in the hopes of promoting tumor regression and delaying disease progression. However, 2 of the selective mTOR inhibitors, temsirolimus (CCI-779) and everolimus (RAD001), had only minimal clinical activity in patients with advanced melanoma (27,74). In addition, temsirolimus in combination with sorafenib had only minimal antitumor efficacy in 2 phase II clinical trials (75). Similarly, a combination of everolimus and bevacizumab had modest activity in a phase II study of patients with metastatic melanoma (16).

Despite the discouraging results of these clinical studies, mTOR inhibition may prove important in certain settings. For example, durable activation of the mTOR signaling pathway was observed in BRAF-mutant human melanoma cell lines with de novo resistance to vemurafenib (76). In those cells, targeting both mTOR and AKT, not mTOR alone, led to cell death, thereby implying a complex feedback mechanism of the AKT/mTOR pathway (76). Thus, 1 effective future strategy may be to combine AKT and mTOR inhibitors with MAPK inhibitors to treat BRAF-mutant melanoma.

Cyclin-Dependent Kinase 4

Cyclin-dependent kinase 4 (CDK4) is a member of the cyclin-dependent protein kinase family and is involved in the control of cell proliferation during the G1 phase of the cell cycle (77). CDK4 mediates phosphorylation of the retinoblastoma (Rb) protein that drives cells into the G1/S phase transition by releasing E2F transcription factor (78). In addition, the complex formed by CDK4 and cyclin D1 has been implicated in the control of cell proliferation (79). Phosphorylation of the Rb protein by CDK4 is inhibited by cyclin-dependent kinase inhibitor 2A (CDKN2A), which is implicated in the genetic risk for familial malignant melanoma when it is mutated (80,81). When CDKN2A is mutated or deleted through hypermethylation, CDK4-mediated phosphorylation of Rb is not inhibited, and cell division is not regulated. Therefore, this CDKN2A/CDK4/Rb pathway is a vital gatekeeper in cell-cycle progression and plays a role in melanoma tumorigenesis and senescence. In a previous study, cyclin D1 protein expression was increased in 1/3 of melanoma cases, which further supports the CDK4-cyclin D1 complex as an attractive target for melanoma treatment (82).

P276–00 is a novel potent small-molecule inhibitor of CDK4-D1, CDK1-B, and CDK9-T that was shown to have significant and selective antiproliferative activity by inducing G0-G1 arrest in vivo (82) and in vitro (83). On the basis of the promising preclinical data, a phase II study of P276–00 in patients with advanced melanoma containing cyclin D1-positive protein expression profiles is under way. Likewise, several CDK inhibitors are being evaluated as single agents or in combination with other approved agents on the basis of their anti-tumor activity in animal models. In a phase I study, PD 0332991, an oral CDK4 and CDK6 (CDK4/6) inhibitor, was well tolerated by patients with solid tumors, including melanoma (84). Phase I studies of LEE011 and LY2835219, 2 other oral CDK4/6 inhibitors, are currently recruiting patients with advanced solid tumors.

Emerging Targets for Uveal Melanoma

Uveal melanoma is the most common intraocular malignancy in adults and accounts for approximately 5% of all melanoma diagnoses (85). Despite its embryologic similarities to cutaneous melanoma, it is a biologically distinct subtype of this disease. Mutations in BRAF and NRAS do not exist in uveal melanoma. Rather, most of these tumors harbor individual gene mutations in G-proteins *GNAQ* and *GNA11* (86,87). The first reports of these alterations linked to uveal melanoma showed that mutations in *GNAQ* and *GNA11* were found in 46% and 32% of uveal melanomas, respectively (86,87). However, these mutations are also often found in benign blue nevi and are therefore insufficient to singularly induce malignancy. *GNAQ* and *GNA11* mutations lead to impaired GTPase function and keep guanosine triphosphate bound to the alpha subunit of the protein. This alteration leads to constitutive activation of the downstream MAPK and protein kinase C (PKC) pathways. Because of this finding, clinical trials of MEK inhibitors are in progress.

KIT overexpression and gene amplification have repeatedly been demonstrated in both primary and metastatic uveal melanoma specimens. No driver mutations of KIT, however, have been noted in this subtype. Furthermore, a clinical trial in France using imatinib at a dose of 400 mg twice daily and another in Germany (600 mg daily) failed to demonstrate blockade of wild-type KIT as an effective mechanism to stunt tumor growth in metastatic uveal melanoma (88,89), although KIT was expressed at more than 90% in most metastatic specimens. Another phase II trial in the United Kingdom evaluating imatinib at 400 mg daily in uveal melanoma successfully enrolled 25 patients with KIT-positive metastatic uveal melanoma in 16.6 months (90). Only 2 responses have been confirmed in this trial; thus, KIT inhibition alone is likely insufficient for treating metastatic uveal melanoma. Sunitinib, a multikinase inhibitor that has activity against KIT, is currently being studied in comparison and in combination with chemotherapy in several clinical trials.

Loss of PTEN has also been described in a small proportion (15%) of uveal melanomas (91,92). Preclinical studies have shown that enzastaurin, an inhibitor of various isoforms of PKC, which inhibits the PI3K/AKT PTEN signaling pathway, had notable activity in *GNAQ* mutant cell lines and was further enhanced with concomitant MEK inhibition (93). An international phase I clinical trial evaluating a novel PKC inhibitor, AEB071, is under way in uveal melanoma.

Loss of chromosome 3 has long been associated with a poor prognosis in uveal melanoma (94–96). Whole-exome sequencing of 2 metastatic uveal melanoma of primary tumors known to harbor monosomy 3 revealed a mutation in *BRCA1-associated protein-1 (BAP1)* (97). Further evaluation of 57 primary uveal melanomas revealed *BAP1* mutations in 47% of the cases, the majority of which occurred almost exclusively in the metastatic tumors (84%) and in those with monosomy 3. *BAP1* encodes for a tumor suppressor gene involved in histone complexing (98). Loss of *BAP1*, as seen in *BAP1*-mutant uveal melanomas, leads to deubiquitination of histone H2A that helps regulate cellular transcription. This has been most clearly delineated in the Drosophila *BAP1* homologue, *calypso* (99). Overcoming the loss of *BAP1* function may be achieved through the use of histone deacetylase inhibitors, several of which are clinically available and used to treat myelodysplastic syndrome and T-cell lymphomas. A phase II clinical trial of vorinostat, a histone deacetylase inhibitor, for metastatic uveal melanoma is enrolling patients in the United States. The use of this class of agents in an adjuvant setting to prevent metastatic disease represents a gap in clinical research and knowledge, as no clinical trial has targeted *BAP1* in high-risk patients with uveal melanoma in the adjuvant setting.

Immunhistochemical analysis has revealed the expression of insulin-like growth factor-1 receptor (IGF-1R) in primary uveal melanomas (100,101). Furthermore, IGF-1R expression was associated with uveal melanoma-specific mortality in multivariate analysis (P = 0.004) (102). The ligand for IGF-1R is IGF-1, a soluble factor produced in the liver, may contribute to the hepatic tropism of uveal melanoma. Successful inhibition of IGF-1R was demonstrated using picopodophyllin in 4 uveal melanoma cell lines and a subcutaneous xenograft model (103). Two clinical trials investigating this pathway are in progress in the United States: one using a monoclonal antibody against IGF-1R, cixutumumab (IMC-A12) and the other using a somatostatin analogue, pasireotide.

Similar to IGF-1R, c-MET expression has been noted in primary uveal melanomas and correlates with liver metastasis (P = 0.0009) and decreased survival (P < 0.03) (102,104). Several phase I studies of c-MET inhibitors have enrolled small numbers of patients with uveal melanoma, but whether inhibition of this receptor alone is sufficient to slow tumor migration and growth remains to be seen.

Bcl-2 is an antiapoptotic protein expressed in uveal melanoma specimens that may confer resistance to programmed cell death. However, expression of Bcl-2 does not seem to correlate with tumor growth or metastasis (105,106). Inhibition of Bcl-2 using an antisense DNA approach may increase the susceptibility of uveal melanoma tumors to apoptosis after the administration of cytotoxic chemotherapy.

■ CONCLUSION

In addition to BRAF, many other molecular targets are of interest for melanoma treatment. In particular, KIT mutations are attractive targets, because several phase II studies have shown the promising clinical efficacy of imatinib in patients with acral lentiginous or mucosal melanoma harboring a KIT mutation. However, the true clinical benefit of the KIT inhibitors will not be apparent until a larger randomized phase III trial is conducted. The practicality of conducting such a large phase III study is debatable because of the relatively low frequency of KIT mutations in melanoma. Encouraging preclinical data have established the rationale for using other molecular targets as therapy for melanoma. More robust preclinical studies and translational biomarker evaluations will be necessary to design more novel and truly personalized clinical trials of these targeted agents and to select appropriate patients with predictive biomarkers for each of these trials.

■ REFERENCES

1. Chapman PB, Hauschild A, Robert C, et al.; BRIM-3 Study Group. Improved survival with vemurafenib in melanoma with BRAF V600E mutation. *N Engl J Med.* 2011;364(26):2507–2516.
2. Hauschild A, Grob JJ, Demidov LV, et al. Phase III, randomized, open-label, multicenter trial (BREAK-3) comparing the BRAF kinase inhibitor dabrafenib (GSK2118436) with dacarbazine (DTIC) in patients with BRAF^{V600E}-mutated melanoma. *J Clin Oncol.* 2012;30:(suppl; abstr LBA8500)
3. Klasa RJ, Gillum AM, Klem RE, Frankel SR. Oblimersen Bcl-2 antisense: facilitating apoptosis in anticancer treatment. *Antisense Nucleic Acid Drug Dev.* 2002;12(3):193–213.
4. Jansen B, Wacheck V, Heere-Ress E, et al. Chemosensitisation of malignant melanoma by BCL2 antisense therapy. *Lancet.* 2000;356(9243):1728–1733.
5. Bedikian AY, Millward M, Pehamberger H, et al. Oblimersen Melanoma Study Group. Bcl-2 antisense (oblimersen sodium) plus dacarbazine in patients with advanced melanoma: the Oblimersen Melanoma Study Group. *J Clin Oncol.* 2006;24(29):4738–4745.
6. Folkman J. Angiogenesis. *Annu Rev Med.* 2006;57:1–18.
7. St Croix B, Rago C, Velculescu V, et al. Genes expressed in human tumor endothelium. *Science.* 2000;289(5482):1197–1202.
8. Hillen F, van de Winkel A, Creytens D, Vermeulen AH, Griffioen AW. Proliferating endothelial cells, but not microvessel density, are a prognostic parameter in human cutaneous melanoma. *Melanoma Res.* 2006;16(5):453–457.
9. Ugurel S, Rappl G, Tilgen W, Reinhold U. Increased serum concentration of angiogenic factors in malignant melanoma patients correlates with tumor progression and survival. *J Clin Oncol.* 2001;19(2):577–583.
10. Helfrich I, Schadendorf D. Blood vessel maturation, vascular phenotype and angiogenic potential in malignant melanoma: one step forward for overcoming anti-angiogenic drug resistance? *Mol Oncol.* 2011;5(2):137–149.
11. Varker KA, Biber JE, Kefauver C, et al. A randomized phase 2 trial of bevacizumab with or without daily low-dose interferon alfa-2b in metastatic malignant melanoma. *Ann Surg Oncol.* 2007;14(8):2367–2376.

12. von Moos R, Seifert B, Simcock M, et al.; Swiss Group for Clinical Cancer Research (SAKK). First-line temozolomide combined with bevacizumab in metastatic melanoma: a multicentre phase II trial (SAKK 50/07). *Ann Oncol.* 2012;23(2):531–536.

13. González-Cao M, Viteri S, Díaz-Lagares A, et al. Preliminary results of the combination of bevacizumab and weekly Paclitaxel in advanced melanoma. *Oncology.* 2008;74(1–2):12–16.

14. Perez DG, Suman VJ, Fitch TR, et al. Phase 2 trial of carboplatin, weekly paclitaxel, and biweekly bevacizumab in patients with unresectable stage IV melanoma: a North Central Cancer Treatment Group study, N047A. *Cancer.* 2009;115(1):119–127.

15. Vihinen PP, Hernberg M, Vuoristo MS, et al. A phase II trial of bevacizumab with dacarbazine and daily low-dose interferon-alpha2a as first line treatment in metastatic melanoma. *Melanoma Res.* 2010;20(4):318–325.

16. Hainsworth JD, Infante JR, Spigel DR, et al. Bevacizumab and everolimus in the treatment of patients with metastatic melanoma: a phase 2 trial of the Sarah Cannon Oncology Research Consortium. *Cancer.* 2010; 116(17):4122–4129.

17. Kim KB, Sosman JA, Fruehauf JP, et al. BEAM: a randomized phase II study evaluating the activity of bevacizumab in combination with carboplatin plus paclitaxel in patients with previously untreated advanced melanoma. *J Clin Oncol.* 2012;30(1):34–41.

18. Biswas S, Wrigley J, East C, et al. A randomised trial evaluating bevacizumab as adjuvant therapy following resection of AJCC stage IIB, IIC and III cutaneous melanoma: an update. *Ecancermedicalscience.* 2008;2:108.

19. Tarhini AA, Frankel P, Margolin KA, et al. Aflibercept (VEGF Trap) in inoperable stage III or stage iv melanoma of cutaneous or uveal origin. *Clin Cancer Res.* 2011;17(20):6574–6581.

20. Wilhelm SM, Carter C, Tang L, et al. BAY 43–9006 exhibits broad spectrum oral antitumor activity and targets the RAF/MEK/ERK pathway and receptor tyrosine kinases involved in tumor progression and angiogenesis. *Cancer Res.* 2004;64(19):7099–7109.

21. Eisen T, Ahmad T, Flaherty KT, et al. Sorafenib in advanced melanoma: a Phase II randomised discontinuation trial analysis. *Br J Cancer.* 2006;95(5):581–586.

22. Eisen T, Marais R, Affolter A, et al. Sorafenib and dacarbazine as first-line therapy for advanced melanoma: phase I and open-label phase II studies. *Br J Cancer.* 2011;105(3):353–359.

23. Amaravadi RK, Schuchter LM, McDermott DF, et al. Phase II Trial of Temozolomide and Sorafenib in Advanced Melanoma Patients with or without Brain Metastases. *Clin Cancer Res.* 2009;15(24):7711–7718.

24. Flaherty KT, Schiller J, Schuchter LM, et al. A phase I trial of the oral, multikinase inhibitor sorafenib in combination with carboplatin and paclitaxel. *Clin Cancer Res.* 2008;14(15):4836–4842.

25. Flaherty KT, Lee SJ, Schuchter LM, et al. Final results of E2603: A double-blind, randomized phase III trial comparing carboplatin (C)/paclitaxel (P) with or without sorafenib (S) in metastatic melanoma. *J Clin Oncol.* 2010;28(Suppl:Abstract 8511).

26. Hauschild A, Agarwala SS, Trefzer U, et al. Results of a phase III, randomized, placebo-controlled study of sorafenib in combination with carboplatin and paclitaxel as second-line treatment in patients with unresectable stage III or stage IV melanoma. *J Clin Oncol.* 2009;27(17):2823–2830.

27. Margolin KA, Moon J, Flaherty LE, et al. Randomized phase II trial of sorafenib with temsirolimus or tipifarnib in untreated metastatic melanoma (S0438). *Clin Cancer Res.* 2012;18(4):1129–1137.

28. Rini BI, Escudier B, Tomczak P, et al. Comparative effectiveness of axitinib versus sorafenib in advanced renal cell carcinoma (AXIS): a randomised phase 3 trial. *Lancet.* 2011;378(9807):1931–1939.

29. Fruehauf J, Lutzky J, McDermott D, et al. Multicenter, phase II study of axitinib, a selective second-generation inhibitor of vascular endothelial growth factor receptors 1, 2, and 3, in patients with metastatic melanoma. *Clin Cancer Res.* 2011;17(23):7462–7469.

30. Fruehauf JP, Alger B, Parmakhtiar B, et al. A phase II single arm study of pazopanib and paclitaxel as first-line treatment for unresectable stage III and stage IV melanoma: Interim analysis. *J Clin Oncol.* 2012;30:(Suppl; Abstract 8524)

31. Meier F, Caroli U, Satyamoorthy K, et al. Fibroblast growth factor-2 but not Mel-CAM and/or beta3 integrin promotes progression of melanocytes to melanoma. *Exp Dermatol.* 2003;12(3):296–306.

32. Schulze D, Plohmann P, Höbel S, Aigner A. Anti-tumor effects of fibroblast growth factor-binding protein (FGF-BP) knockdown in colon carcinoma. *Mol Cancer.* 2011;10:144.

33. Casanovas O, Hicklin DJ, Bergers G, Hanahan D. Drug resistance by evasion of antiangiogenic targeting of VEGF signaling in late-stage pancreatic islet tumors. *Cancer Cell.* 2005;8(4):299–309.

34. Kim KB, Chesney J, Robinson D, Gardner H, Shi MM, Kirkwood JM. Phase I/II and pharmacodynamic study of dovitinib (TKI258), an inhibitor of fibroblast growth factor receptors and VEGF receptors, in patients with advanced melanoma. *Clin Cancer Res.* 2011;17(23):7451–7461.

35. Hong DS, Andresen C, Mink J, et al. A phase IB study of lenvatinib (E7080) in combination with temozolomide for treatment of advanced melanoma. *J Clin Oncol.* 2012;30:(Suppl; Abstract 8594).

36. Senger DR, Ledbetter SR, Claffey KP, Papadopoulos-Sergiou A, Peruzzi CA, Detmar M. Stimulation of endothelial cell migration by vascular permeability factor/vascular endothelial growth factor through cooperative mechanisms involving the alphavbeta3 integrin, osteopontin, and thrombin. *Am J Pathol.* 1996;149(1):293–305.

37. Eliceiri BP, Cheresh DA. Role of alpha v integrins during angiogenesis. *Cancer J.* 2000;6 Suppl 3:S245–S249.

38. Tentori L, Dorio AS, Muzi A, et al. The integrin antagonist cilengitide increases the antitumor activity of temozolomide against malignant melanoma. *Oncol Rep.* 2008;19(4):1039–1043.

39. Kim KB, Prieto V, Joseph RW, et al. A randomized phase II study of cilengitide (EMD 121974) in patients with metastatic melanoma. *Melanoma Res.* 2012;22(4):294–301.

40. Hersey P, Sosman J, O'Day S, et al.; Etaracizumab Melanoma Study Group. A randomized phase 2 study of etaracizumab, a monoclonal antibody against integrin alpha(v)beta(3), + or - dacarbazine in patients with stage IV metastatic melanoma. *Cancer.* 2010;116(6):1526–1534.

41. Cranmer LD, Bedikian AY, Ribas A, et al. Phase II study of volociximab (M200), an α5β1 anti-integrin antibody in metastatic melanoma. *J Clin Oncol.* 2006;24(18S::Abstract 8011).

42. Mackenzie MA, Jordan SA, Budd PS, Jackson IJ. Activation of the receptor tyrosine kinase Kit is required for the proliferation of melanoblasts in the mouse embryo. *Dev Biol.* 1997;192(1):99–107.

43. Wehrle-Haller B. The role of Kit-ligand in melanocyte development and epidermal homeostasis. *Pigment Cell Res.* 2003; 16(3):287–296.

44. Grichnik JM, Burch JA, Burchette J, Shea CR. The SCF/KIT pathway plays a critical role in the control of normal human melanocyte homeostasis. *J Invest Dermatol.* 1998;111(2):233–238.

45. Natali PG, Nicotra MR, Winkler AB, Cavaliere R, Bigotti A, Ullrich A. Progression of human cutaneous melanoma is associated with loss of expression of c-kit proto-oncogene receptor. *Int J Cancer.* 1992;52(2):197–201.

46. Shen SS, Zhang PS, Eton O, Prieto VG. Analysis of protein tyrosine kinase expression in melanocytic lesions by tissue array. *J Cutan Pathol.* 2003;30(9):539–547.

47. Huang S, Luca M, Gutman M, et al. Enforced c-KIT expression renders highly metastatic human melanoma cells susceptible to stem cell factor-induced apoptosis and inhibits their tumorigenic and metastatic potential. *Oncogene.* 1996;13(11):2339–2347.

48. McGary EC, Onn A, Mills L, et al. Imatinib mesylate inhibits platelet-derived growth factor receptor phosphorylation of melanoma cells but does not affect tumorigenicity in vivo. *J Invest Dermatol.* 2004;122(2):400–405.

49. Ugurel S, Hildenbrand R, Zimpfer A, et al. Lack of clinical efficacy of imatinib in metastatic melanoma. *Br J Cancer.* 2005;92(8):1398–1405.

50. Wyman K, Atkins MB, Hubbard F, et al. A phase II trial of imatinib mesylate at 800 mg daily in metastatic melanoma: lack of clinical efficacy with significant toxicity. *Proc. Amer. Soc. Clin. Oncol.* 2003;22:713(Abstract 2865).

51. Kim KB, Eton O, Davis DW, et al. Phase II trial of imatinib mesylate in patients with metastatic melanoma. *Br J Cancer.* 2008;99(5):734–740.

52. Curtin JA, Busam K, Pinkel D, Bastian BC. Somatic activation of KIT in distinct subtypes of melanoma. *J Clin Oncol.* 2006;24(26):4340–4346.

53. Beadling C, Jacobson-Dunlop E, Hodi FS, et al. KIT gene mutations and copy number in melanoma subtypes. *Clin Cancer Res.* 2008;14(21):6821–6828.

54. Corless CL, Fletcher JA, Heinrich MC. Biology of gastrointestinal stromal tumors. *J Clin Oncol.* 2004;22(18):3813–3825.

55. Hodi FS, Friedlander P, Corless C, et al. Phase II Trial of Imatinib in KIT Mutant/Amplified Melanoma. 6th Annual International Melanoma Congress; 1–4, 2009; Boston, MA.

56. Guo J, Si L, Kong Y, et al. Phase II, open-label, single-arm trial of imatinib mesylate in patients with metastatic melanoma harboring c-Kit mutation or amplification. *J Clin Oncol.* 2011;29(21):2904–2909.

57. Carvajal RD, Antonescu CR, Wolchok JD, et al. KIT as a therapeutic target in metastatic melanoma. *JAMA.* 2011;305(22):2327–2334.

58. Russo AE, Torrisi E, Bevelacqua Y, et al. Melanoma: molecular pathogenesis and emerging target therapies (Review). *Int J Oncol.* 2009;34(6):1481–1489.

59. Stahl JM, Sharma A, Cheung M, et al. Deregulated Akt3 activity promotes development of malignant melanoma. *Cancer Res.* 2004;64(19):7002–7010.

60. Lu Y, Lin YZ, LaPushin R, et al. The PTEN/MMAC1/TEP tumor suppressor gene decreases cell growth and induces apoptosis and anoikis in breast cancer cells. *Oncogene.* 1999;18(50):7034–7045.

61. Robertson GP. Functional and therapeutic significance of Akt deregulation in malignant melanoma. *Cancer Metastasis Rev.* 2005;24(2):273–285.

62. Bandura L, Drukala J, Wolnicka-Glubisz A, Björnstedt M, Korohoda W. Differential effects of selenite and selenate on human melanocytes, keratinocytes, and melanoma cells. *Biochem Cell Biol.* 2005;83(2):196–211.

63. Keum YS, Jeong WS, Kong AN. Chemoprevention by isothiocyanates and their underlying molecular signaling mechanisms. *Mutat Res.* 2004;555(1–2):191–202.

64. Sharma A, Sharma AK, Madhunapantula SV, et al. Targeting Akt3 signaling in malignant melanoma using isoselenocyanates. *Clin Cancer Res.* 2009;15(5):1674–1685.

65. Feng Y, Barile E, De SK, et al. Effective inhibition of melanoma by BI-69A11 is mediated by dual targeting of the AKT and NF-?B pathways. *Pigment Cell Melanoma Res.* 2011;24(4):703–713.

66. Van Ummersen L, Binger K, Volkman J, et al. A phase I trial of perifosine (NSC 639966) on a loading dose/maintenance dose schedule in patients with advanced cancer. *Clin Cancer Res.* 2004;10(22):7450–7456.

67. Yap TA, Yan L, Patnaik A, et al. First-in-man clinical trial of the oral pan-AKT inhibitor MK-2206 in patients with advanced solid tumors. *J Clin Oncol.* 2011; 29(35):4688–4695.

68. Burris HA, Siu LL, Infante JR, et al. Safety, pharmacokinetics (PK), pharmacodynamics (PD), and clinical activity of the oral AKT inhibitor GSK2141795 (GSK795) in a phase I first-in-human study. *J Clin Oncol.* 2011;29:(Suppl; Abstract 3003)

69. Atefi M, von Euw E, Attar N, et al. Reversing melanoma cross-resistance to BRAF and MEK inhibitors by co-targeting the AKT/mTOR pathway. *PLoS ONE.* 2011;6(12):e28973.

70. Gopal YN, Deng W, Woodman SE, et al. Basal and treatment-induced activation of AKT mediates resistance to cell death by AZD6244 (ARRY-142886) in Braf-mutant human cutaneous melanoma cells. *Cancer Res.* 2010;70(21):8736–8747.

71. Nathanson KL, Martin A, Letrero R, et al. Tumor genetic analyses of patients with metastatic melanoma treated with the BRAF inhibitor GSK2118436 (GSK436). *J Clin Oncol.* 2011;29:(suppl; abstr 8501)

72. Mitsiades N, Chew SA, He B, et al. Genotype-dependent sensitivity of uveal melanoma cell lines to inhibition of B-Raf, MEK, and Akt kinases: rationale for personalized therapy. *Invest Ophthalmol Vis Sci.* 2011;52(10):7248–7255.

73. Granville CA, Memmott RM, Gills JJ, Dennis PA. Handicapping the race to develop inhibitors of the phosphoinositide 3-kinase/Akt/mammalian target of rapamycin pathway. *Clin Cancer Res.* 2006;12(3 Pt 1): 679–689.

74. Rao RD, Windschitl HE, Allred JB, et al. Phase II trial of the mTOR inhibitor everolimus (RAD-001) in metastatic melanoma. *J Clin Oncol.* 2006;24:(Suppl; Abstract 8043).

75. Davies MA, Fox PS, Papadopoulos NE, et al. Phase I study of the combination of sorafenib and temsirolimus in patients with metastatic melanoma. *Clin Cancer Res.* 2012;18(4):1120–1128.

76. Deng W, Gopal YN, Scott A, Chen G, Woodman SE, Davies MA. Role and therapeutic potential of PI3K-mTOR signaling in de novo resistance to BRAF inhibition. *Pigment Cell Melanoma Res.* 2012;25(2):248–258.

77. Harbour JW, Dean DC. The Rb/E2F pathway: expanding roles and emerging paradigms. *Genes Dev.* 2000;14(19):2393–2409.

78. Sherr CJ. The INK4a/ARF network in tumour suppression. *Nat Rev Mol Cell Biol.* 2001;2(10):731–737.

79. Harbour JW, Luo RX, Dei Santi A, Postigo AA, Dean DC. Cdk phosphorylation triggers sequential intramolecular interactions that progressively block Rb functions as cells move through G1. *Cell.* 1999;98(6):859–869.

80. Hussussian CJ, Struewing JP, Goldstein AM, et al. Germline p16 mutations in familial melanoma. *Nat Genet.* 1994;8(1):15–21.

81. Goldstein AM, Chan M, Harland M, et al.; Lund Melanoma Study Group; Melanoma Genetics Consortium (GenoMEL). Features associated with germline CDKN2A mutations: a GenoMEL study of melanoma-prone families from three continents. *J Med Genet.* 2007;44(2):99–106.

82. Joshi KS, Rathos MJ, Joshi RD, et al. *In vitro* antitumor properties of a novel cyclin-dependent kinase inhibitor, P276–00. *Mol Cancer Ther.* 2007;6(3):918–925.

83. Joshi KS, Rathos MJ, Mahajan P, et al. P276–00, a novel cyclin-dependent inhibitor induces G1-G2 arrest, shows antitumor activity on cisplatin-resistant cells and significant *in vivo* efficacy in tumor models. *Mol Cancer Ther.* 2007;6(3):926–934.

84. Schwartz GK, LoRusso PM, Dickson MA, et al. Phase I study of PD 0332991, a cyclin-dependent kinase inhibitor, administered in 3-week cycles (Schedule 2/1). *Br J Cancer.* 2011;104(12):1862–1868.

85. Singh AD, Topham A. Incidence of uveal melanoma in the United States: 1973–1997. *Ophthalmology.* 2003;110(5):956–961.

86. Van Raamsdonk CD, Bezrookove V, Green G, et al. Frequent somatic mutations of GNAQ in uveal melanoma and blue naevi. *Nature.* 2009;457(7229):599–602.

87. Van Raamsdonk CD, Griewank KG, Crosby MB, et al. Mutations in GNA11 in uveal melanoma. *N Engl J Med.* 2010;363(23):2191–2199.

88. Penel N, Delcambre C, Durando X, et al. O-Mel-Inib: a Cancéro-pôle Nord-Ouest multicenter phase II trial of high-dose imatinib mesylate in metastatic uveal melanoma. *Invest New Drugs.* 2008;26(6):561–565.

89. Hofmann UB, Kauczok-Vetter CS, Houben R, Becker JC. Overexpression of the KIT/SCF in uveal melanoma does not translate into clinical efficacy of imatinib mesylate. *Clin Cancer Res.* 2009;15(1):324–329.

90. Nathan PD, Marshall E, Smith CT, et al. A Cancer Research UK two-stage multicenter phase II study of imatinib in the treatment of patients with c-kit positive metastatic uveal melanoma (ITEM). *J Clin Oncol.* 2012;30:(Suppl; Abstract 8523).

91. Abdel-Rahman MH, Yang Y, Zhou XP, Craig EL, Davidorf FH, Eng C. High frequency of submicroscopic hemizygous deletion is a major mechanism of loss of expression of PTEN in uveal melanoma. *J Clin Oncol.* 2006;24(2):288–295.

92. Ehlers JP, Worley L, Onken MD, Harbour JW. Integrative genomic analysis of aneuploidy in uveal melanoma. *Clin Cancer Res.* 2008;14(1):115–122.

93. Wu X, Zhu M, Fletcher JA, Giobbie-Hurder A, Hodi FS. The protein kinase C inhibitor enzastaurin exhibits antitumor activity against uveal melanoma. *PLoS ONE.* 2012;7(1):e29622.

94. Prescher G, Bornfeld N, Hirche H, Horsthemke B, Jöckel KH, Becher R. Prognostic implications of monosomy 3 in uveal melanoma. *Lancet.* 1996;347(9010):1222–1225.

95. Scholes AG, Damato BE, Nunn J, Hiscott P, Grierson I, Field JK. Monosomy 3 in uveal melanoma: correlation with clinical and histologic predictors of survival. *Invest Ophthalmol Vis Sci.* 2003;44(3):1008–1011.

96. Shields CL, Ganguly A, Bianciotto CG, Turaka K, Tavallali A, Shields JA. Prognosis of uveal melanoma in 500 cases using genetic testing of fine-needle aspiration biopsy specimens. *Ophthalmology.* 2011;118(2):396–401.

97. Harbour JW, Onken MD, Roberson ED, et al. Frequent mutation of BAP1 in metastasizing uveal melanomas. *Science.* 2010;330(6009):1410–1413.

98. Jensen DE, Proctor M, Marquis ST, et al. BAP1: a novel ubiquitin hydrolase which binds to the BRCA1 RING finger and enhances BRCA1-mediated cell growth suppression. *Oncogene.* 1998;16(9):1097–1112.

99. Scheuermann JC, de Ayala Alonso AG, Oktaba K, et al. Histone H2A deubiquitinase activity of the Polycomb repressive complex PR-DUB. *Nature.* 2010;465(7295): 243–247.

100. All-Ericsson C, Girnita L, Seregard S, Bartolazzi A, Jager MJ, Larsson O. Insulin-like growth factor-1 receptor in uveal

melanoma: a predictor for metastatic disease and a potential therapeutic target. *Invest Ophthalmol Vis Sci.* 2002;43(1):1–8.

101. Mallikarjuna K, Pushparaj V, Biswas J, Krishnakumar S. Expression of insulin-like growth factor receptor (IGF-1R), c-Fos, and c-Jun in uveal melanoma: an immunohistochemical study. *Curr Eye Res.* 2006;31(10):875–883.

102. Economou MA, All-Ericsson C, Bykov V, et al. Receptors for the liver synthesized growth factors IGF-1 and HGF/SF in uveal melanoma: intercorrelation and prognostic implications. *Invest Ophthalmol Vis Sci.* 2005;46(12):4372–4375.

103. Economou MA, Andersson S, Vasilcanu D, et al. Oral picropodophyllin (PPP) is well tolerated *in vivo* and inhibits IGF-1R expression and growth of uveal melanoma. *Invest Ophthalmol Vis Sci.* 2008;49(6):2337–2342.

104. Mallikarjuna K, Pushparaj V, Biswas J, Krishnakumar S. Expression of epidermal growth factor receptor, ezrin, hepatocyte growth factor, and c-Met in uveal melanoma: an immunohistochemical study. *Curr Eye Res.* 2007;32(3):281–290.

105. Chana JS, Wilson GD, Cree IA, et al. c-myc, p53, and Bcl-2 expression and clinical outcome in uveal melanoma. *Br J Ophthalmol.* 1999;83(1):110–114.

106. Sulkowska M, Famulski W, Bakunowicz-Lazarczyk A, Chyczewski L, Sulkowski S. Bcl-2 expression in primary uveal melanoma. *Tumori.* 2001;87(1):54–57.

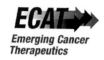

Ipilimumab: The New Frontier of T-Cell Antibodies: A Paradigm Shift in Immuno-Oncology

Steven J. O'Day

The Los Angeles Skin Cancer Institute, Department of Medical Oncology, Beverly Hills Cancer Center, Beverly Hills, CA

■ ABSTRACT

The discovery of cytotoxic T-lymphocyte associated antigen-4 (CTLA-4) as a critical immune target led to the development of ipilimumab, a novel anti-CTLA-4 monoclonal antibody for metastatic melanoma. Ipilimumab is a major breakthrough in the field of immuno-oncology. This chapter focuses on the development of ipilimumab, the early clinical success, and the pivotal phase III trials that led to the U.S. Food and Drug Administration (FDA) approval in 2011. Emphasis is placed on its novel mechanism of action, immune-related toxicity profile, and detailed toxicity management guidelines. The differences between tumor-directed cytotoxic therapies and immune therapies are highlighted. Ipilimumab is the first of a new class of T-cell antibodies that are shifting the paradigm of cancer treatment. These novel immunotherapies are opening the door for possible success across a wide variety of cancers.

Keywords: melanoma, immunotherapy, ipilimumab, T cell

*Corresponding author, Department of Medical Oncology, The Beverly Hills Cancer Center, 8900 Wilshire Blvd., Beverly Hills, CA

E-mail address: soday@bhcancercenter.com

Emerging Cancer Therapeutics 3:3 (2012) 517–530.
DOI: 10.5003/2151–4194.3.3.517

INTRODUCTION

The discovery of cytotoxic T-lymphocyte associated antigen-4 (CTLA-4), its recognition as a critical immunotherapy target, and the development of the novel oncology drug ipilimumab is a remarkable story. Ipilimumab, a human monoclonal antibody blocking CTLA-4, was approved by the U.S. Food and Drug Administration (FDA) for the treatment of metastatic melanoma in March 2011. The success of ipilimumab revitalized the field of immuno-oncology and expanded the scope of immunotherapy beyond melanoma. Investigators have launched clinical studies with ipilimumab across a wide variety of solid tumors.

CYTOTOXIC T-LYMPHOCYTE ASSOCIATED ANTIGEN-4 AS AN IMMUNE TARGET

CTLA-4 is a T-cell receptor (TCR). It is a naturally occurring, negative regulator of the immune system. CTLA-4 has a central role both in shaping T-cell responses and maintaining peripheral tolerance, thereby preventing autoimmune disease. CTLA-4 is important in limiting antitumor responses during tumor genesis and progression (1,2). CTLA-4 is expressed on activated helper T-cells and cytotoxic T lymphocytes (CTL). It inhibits T-cell activation and proliferation by binding to the B7 molecule on the surface of the antigen presenting cell (APC) with higher affinity than CD28. By this process, CTLA-4 operates as a brake on T-cell proliferation (3).

T-CELL ACTIVATION AND INHIBITION

T-cell activation is a multistep process. The first step is the binding of the peptide-major histocompatibility complex (MHC), displayed by APCs, to the TCR on its surface. This step is required but not sufficient for activation. The second or costimulatory signal is also required. During signal 2, CD28, expressed on T-cells binds to the B7 molecules expressed on the APCs surface. This results in T-cell activation and proliferation, and secondary cytokine release initiating the adaptive immune response.

Forty-eight to seventy-two hours after T-cell activation, CTLA-4 moves from the T-cell cytoplasm to the surface, binding to B7 on the APC with higher affinity than CD28 and inducing an inhibitory effect on T-cell activation and proliferation. Deactivated T-cells then go into memory and wait for the next antigenic challenge. This on/off function of T-cells is exquisitely balanced to efficiently clear foreign antigens while preventing autoimmunity (1) (Figure 1).

IPILIMUMAB: HUMAN ANTI-CTLA-4 ANTIBODY

Ipilimumab is a fully human IgG1 anti-CTLA-4 monoclonal antibody that fixes complement. Unlike immune cytokines that are indirect in the immune activation, ipilimumab has a direct endogenous effect on T-cells. Blocking CTLA-4 induces targeted T-cell activation and proliferation. This prolongs and potentiates T-cell activity against tumor cells (4,5).

Ipilimumab Preclinical Data

Antitumor activity of CTLA-4 blockade has been demonstrated in multiple murine tumor models (6,7). CTLA-4 blockade elicits an effective antitumor response and rejection of preestablished tumors. It is important to note that this blockade inhibits tumor growth in a variety of tumor types. The immune response to CTLA-4

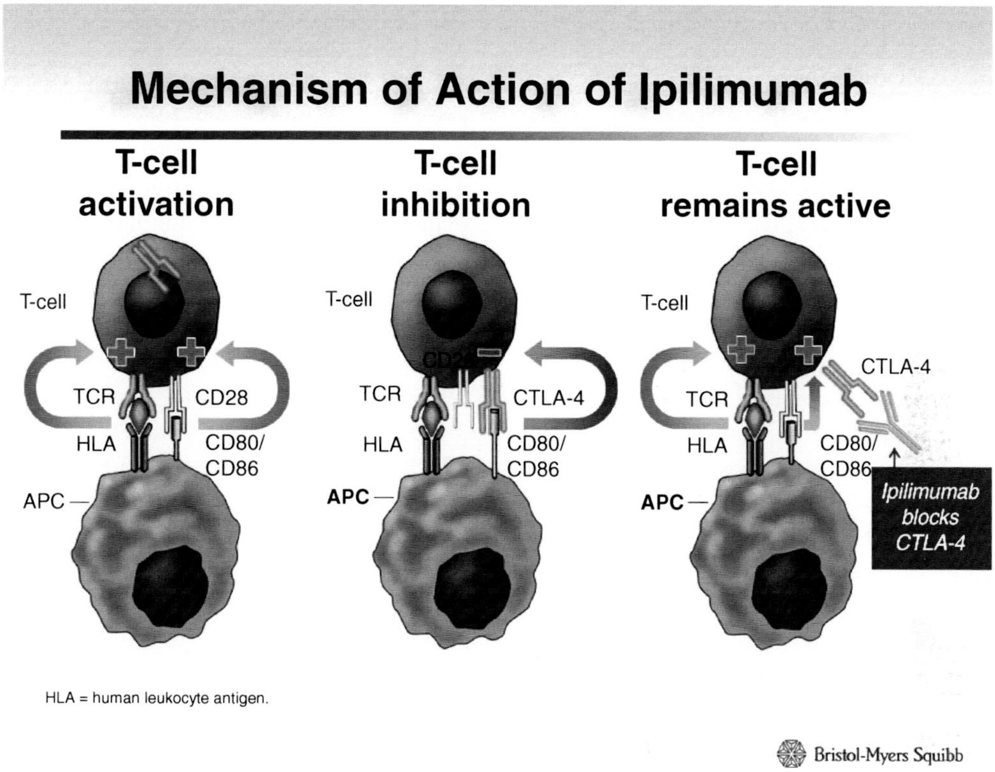

Mechanism of Action of Ipilimumab

FIGURE 1
Mechanism of action of ipilimumab.
Adapted from O'Day S, et al. Presented at: ASCO Annual Meeting; June 4–8, 2010; Chicago, IL.

blockade in murine models results in T-cell proliferation and an increased ratio of effector to regulatory T-cells. Effector T-cells are the primary target of CTLA-4 blockade. CTLA-4 knockout mice develop overwhelming lymphocytosis, organ infiltration, and death. Immunity to a secondary exposure to tumor cells suggests the presence of memory T-cells (8).

Ipilimumab Early Phase I and II Trials

In 1999, the first fully human monoclonal antibody to block CTLA-4 was developed by Medarex, and this led to the first human trial in 2000. Early phase I/II studies with ipilimumab were performed at the National Cancer Institute (NCI) and other selected melanoma centers from 2000 to 2004. These studies included both single- and multiple-dose regimens. In addition, ipilimumab combinations with GP100 peptide vaccine, high-dose interleukin-2 (IL-2), and dacarbazine (DTIC) were initiated. Ipilimumab monotherapy dose levels ranged from 0.1 to 20 mg/kg. Multidose safety was established at doses of 3 mg/kg in combination with vaccine and high-dose bolus IL-2. Immune-related toxicity was observed in a subgroup of patients, the most important being immune colitis (9,10).

Two other early phase I and II studies of note were performed. The first was a 3 arm PHASE I/II study evaluating both dose and schedule. Single doses of ipilimumab were escalated from 7.5 to 20 mg/kg safely. Multiple doses were evaluated at a 3 and an 8 week schedule. The optimal dose and schedule seemed to be 10 mg/kg dose given at 3 week intervals for 4 doses. Complete and partial responses were demonstrated, and a favorable disease control rate ([DCR]; complete remission [CR], partial remission [PR], stable disease [SD] of 39% was observed (11). The second study was a small multicenter randomized phase II trial with ipilimumab dosed at 3 mg/kg in combination with dacarbazine. Objective responses were observed in both arms, but there seemed to be more activity in the combination arm. No new toxicity signals were noted with the combination (12).

The phase I and II trials were too small to make any firm conclusions about efficacy, but there was clearly a strong early positive signal. Objective tumor responses were observed in approximately 15% of the patients and included both complete and partial responses. The vast majority of these responses were durable, with ongoing responses noted from 11+ to 34+ months. Many responders were beyond 1 year, and 2 year responders were also reported. In marked contrast with the high-dose IL-2 experience at the NCI, partial responses from ipilimumab were as durable as complete responses. Stable disease was equally durable in the majority of patients. Immune-related toxicities were apparent in a subset of patients. These could be life threatening, particularly colitis and hepatitis. Treatment-related deaths were reported in a small number of patients. The use of high-dose steroids for severe toxicity management was successful in the vast majority of cases.

Ipilimumab Late Phase II Trials

A series of important larger phase II trials were performed, which further defined the efficacy and toxicity profile of ipilimumab. These studies investigated the dose response and the concept of maintenance therapy. The first, Bristol Myer Squibb protocol 022 (BMS022), was a randomized phase II study of ipilimumab at 3 dose levels 0.3, 3, and 10 mg/kg given every 3 weeks for 4 doses (induction therapy), followed by maintenance dosing at 3 month intervals in responding patients. Two hundred seventeen patients were randomized. There was clear evidence of dose response, with objective response rates of 0%, 4.2%, and 11.1%, respectively, with 0.3, 3, and 10 mg/kg ($P = .0015$). The DCR was 13.7%, 26.4%, and 29.2%, respectively. Two year survival was 18.4%, 24.2%, and 29.8%, respectively. The conclusions from this study were that there was a clear dose response with ipilimumab for the overall response and disease control, favoring the 10 mg dose level. Two year overall survival differences were less impressive for 10 mg compared with 3 mg, although a trend was present. The spectrum of toxicity was similar between 3 and 10 mg, but the overall toxicity was slightly increased at the 10 mg dose level (13).

A larger multicenter global phase II ipilimumab study was performed in second-line metastatic treatment ($N = 155$) using 10 mg/kg induction, followed by maintenance therapy every 3 months. The objective response rate for this trial was only 5.8%, but the DCR was approximately 30%, and the median overall survival was 10.2 months, with 2 year overall survival of 32.8%. This 2 year survival data was impressive in a poor-risk group of advanced melanoma patients (14).

Another randomized placebo-controlled phase II trial ($N = 115$) was performed, combining budesonide with ipilimumab in efforts to reduce immune-related colitis. Budesonide is an oral corticosteroid with minimal systemic absorption. Ipilimumab was dosed at 10 mg/kg. Budesonide did not reduce immune-related gastrointestinal toxicity and did not affect efficacy.

Objective tumor response and DCRs were consistent with previous studies. The median overall survival of 18 to 19 months was impressive, as was the 2 year survival of 40% to 45% (15).

Ipilimumab Phase III Trials

The first large phase III ipilimumab trial results were presented at the plenary session of the American Society of Clinical Oncology (ASCO) 2010 and simultaneously published in the *New England Journal of Medicine* (NEJM) (16). Six hundred seventy-six patients with previously treated metastatic melanoma were randomized to 1 of the following 3 treatment arms: (a) ipilimumab 3 mg/kg with gp100 vaccine; (b) ipilimumab 3 mg/kg/placebo; or (c) gp100 vaccine/placebo. All patients were required to be human leukocyte antigen 201 (HLA201) because of HLA restrictions of the vaccine. The primary study end point was overall survival.

This landmark study was the first, large, randomized, placebo-controlled trial in metastatic melanoma to demonstrate an improvement in overall survival. The

design was a 3:1:1 randomization favoring the combination arm based on preclinical rationale. No maintenance ipilimumab dosing was allowed. Reinduction of ipilimumab was allowed if patients progressed after initial disease control. Tumor assessment was conducted at weeks 12 and 24 and then every 3 months thereafter.

The 2 ipilimumab arms resulted in a median overall survival of 10 months compared with 6 months for vaccine monotherapy. Two year overall survival in the ipilimumab arms was 24% compared with 14% for the vaccine. The results were both clinically meaningful and highly statistically significant (hazard ratio [HR] 0.66; P = .0026; Figure 2). The survival benefit in this study was consistent across all patient subgroups, including M stage and lactate dehydrogenase. These impressive survival results were achieved despite a statistically significant but relatively low overall response rate of 5% to 10% in the ipilimumab arms compared with 1.5% in the vaccine arm. Complete responses were rare, but the duration of complete or partial responses was impressive. The duration of response in the ipilimumab arms was

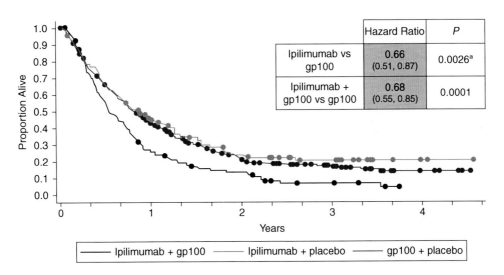

FIGURE 2
Ipilimumab overall survival.

23 and 15 months compared with 3 months in the vaccine arm.

Overall, ipilimumab was well tolerated, but severe immune-related adverse events did occur. The percentage of drug-related grade 3 or 4 adverse events was 17% to 23% in the ipilimumab arms compared with 11% in the vaccine arm. There was also a small increase in drug-related deaths: 3.1% and 2.1% in the ipilimumab arms versus 1.5% in the vaccine arm. The most common sites for immune-related adverse events were skin, gastrointestinal tract, liver, and endocrine organs. Treatment-related deaths were almost exclusively secondary to colitis and hepatitis.

One year after the landmark publication of the ipilimumab study, the results of a second large phase III study was reported in another ASCO plenary session and simultaneously published in *NEJM* (17). This phase III trial randomized 502 first-line metastatic melanoma patients to ipilimumab 10 mg/kg/dacabazine compared with dacarbazine/placebo in a 1:1 fashion. Patients were eligible for maintenance ipilimumab/placebo at 3 month intervals if there was clinical benefit after induction therapy.

The ipilimumab/DTIC combination improved median survival from 9.1 to 11.2 months and 3 year survival from 12.2% to 20.8% (HR for death $P < .001$). Grade 3 or 4 adverse events occurred in 56.3% of the ipilimumab arm versus 27.5% of the chemotherapy-alone arm. The spectrum of ipilimumab toxicities was similar to previous studies, but the incidence of liver function abnormalities was significantly higher in this study. This may have been a result of an ipilimumab interaction with dacarbazine, which has known potential deleterious hepatic effects. On the contrary, the incidence of gastrointestinal events was lower in the ipilimumab/DTIC combination than previous ipilimumab monotherapy studies. No drug-related deaths or gastrointestinal perforations occurred. The study clearly established the role of ipilimumab as first-line therapy in metastatic melanoma and complemented the second-line study previously reported, demonstrating both a median and long-term survival advantage for ipilimumab.

Ipilimumab Adjuvant Therapy

Ipilimumab's improvement of overall survival in the metastatic setting led to great interest in studying its effects in the adjuvant setting where risk of recurrence and death remains high. High-dose interferon is the only FDA-approved drug for high-risk American Joint Cancer Commission stage IIB and III melanoma patients. Despite a consistent disease-free survival (DFS) benefit for interferon multiple studies, interferon has failed to consistently produce an overall survival benefit. When present, the absolute survival benefit has been small and associated with considerable toxicity and extended therapy (18) A large ipilimumab phase III adjuvant trial in high-risk stage III melanoma has completed accrual in 2011. It was conducted by the European Organization for Research and Treatment of Cancer (EROTC) and was a global effort. Initial results are anticipated in the next 12 to 18 months.

Ipilimumab Immune-Related Adverse Events

Early in the course of the development of ipilimumab, it was noted that toxicity was related to the drug's mechanism of action. In addition to the desired tumor inflammation, it was clear that, in some cases, T-cells lost tolerance to self-antigens and normal tissues. These tissues then became the unintended source of an immune inflammatory attack. The majority of toxicity is mild to moderate grade 1 and 2 and can symptomatically be managed with supportive care. However, approximately 15% to 20% of the patients will experience more severe grade 3 or 4 toxicity (19–21). The most common sites of tissue inflammation are skin, gastrointestinal tract, liver, and endocrine organs, particularly the pituitary gland. However, any tissue or organ site seems vulnerable to immune inflammation. Therefore, a high level of clinical suspicion is required for good toxicity management. Skin toxicity generally seems earliest usually after the first or second treatment. Gastrointestinal, liver, and endocrine toxicities more commonly appear after the third or fourth dose. It is important to note that some toxicity may begin after the completion of treatment between weeks 12 and 18. Close toxicity follow-up management during this time is imperative. If appropriate toxicity treatment is not initiated or significantly delayed, these immune-related adverse events can become life threatening. Drug-related deaths were 2% to 3% in many of the ipilimumab studies. Because toxicity management guidelines were developed in the later trials, treatment-related morbidity and mortality substantially decreased (22).

Dermatitis

Immune-mediated rash is a common side effect of ipilimumab treatment occurring in approximately 1/3 of patients. The skin toxicity can have a wide array of presentations. Pruritus without rash is not uncommon. The rash, when it presents, is typically a maculopapular eruption that is often pruritic. It most commonly involves the trunk and extremities and usually spares the face. It is rarely actiniform. Most rashes are grade 1 or 2 in severity, with <5% grade 3 or 4. Rarely (<1%) more severe skin reactions, including toxic epidermal necrolysis or Stevens Johnson Syndrome, have been reported.

If the dermatitis is mild, symptomatic treatment with oral antipruritic or topical steroids to affected areas can be used. If more extensive or symptomatic, a short course of oral steroids may be necessary. Very rarely do high-dose steroids ever need to be used or therapy discontinued because of skin toxicity.

Gastrointestinal

Ipilimumab can affect any portion of the gastrointestinal tract, but the colon is, by far, the most common and important site for management. Diarrhea is the presenting symptom and occurs in approximately 30% of patients. Half of these cases are grade 1 or 2, and the other half is grade 3 or 4. The onset of diarrhea typically occurs after the third or fourth dose, but it can occur even after treatment is complete. The clinical presentation is typically watery diarrhea with some mild abdominal cramping. It can rapidly escalate from several loose bowel moments to 7 to 8 watery bowel movements daily. Bloody or mucous involvement is much less frequent. Fever or peritoneal signs are of concern for more severe colitis or perforation and must aggressively be managed. Stool cultures should be obtained at the onset of diarrhea to rule out infectious etiologies or clostridium difficile colitis. Flexible sigmoidoscopy or colonoscopies were routinely done in the early development of ipilimumab to document immune colitis but should now be reserved for diagnostic dilemmas or specific clinical indications.

If diarrhea is judged to be consistent with immune colitis, and grade 1 or 2 in severity, symptomatic treatment with antimotility agents, dietary modifications, and oral or intravenous rehydration and electrolyte repletion are recommended. If grade 2 diarrhea persists for more than 1 week or becomes clinically significant, intermediate dose corticosteroids

(0.5 mg/kg prednisone) are recommended, with a short taper when symptoms improve. Patients can continue treatment with ipilimumab if grade 2 toxicity resolves to grade 1 or less and corticosteroids have successfully been tapered to less than 7.5 mg prednisone day. If patients develop grade 3 toxicity, high-dose corticosteroids (1–2 mg/kg prednisone) should promptly be initiated. Symptoms should improve in 48 to 72 hours. Once the patient responds to high-dose corticosteroids, it is critical that the dose is slowly tapered over 4 to 6 weeks, because more abrupt tapers lead to relapse of the colitis in a high percentage of patients. Fluid and electrolyte management is critical during this period, and a combination of intensive outpatient follow-up or inpatient treatment may be required. If the patient does not respond to oral corticosteroids, they should be admitted for intravenous (IV) corticosteroids after 48 to 72 hours. Approximately 90% of patients with grade 3 or 4 colitis will respond to oral or IV high-dose corticosteroid therapy. In patients that do not, tumor necrosis factor inhibitors such as infliximab have been highly effective at a single dose of 5 mg/kg. A second dose may need to be repeated 4 to 6 weeks later. Patients who experience grade 3 or 4 colitis even if effectively managed should not be retreated with ipilimumab and should permanently be discontinued for therapy.

Hepatitis

Immune hepatitis is an uncommon side effect from ipilimumab but can rapidly develop and requires careful monitoring. Immune hepatitis presents with a classic transaminitis that may otherwise be asymptomatic or can involve right upper quadrant or upper gastrointestinal symptoms. It occurs in approximately 5% of cases and is more typical after the third or fourth dose. However, it can occur anytime during or immediately after completion of ipilimumab treatment. Viral etiologies, medication interactions, or tumor causes for the hepatitis should be excluded at the time of initial rise of liver function tests (LFT). If grade 1 or 2 elevations occur, supportive care alone is recommended. If grade 2 elevations persist beyond 1 week, intermediate-dose corticosteroids may be used (0.5 mg/kg prednisone) with a short taper. Patients may continue ipilimumab treatment if the toxicity reduces to grade 1 or less and dose of prednisone is 7.5 mg or less at the time of the next dose. If grade 3 or 4 elevations occur, ipilimumab should permanently be discontinued, and high-dose corticosteroids (1–2 mg/kg prednisone) should promptly be initiated. LFT should stabilize within 48 to 72 hours. If not, patients should be hospitalized for IV steroids. After hepatic toxicity has decreased to grade 1 or less, steroids should be tapered over 4 to 6 weeks. About 90% of patients will respond to high-dose corticosteroids. Patients who are corticosteroid refractory usually respond to second-line treatment with the immunosuppressive drug mycophenolate mofetil. If second-line treatment is required, corticosteroids should still be continued and tapered over 4 to 6 weeks. It is very important that LFT be checked before each dose of ipilimumab, because a rapid LFT rise can occur with little or no symptoms, and rare deaths from hepatic failure because of immune hepatitis have occurred.

Endocrinopathies

Immune-mediated endocrinopathies were an unanticipated consequence of ipilimumab therapy in approximately 5% of patients. In the early clinical trials, these patients presented with profound fatigue, frontal headaches, mental status changes, and even double vision. Magnetic resonance imaging of the brain revealed enlarged, edematous pituitary glands without hemorrhage. Blood evaluation generally revealed evidence of pan-hypopituitarism with low adrenocorticotrophic hormone (ACTH), thyroid stimulating hormone (TSH) , free T4 (FT4) and cortisol. Low testosterone was seen in men, resulting in decreased libido and erectile dysfunction. Some patients have additional isolated or concomitant endocrinopathies such as adrenal insufficiency, hypogonadism, hypothyroidism, or hyperthyroidism. Median time to onset in the large phase III trial was 11 weeks and ranged up to 19.3 weeks after the initiation of ipilimumab (16). If the patient presents with headache and acute symptoms, a short course of high-dose steroids followed by endocrine replacement therapy is recommended. Some cases of endocrinopathy will completely resolve, whereas other patients will require long-term hormone replacement.

Although only 5% of patients present with acute endocrine dysfunction, there is a larger group of patients that have mild nonspecific constitutional symptoms. Many of these patients, when evaluated, have more subacute or isolated endocrine dysfunction. These patients can avoid high-dose steroids and successfully be treated with endocrine replacement therapy alone. Baseline endocrine tests should be performed before starting ipilimumab and at 12 week intervals. Endocrine levels can more frequently be checked if more subtle endocrine signs and symptoms appear, particularly nonspecific constitutional symptoms such as fatigue and sexual dysfunction. Patients can safely continue treatment with ipilimumab after diagnosis and endocrine replacement therapy, as long as the prednisone dose is 7.5 mg or less.

In addition to the 4 most common immune-related toxicities of ipilimumab previously outlined, a wide spectrum of rarer toxicities have been reported, including meningitis, Guillain–Barre syndrome, myocarditis, pericarditis, sarcoid, temporal arteritis, nephritis, pneumonitis, uveitis, hemolytic anemia, psoriasis, pancreatitis, and arthritis. The principles of management remain the same: early recognition, symptomatic management, and early use of corticosteroids for more clinically significant toxicities.

Summary: Ipilimumab Immune Toxicity Management Guidelines

Immune toxicity management guidelines have been established and are summarized below:

Grade 1: Symptomatic management and close clinical follow-up. Continue ipilimumab dosing on schedule.

Grade 2: Symptomatic management initially. If prolonged more than 1 week or clinically significant, consider intermediate dose steroid 0.5 mg/kg prednisone equivalent day. Hold ipilimumab doses until prednisone dose is less than or equal to 7.5 mg a day and toxicity has reduced to grade 1 or less. Delivery of all 4 ipilimumab doses within 16 weeks.

Grade 3 or 4: Discontinue ipilimumab and initiate high-dose steroids 1 to 2 mg/kg prednisone equivalent followed by a minimum 4 week taper after toxicity has resolved to grade 1 or less. Patients with endocrine or skin toxicity may be considered for further treatment in select cases. Patients with liver or gastrointestinal grade 3 or 4 immune-related toxicity should permanently be discontinued from ipilimumab treatment.

Immuno-Oncology Paradigm Shift

Recent advances in specific T-cell antibody therapies, in particular the successful development of ipilimumab, has led to a remarkable shift in the cancer treatment paradigm. This shift is manifest in a new appreciation for clinically meaningful efficacy end points in immunotherapy drug development, an appreciation for the kinetics of the immune response, and the relationship between mechanism of action, toxicity, and clinical benefit.

The traditional treatment of advanced solid tumors focuses on tumor directed cytotoxic treatments. These therapies result in variable short-term tumor regression but marginal, if any, benefit in survival. Complete remissions and long-term survival are rare. Tumor heterogeneity and early treatment resistance are formidable challenges. Combinations or high doses of these treatment strategies generally fail to improve long-term outcome.

Ipilimumab, by contrast, elegantly targets a critical off-tumor target, effector T-cells of the human immune system. In contrast with traditional tumor directed therapies, overt tumor regression is relatively infrequent. Nevertheless, ipilimumab has profound effects on median and long-term survival. This is because ipilimumab results in durable disease control and stabilization in approximately 1/3 of patients. DCRs at 6 and 12 months are far better surrogates of overall and long-term survival and should correlate better with overall survival in future immunotherapy trials. The gold standard remains 2 and 3 year survival rates, which frequently reflect the "tail" or "plateau" of survival curve. Because a relative minority of patients seems to have a profound effect on the survival curves, there is tremendous need for predictive markers of clinical benefit. To date, reliable markers remain elusive but continue to be an intensive area of research.

Understanding and appreciating the kinetics and patterns of the immune response are additional valuable contributions arising from the successful development of ipilimumab. In general, the immune response takes months, not weeks, to fully develop. This is understandable, given that an army of T-cells need to proliferate, activate, and reach the tumor microenvironment. Once in the microenvironment, T-cells must overcome a plethora of tumor directed immune defenses. An understanding of the kinetics of tumor responses to ipilimumab evolved over the course of the early and late phase I/II studies and was further confirmed in the larger phase III trials. A keen awareness of the biology of the individual melanoma and the pace and sites of metastases are critical to making the most informed decisions about changing to an alternative treatment between week 12 and 24 weeks after ipilimumab therapy (23–26). Several different response patterns have been identified to date. The first is a relatively classic early durable response in the first 12 weeks. These patients are straightforward to manage. Approximately 5% to 10% of patients will have this favorable pattern. Another 15% to 20% of patients will have minor regression, stable disease, minor progression, or a mixed response at week 12. In these cases, it is extremely helpful to understand the pace of their disease and the pattern of their metastases before commencing ipilimumab to make optimal treatment decisions. Observation alone during the critical weeks 12 to 24 may be the best approach for these patients to allow the immune response to declare itself fully. It is important to note that many patients in this subgroup will stop developing new sites of metastases during this timeframe. Last, there are approximately 5% to 10% of patients with frank progressive disease at week 12 who, by week 24, will stabilize, and many will have long-term disease control equal to rapid responders.

These patients have been described as "late responders." The second and third categories of immune responses led to the immune-related response criteria, a modification of the response evaluation criteria in solid tumors assessment (27).

Early in the development of ipilimumab, there was recognition of the relationship between mechanism of action and immune-related adverse events. This facilitated toxicity management and the development of toxicity management guidelines. Later in the development, there was confirmation that immune-related events against normal tissues were associated with improved clinical benefit. This has been recognized in immunotherapy trials, particularly with high-dose interferon in the adjuvant and IL-2 and biochemotherapy in the metastatic setting (28–30).

Lutzky et al. evaluated the patients who developed an immune-related adverse event from 2 large Phase II trials (Bristol Myer Squibb protocol 008 [BMS008], 022); patients who had an immune event had a median overall survival of 14.8 months versus 8.21 months for patients who did not have an immune-related adverse event (31).

More prospective clinical trials need to be designed, evaluating the relationship between toxicity and outcome. Although not a predictive maker, immune-related adverse events may be helpful as a dynamic, intermediate marker of clinical benefit in future trials.

Associating autoimmunity with clinical benefit was a relatively easy observation based on previous immunotherapy experience. However, the observation that corticosteroid rescue of immune toxicity would not interfere with the antitumor immune response was a more challenging lesson to learn. There was a strong bias to withhold steroids for moderate or severe toxicity in the early clinical experience with ipilimumab because of concern that steroids would nullify the antitumor effects and lead to a more rapid progression and death from melanoma. This approach was based on an extensive clinical experience with corticosteroids and melanoma. It is well known that immunosuppressed patients have a higher incidence of melanoma and a more virulent clinical course after developing melanoma. Because of this concern, administration of steroids frequently was delayed in early management, particularly in the setting of colitis. This delay could have led to more severe bowel involvement and perforation. When studies reported deaths from colitis and bowel perforation, earlier intervention was advised, and a higher vigilance ensued. The death rate from colitis complications considerably decreased, and overall toxicity management was improved.

With the transition to early and more aggressive use of steroids for more severe immune-related toxicities came the clinical observation that ongoing tumor responses did not seem to be affected by the corticosteroids. It seems that, once significant immune toxicity develops, T-cells directed against tumor antigens are more resistant to the apoptotic effects of corticosteroids compared with T-cells directed at self antigens. It must be noted that more rigorous immunological translational studies will be necessary to corroborate these clinical observations.

Future Ipilimumab Clinical Questions and New Combination Trials

Important questions of dose and schedule and the value of ipilimumab maintenance therapy are actively being addressed in current and planned trials. A large international phase III study recently completed accrual, comparing 3 mg with 10 mg/kg dosing. Although maintenance ipilimumab remains an open clinical question, reinduction of ipilimumab after clinical benefit seems effective, with 50% to 75% of these patients obtaining a second clinical benefit from ipilimumab that is often durable (16).

The most exciting new T-cell antibody that has emerged in recent years is anti-PD-1 antibody (32,33). Phase I and II studies have recently procupdated at ASCO 2012 and are highly encouraging (34). Programed death-1 (PD-1), like CTLA-4, is an inhibitory TCR. B blocking it has led to tumor regression and disease control, which has been remarkably durable not only in patients with melanoma but also in patients with renal cell carcinoma, non–small cell lung cancer, and a variety of other solid tumors. Objective tumor regression in melanoma with PD-1 is higher than seen with ipilimumab to date. Although the follow-up is certainly shorter than ipilimumab, the majority of PD-1 responses have been durable and some extend beyond 2 years at present. PD-1 responses have been seen in ipilimumab failures, and vice versa. Toxicity, overall, has considerably been less than seen with ipilimumab, although a similar spectrum of immune-related toxicities have been observed. Phase III trials are rapidly being planned with this new target of the immune system.

In addition to rapid development of PD1 as monotherapy, there is great interest in combining PD-1 with ipilimumab, and a phase I study has recently begun. In addition to inhibitory antibodies such as anti-CTLA-4 and anti-PD1, agonistic stimulatory antibodies to CD137 and CD40 on T-cells have been developed and are entering early human trials. Soon, we will be able to manipulate the immune system *in vivo* with cocktails of T-cell antibodies, both stimulatory and inhibitory.

The success of ipilimumab in metastatic melanoma has closely been tied with the success of a second FDA-approved drug for metastatic melanoma, vemurafinib, a selective serine-threonine protein kinase (BRAF) inhibitor. BRAF mutations are present in approximately 50% of cutaneous melanoma. Inhibition of the BRAF pathway leads to rapid, remarkable tumor regression and disease control in almost 90% of patients. This has led to improvement in the overall survival in randomized trials and rapid approval by the FDA in late September 2011 (35).

Ipilimumab and vemurafinib both have improved survivals in metastatic melanoma. Nevertheless, that is where the similarity ends. The 2 drugs could not be more different in terms of the following factors: (a) the percentage of patients with tumor regression; (b) the kinetics of the response; (c) predictive markers; (e) durability of response; (f) target of attack; and (g) duration of treatment. Vemurafinib leads to rapid tumor regression within days to weeks, but the durability of responses are relatively short (median 6 months), often with rapid progression and death thereafter. Early resistance is being aggressively studied, and activation of BRAF's MAP kinase (MAPK) pathway through MEK seems to contribute to early resistance in a large number of cases. MEK inhibitors added to BRAF inhibitors seem very promising and may prevent early resistance and improve outcomes.

In BRAF-mutant melanoma, the important clinical question is whether combining ipilimumab with vemurafinib is better than sequential treatment. If sequential treatment is better, one important question will be which sequence is optimal. These studies are underway. Obviously, in patients with multifocal, rapidly progressive disease that is symptomatic, BRAF inhibition is a straightforward clinical decision. In less symptomatic patients, who have time to develop an immune response, the proper sequence of drugs is much more complex.

■ FINAL THOUGHTS

The successful development and FDA approval of ipilimumab in metastatic melanoma has been a paradigm-shifting revolution in immuno-oncology. It has ushered in the brave new world of T-cell human monoclonal antibodies. It has shattered the myth that immunotherapies must be limited to the minimal-disease-burden setting or to low-volume, highly selected metastatic disease. Now, patients with widespread disease can be considered for treatment. These treatments can safely be given in the outpatient clinic and evaluated in rigorous clinical trials. We have understood the kinetics and patterns of an immune response better. Moreover, ipilimumab has informed us about the relationship between mechanism of action, toxicity, and clinical benefit. Corticosteroid management of severe toxicity has improved safety and has not interfered with tumor control. The field is now open to the possibility that melanoma and renal cell carcinoma are not the only solid tumors that can benefit from immunotherapy treatment strategies. Ultimately, rigorous clinical trials are required to determine benefit across nonmelanoma solid tumors. It is also important to note that the intellectual capital invested collaboratively by the industry and academia in the development of ipilimumab should well serve the future development of other exciting immunotherapies.

■ REFERENCES

1. Gabriel EM, Lattime EC. Anti-CTL-associated antigen 4: are regulatory T cells a target? *Clin Cancer Res.* 2007;13(3):785–788.

2. Queirolo P, Acquati M. Targeted therapies in melanoma. *Cancer Treat Rev.* 2006;32(7):524–531.

3. Sharpe AH, Abbas AK. T-cell costimulation–biology, therapeutic potential, and challenges. *N Engl J Med.* 2006;355(10):973–975.

4. Fong L, Small EJ. Anti-cytotoxic T-lymphocyte antigen-4 antibody: the first in an emerging class of immunomodulatory antibodies for cancer treatment. *J Clin Oncol.* 2008;26(32):5275–5283.

5. Hoos A, Ibrahim R, Korman A, et al. Development of ipilimumab: contribution to a new paradigm for cancer immunotherapy. *Semin Oncol.* 2010;37(5):533–546.

6. Leach DR, Krummel MF, Allison JP. Enhancement of antitumor immunity by CTLA-4 blockade. *Science.* 1996;271(5256):1734–1736.

7. Korman AJ, Peggs KS, Allison JP. Checkpoint blockade in cancer immunotherapy. *Adv Immunol.* 2006;90:297–339.

8. Peggs KS, Quezada SA, Chambers CA, Korman AJ, Allison JP. Blockade of CTLA-4 on both effector and regulatory T cell compartments contributes to the antitumor activity of anti-CTLA-4 antibodies. *J Exp Med.* 2009;206(8):1717–1725.

9. Attia P, Phan GQ, Maker AV, et al. Autoimmunity correlates with tumor regression in patients with metastatic melanoma treated with anti-cytotoxic T-lymphocyte antigen-4. *J Clin Oncol.* 2005;23(25):6043–6053.

10. Maker AV, Phan GQ, Attia P, et al. Tumor regression and autoimmunity in patients treated with cytotoxic T lymphocyte-associated antigen 4 blockade and interleukin 2: a phase I/II study. *Ann Surg Oncol.* 2005;12(12):1005–1016.

11. Weber JS, O'Day S, Urba W, et al. Phase I/II study of ipilimumab for patients with metastatic melanoma. *J Clin Oncol.* 2008;26(36):5950–5956.

12. Fischkoff SA, Hersh E, Weber J, et al. Durable responses and long-term progression-free survival observed in a phase II study of MDX-010 alone or in combination with dacarbazine (DTIC) in metastatic melanoma. *J Clin Oncol.* 2005;23(Suppl 16). Abstract 7525.

13. Wolchok JD, Neyns B, Linette G, et al. Ipilimumab monotherapy in patients with pretreated advanced melanoma: a randomised, double-blind, multicentre, phase 2, dose-ranging study. *Lancet Oncol.* 2010;11(2):155–164.

14. O'Day SJ, Maio M, Chiarion-Sileni V, et al. Efficacy and safety of ipilimumab monotherapy in patients with pretreated advanced melanoma: a multicenter single-arm phase II study. *Ann Oncol.* 2010;21(8):1712–1717.

15. Weber J, Thompson JA, Hamid O, et al. A randomized, double-blind, placebo-controlled, phase II study comparing the tolerability and efficacy of ipilimumab administered with or without prophylactic budesonide in patients with unresectable stage III or IV melanoma. *Clin Cancer Res.* 2009; 15(17):5591–5598.

16. Hodi FS, O'Day SJ, McDermott DF, et al. Improved survival with ipilimumab in patients with metastatic melanoma. *N Engl J Med.* 2010;363(8):711–723.

17. Robert C, Thomas L, Bondarenko I, et al. Ipilimumab plus dacarbazine for previously untreated metastatic melanoma. *N Engl J Med.* 2011;364(26):2517–2526.

18. Kirkwood JM, Manola J, Ibrahim J, Sondak V, Ernstoff MS, Rao U. A pooled analysis of eastern cooperative oncology group and intergroup trials of adjuvant high-dose interferon for melanoma. *Clin Cancer Res.* 2004;10(5):1670–1677.

19. Beck KE, Blansfield JA, Tran KQ, et al. Enterocolitis in patients with cancer after antibody blockade of cytotoxic T-lymphocyte-associated antigen 4. *J Clin Oncol.* 2006;24(15):2283–2289.

20. Agarwala SS. Current systemic therapy for metastatic melanoma. *Expert Rev Anticancer Ther.* 2009;9(5):587–595.

21. Weber J. Ipilimumab: controversies in its development, utility and autoimmune adverse events. *Cancer Immunol Immunother.* 2009; 58(5):823–830.

22. Hamid O, Hwu WJ, Richards JM, et al. Ipilimumab Expanded Access Program (EAP) for patients with stage III/IV melanoma: 10 mg/kg cohort interim results. Presented at: the American Society of Clinical Oncology (ASCO) Annual Meeting: Collaborating to Conquer Cancer; June 1–5, 2012; Chicago, IL.

23. Finn OJ. Molecular origins of cancer: cancer immunology. *New Engl J Med.* 2008;358:2704–2715.

24. Hoos A, Parmiani G, Hege K, et al. A clinical development paradigm for cancer vaccines and related biologics. *J Immunother.* 2007;30(1):1–15.

25. Fong L, Small EJ. Anti-cytotoxic T-lymphocyte antigen-4 antibody: the first in an emerging class of immunomodulatory antibodies for cancer treatment. *J Clin Oncol.* 2008; 26(32):5275–5283.

26. Weber JS, O'Day S, Urba W, et al. Phase I/II study of ipilimumab for patients with metastatic melanoma. *J Clin Oncol.* 2008;26(36):5950–5956.

27. Wolchuk JD, Hoos A, O'Day S, et al. Guidelines for the evaluation of immune therapy activity in solid tumors: immune-related response criteria. *Clin Cancer Res.* 2009;15(23):7412–7420.

28. Gogas H, Ioannovich J, Dafni U, et al. Prognostic significance of autoimmunity during treatment of melanoma with interferon. *N Engl J Med.* 2006;354(7):709–718.

29. Atkins MB, Mier JW, Parkinson DR, Gould JA, Berkman EM, Kaplan MM. Hypothyroidism after treatment with interleukin-2 and lymphokine-activated killer cells. *N Engl J Med.* 1988;318(24):1557–1563.

30. Boasberg PD, Hoon DS, Piro LD, et al. Enhanced survival associated with vitiligo expression during maintenance biotherapy for metastatic melanoma. *J Invest Dermatol.* 2006;126(12):2658–2663.

31. Lutzky J, Wolchok J, Hamid O, et al. Association between immune-related adverse events (irAEs) and disease control or overall survival in patients (pts) with advanced melanoma treated with 10 mg/kg ipilimumab in three phase II clinical trials. Presented at: the American Society of Clinical Oncology (ASCO) Annual Meeting; May 29–June 2, 2009; Orlando, FL. *J Clin Oncol.* 2009;27(15s):Suppl; Abstract 9034.

32. Nurieva RI, Liu X, Dong C. Yin-Yang of costimulation: crucial controls of immune tolerance and function. *Immunol Rev.* 2009;229(1):88–100.

33. Hamanishi J, Mandai M, Iwasaki M, et al. Programmed cell death 1 ligand 1 and tumor-infiltrating CD8+ T lymphocytes are prognostic factors of human ovarian cancer. *Proc Natl Acad Sci USA.* 2007;104(9):3360–3365.

34. Topalian SL, Hodi FS, Brahmer JR, et al. Safety, activity, and immune correlates of anti-PD-1 antibody in cancer. *N Engl J Med.* 2012;366(26):2443–2454.

35. Flaherty KT, Robert C, Hersey P, et al. Improved survival with MEK inhibition in BRAF-mutated melanoma. *N Engl J Med.* 2012;367(2):107–114.

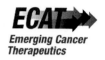

Adoptive Cell Transfer Immunotherapy for Patients With Metastatic Melanoma

Crystal J. Hessman,* Ashley A. Stewart, Akemi D. Miller, James C. Yang, and Steven A. Rosenberg

Surgery Branch, National Cancer Institute, Bethesda, MD

■ ABSTRACT

Cancer immunotherapy using adoptive cell transfer (ACT) of autologous tumor-infiltrating lymphocytes (TIL) has emerged as one of the most effective therapies for patients with metastatic melanoma, resulting in objective tumor regression in 49% to 72% of patients when administered in combination with a lymphodepleting preparative regimen. With increased lymphodepletion, complete tumor regression has been achieved in up to 40% of patients with ongoing durable responses beyond 3 to 7 years. New approaches to cell transfer using genetically engineered peripheral blood lymphocytes (PBL) that express conventional or chimeric T-cell receptors (TCRs) have increased the applicability of ACT and mediated significant regression in patients with metastatic melanoma, synovial sarcoma, and refractory lymphoma. This chapter will discuss the development of ACT and the more recent advances that are currently under investigation.

Keywords: adoptive cell therapy, tumor infiltrating lymphocytes, immunotherapy, metastatic melanoma

*Corresponding author, Surgery Branch, National Cancer Institute, 10 Center Drive, CRC, Building 10, Room 3–1730, Bethesda, MD

E-mail address: crystal.hessman@gmail.com

Emerging Cancer Therapeutics 3:3 (2012) 531–546.
© 2012 Demos Medical Publishing LLC. All rights reserved.
DOI: 10.5003/2151–4194.3.3.531

■ INTRODUCTION

Cancer immunotherapy for treatment of patients with metastatic melanoma aims at enhancing or inducing effector cells of the immune system to recognize and eradicate melanoma tumor cells. It can be divided into 4 broad categories based on the mechanism of action: nonspecific stimulation of the immune system, immune checkpoint blockade by antibodies, active immunization against tumor antigens through vaccines, and adoptive transfer of antitumor lymphocytes. Stimulation of the immune system can be achieved through either nonspecific activation of immune cells, as seen after the administration of interleukin-2 (IL-2), or a blockade of inhibitory signals to immune cells, as achieved by monoclonal antibodies against cytotoxic T lymphocyte-associated antigen 4 (CTLA-4) or programmed death 1 (PD-1) (1). These immune therapies have been shown to mediate tumor regression in approximately 10% to 15% of patients with metastatic melanoma (2,3). Active immunization against melanoma-related antigens has been performed using vaccination with peptides, dendritic cells, recombinant viruses encoding tumor-associated antigens, and whole tumor cells (3,4). Many attempts have been made to develop effective vaccines against melanoma, but no approach that can reproducibly mediate meaningful regression of tumors has yet been developed (5). Transfer of autologous antitumor lymphocytes to a cancer patient, a process known as adoptive cell transfer (ACT), has been shown to be, perhaps, the most effective form of immunotherapy in metastatic melanoma with objective tumor regression in 49% to 72% of patients and complete responses in up to 40% of patients (Table 1) (6). Lymphocytes currently used in ACT can be derived from stroma of resected tumors (tumor-infiltrating lymphocytes [TIL]) or collected from circulating blood (peripheral blood lymphocytes [PBL]) and genetically engineered to express antitumor T-cell receptors (TCRs). In this chapter, we will review the process of ACT and the basic science that led to its development and helped shape its clinical application.

■ EARLY STUDIES OF ADOPTIVE CELL TRANSFER WITH LYMPHOKINE-ACTIVATED KILLER CELLS

ACT is a process that involves the ex vivo identification, expansion, and activation of tumor-specific lymphocytes, followed by the transfer of these lymphocytes back to the tumor-bearing host (Figure 1) (7,8). The landmark discovery of T-cell growth factor (TCGF; IL-2) in 1976 allowed for the expansion of lymphoid cells to numbers sufficient for investigational research (9). However, studies were limited by the availability of IL-2 until 1984, when the human IL-2 gene was successfully cloned using *Escherichia coli*. This finally permitted mass production of the lymphokine for use in the laboratory and the clinic (10).

Early in vitro studies investigating the expansion of murine tumor–derived lymphocytes using IL-2 led to the discovery that incubation of murine splenic lymphocytes in an IL-2 rich medium resulted in the generation of nonspecific cytotoxic cells, known as lymphokine activated killer (LAK) cells, which were capable of mediating the lysis of fresh, syngeneic sarcomas (11,12). Promising results from in vivo murine trials using IL-2 in combination with LAK cell transfer (13–18) led to clinical trials where combining IL-2 and LAK cells resulted in regression of melanoma and renal cell cancer (13–15). However, a subsequent prospective, randomized trial that compares IL-2 alone with IL-2 plus LAK cells in patients with renal

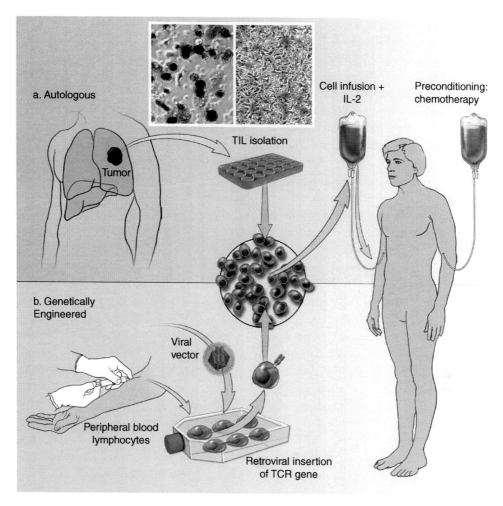

FIGURE 1

Process of adoptive cell therapy using tumor-infiltrating lymphocytes (TIL) (a) or genetically modified peripheral blood lymphocytes (b). The photo inset depicts an enzymatically dispersed melanoma when first cultured (left) and after 2 weeks in interleukin-2 (right). Stromal and tumor cells initially present are replaced by activated proliferating lymphocytes.

cell cancer (N = 97) and melanoma (N = 54) led to the conclusion that tumor responses were largely a result of IL-2 alone (16).

■ ADOPTIVE CELL TRANSFER WITH TUMOR INFILTRATING LYMPHOCYTES

Following work with nonspecific LAK-cell mediated therapy, attention shifted to the identification and isolation of T lymphocytes that can mediate specific, autologous antitumor activity. These lymphocytes are found infiltrating the stroma of tumors and, as such, are referred to as TIL. TIL, unlike LAK cells, are classical T cells with the ability to exhibit lysis and secrete cytokines in response to autologous tumor in a major histocompatibility complex (MHC)-restricted fashion (17–20). In vitro TIL recognition can be blocked by antibodies against the TCR complex or the presenting MHC molecule (21). Subsequent studies demonstrated the ability of some melanoma TIL to recognize other melanomas that shared their restricting human leukocyte antigen (HLA) allele, thereby implying the presence of common tumor antigens among allogeneic melanomas (22,23). In murine models of 3 day old lung and liver metastases from various primaries (sarcoma, carcinoma, and melanoma), the use of TIL resulted in a significant reduction in tumor burden compared with controls after cell infusion (17,18). Similar to LAK cells, coadministered IL-2 augmented tumor response in a dose-dependent manner; however, TIL demonstrated a 50- to 100-fold higher per-cell potency than LAK cells do (18). In cases of macroscopic disease (8 to 14 day old metastases), the TIL/IL-2–mediated antitumor response was further augmented by lymphodepletion using cyclophosphamide before cell infusion (17).

Early on, TIL was generated for ACT from enzymatic digestion of excised tumors into single-cell suspensions that were grown in IL-2 until sufficient cell numbers were attained for transfer (2). TIL were administered, regardless of their antitumor activity as measured by in vitro assays of interferon-γ (IFN-γ) secretion in response to coculture with melanoma cells. However, early analysis demonstrated a significant correlation between clinical response and the in vitro lysis of autologous tumor cells and release of IFN-γ by the administered TIL (24). In response to this, TIL production was modified to use only cultures that were "selected" based on demonstrated in vitro antitumor reactivity.

Compared with endogenous antitumor T cells, ACT has the advantage of overcoming suppressive influences that limit T-cell activity in vivo by allowing for the manipulation of the host environment before cell transfer. In mice, the addition of a lymphodepleting preparative regimen before the transfer of cells led to a dramatic increase in tumor regression. This was first explored in a phase I/II trial that investigated the safety of TIL cells with and without cyclophosphamide in patients with metastatic melanoma (25). At the time of publication in 1994, a total of 86 consecutive patients had been treated (26). Of these 86 patients, 57 received a single dose of cyclophosphamide (25 mg/kg) approximately 36 hours before TIL infusion. After cell infusion, patients received high-dose IL-2 (720,000 IU/kg) through intravenous infusion every 8 hours to a maximum of 15 doses or until the dose-limiting toxicity was reached. Objective responses were observed in 29 patients (34%), with no significant difference in response rates for patients receiving cyclophosphamide (35%) and patients treated without cyclophosphamide (31%). One dose of cyclophosphamide did not result in complete or sustained lymphodepletion. In addition, there was no difference in response rates between patients who had prior IL-2 and those who were IL-2 naive (32% vs. 34%, respectively), implying that these responses were not a result of the IL-2 given with TIL.

These findings led to the investigation of more active regimens, including a nonmyeloablative regimen often used to prepare patients for bone marrow allotransplantation. In this regimen, patients receive cyclophosphamide (60 mg/kg) for 2 consecutive days, followed by fludarabine (25 mg/m²; referred to in this chapter as Cy-Flu) for 5 consecutive days. This Cy-Flu preparative regimen was given to 43 patients with metastatic melanoma before administering TIL and IL-2. Of these patients, 43% had prior chemotherapy, 83% had prior IL-2, and 86% had visceral disease involvement (M1b or M1c disease). These 43 patients had an overall response rate of 49% with a 12% complete response rate, all of which are durable beyond 5 years (6).

Murine studies have shown a direct relationship between the degree of lymphodepletion and the magnitude of in vivo tumor regression after adoptive transfer of TIL (27). The benefit of lymphodepletion is thought to be largely a result of the elimination of suppressive CD4$^+$CD25$^+$T-regulatory lymphocytes (6,28) and the induction of supportive homeostatic cytokine production from nonlymphoid sources (primarily interleukin-7 [IL-7] and IL-15) (8,28). Before Cy-Flu, IL-15 is undetectable in the sera of melanoma patients; however, following Cy-Flu, high levels of IL-15 appear in the blood and provide a growth stimulus to the adoptively transferred lymphocytes (6,8). A murine study by Wrzesinski et al. in 2010 showed a strong correlation between increasing amounts of preparative total body irradiation (TBI) and the regression of large established melanomas when tumor-reactive CD8+ T cells were transferred into a mouse model treated with escalating doses of radiation (with bone marrow support) to a maximum dose of 24 Gy (27). Administering increasing doses of TBI led to greater levels of proinflammatory cytokines, lipopolysaccharide (LPS), and a greater ratio of tumor-reactive CD8+ T cells to endogenous inhibitory T cells. These findings prompted 2 clinical trials that examined increasing levels of lymphodepletion before TIL transfer (6). A total of 50 additional patients with metastatic melanoma were enrolled in the 2 trials. In the first trial, 25 patients received Cy-Flu along with 2-Gy TBI. In a second trial, 25 patients received Cy-Flu along with 12-Gy TBI. Radiation was administered in 2-Gy fractions as either a 1 time dose on the day before cell transfer

(2 Gy arm) or twice daily beginning 3 days before cell transfer (12 Gy arm). Before starting chemotherapy, all TBI patients completed an autologous CD34+ hematopoietic stem cell collection after mobilization with granulocyte colony-stimulating factor. After receiving TBI, patients received autologous TIL cells followed by high-dose IL-2 dosed to tolerance, as done in the prior 43 patients receiving Cy-Flu alone. The CD34+ cells were reinfused 1 or 2 days after TIL transfer. Objective response rates by response evaluation criteria in solid tumors (RECIST) occurred in 49% (21 out of 43) of the patients treated with Cy-Flu alone, whereas 52% (13 out of 52) of the patients in the 2-Gy TBI trial and 72% (18 out of 25) of the patients in the 12-Gy TBI trial achieved partial or complete responses. Complete tumor regression was seen in 12% (5 out of 43) of the patients who received Cy-Flu alone, 20% (5 out of 25) of the patients who received 2-Gy TBI, and 40% (10 out of 25) patients who received 12-Gy TBI. Overall, 19 of the 20 patients with complete regression of tumors had an ongoing response 3 to 7 years later (6). The overall survival of patients in these 3 trials is shown in Figure 2. Tumor regression was seen in all sites of the body, including lung, liver, brain, lymph nodes, subcutaneous tissue, and bone. Examples of these responses are shown in Figure 3. In these 93 patients, there was no effect of prior chemotherapy or immunotherapy on the likelihood of response to TIL.

Despite these promising results, the availability of TIL for treatment in metastatic melanoma may be limited by the complexity of the process required to create, select, and grow individual TIL cultures for each patient. The original process for generating and selecting tumor-reactive TIL requires initial growth of multiple separate microcultures, followed by individualized assays to identify

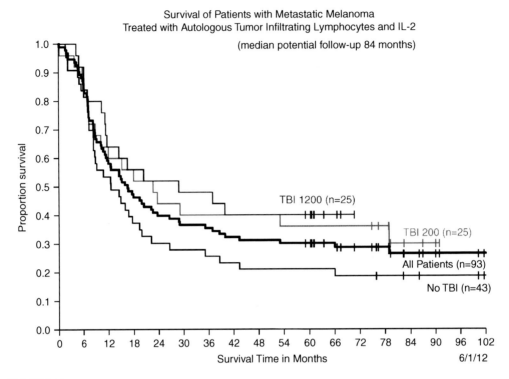

Survival of Patients with Metastatic Melanoma
Treated with Autologous Tumor Infiltrating Lymphocytes and IL-2
(median potential follow-up 84 months)

FIGURE 2

Survival of patients with metastatic melanoma who were treated with adoptive cell therapy in 3 consecutive clinical trials using increasing amounts of lymphodepletion before cell transfer. Forty-three patients received nonmyeloablative (NMA) chemotherapy with Cy-Flu without total body irradiation (TBI), 25 patients received NMA and a single fraction of 200 cGy TBI, and 25 patients received NMA and a total of 1200 cGy TBI. The summary experience with these 93 patients (bold line), after 4.8 to 8 years of follow-up, shows that complete and durable responses could be achieved in approximately 20% of patients.

microcultures with patient-specific tumor recognition by in vitro assay (29). Patients whose TIL fail the test for tumor recognition are ineligible for treatment. Rapid disease progression during the weeks required to grow TIL can also lead to an inability to treat a patient. As reported by Goff et al. (30), the process of producing selected TIL that meet all criteria results in delivering approximately 1 treatment per month and, on the average, only 27% of patients who underwent tumor resection received their TIL product (for a variety of reasons).

The recognition that the complexity of TIL production was a limitation to patient therapy led to the development of "young" TIL. In this process, TIL cultures are minimally manipulated; lymphocytes are grown in bulk rather than microcultures and spend less time in culture (7). Because some assays for tumor recognition can falsely be negative because of poor tumor cell targets, the patient-specific assays for tumor recognition are also eliminated, significantly decreasing time and cost (7). Studies of young TIL have shown that they possess attributes associated with improved

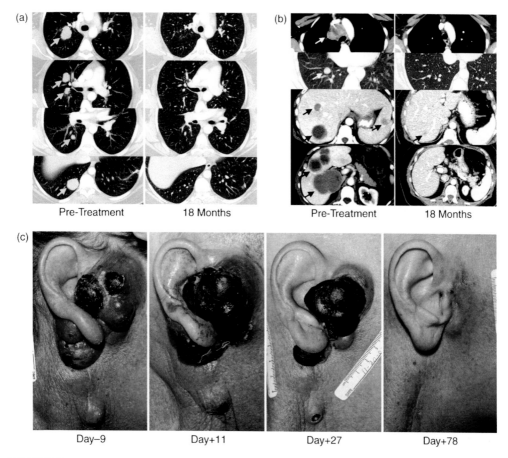

FIGURE 3

Objective tumor regression in patients with metastatic melanoma treated with adoptive cell transfer. (a) Regression of multiple melanoma metastases in the lungs ongoing at 23 months posttreatment. (b) Regression of melanoma metastases in the mediastinum (upper), lungs (middle), and liver (lower) ongoing at 18 months posttreatment. (c) Rapid regression of a large fungating periauricular melanoma metastasis within 76 days after cell transfer.

persistence and response in vivo, including longer telomeres and higher expression of CD27 and CD28 than selected TIL (29,31,32). In a study by Besser et al. (33), young TIL was successfully generated for transfer in 90% of patients and mediated an objective response by RECIST in 50% (10 out of 20) of patients. This included 2 complete responses (ongoing at 4 and 20 months) and 8 partial responses (progression-free survival of 3–18 months).

Dudley et al. (29) also reported a series of melanoma patients treated with young TIL incorporating enrichment of CD8+ T cells, thus eliminating CD4+ T cells and T regulatory cells. In this clinical trial of 56 patients treated with CD8+ enriched young TIL (41% of whom also received 6 Gy TBI), 3 to 4 patients were treated per month, and 53% of patients who underwent tumor resection received TIL therapy. The overall response rate was

54% and included 11 out of 30 objective responders who would have been ineligible for treatment if the "selected" TIL method with tumor recognition had been required. The benefits of the young TIL approach, CD8+ purification, and assaying for in vitro tumor recognition all require further study before widespread acceptance.

ACT using autologous TIL is not feasible for all patients with metastatic melanoma. Patients must have a site of resectable disease that is of sufficient size to generate TIL, generally in the range >1 to 2 cm. In terms of the surgical resection itself, the least morbid procedure is preferred to limit the chance of postoperative complications, which could delay the start of therapy, particularly complications that would be problematic during the neutropenia and thrombocytopenia associated with Cy-Flu or TBI. Patients with untreated brain metastases larger than 1 cm in diameter or greater than 3 in total number are excluded from TIL therapy because of the risk of intracranial bleed during the period of thrombocytopenia after administration of Cy-Flu. Patients with transmural small-bowel involvement are also excluded from therapy because of the risk of significant gastrointestinal bleeding during the thrombocytopenic period, as well as bacterial infection from direct contact of ulcerated tumor surfaces with normal gut flora in the setting of pancytopenia. Patients must have good organ function, tolerate the lymphodepleting chemotherapy, and remain suitable for treatment during the 4 to 6 weeks required to grow the cells in vitro. To be a candidate for TBI, patients must safely tolerate the dose of irradiation and have adequate CD34+ stem cells for collection.

In patients without contraindication whose TIL grow, the immediate toxicity of TIL therapy is largely related to the effects of high-dose IL-2 therapy. These include hypotension, pulmonary congestion secondary to vascular leak syndrome, and mental-status changes. Patients are also vulnerable to infection and bleeding because of bone marrow suppression secondary to the chemotherapy. The overall treatment-related mortality with or without TBI is 1% to 2%, most often because of sepsis. In summary, most human melanoma tumors are populated with tumor-reactive T-cells, which can rapidly be expanded in vitro. When given back to a properly pretreated recipient, they can cause objective tumor regression in 40% to 70% of patients with complete responses maintained for years.

■ ADOPTIVE CELL TRANSFER WITH GENETICALLY MODIFIED LYMPHOCYTES

Although ACT with autologous TIL has shown very promising results, there are limitations to its widespread use in the treatment of melanoma. Only 50% of melanomas reliably produce sufficient reactive TIL for administration (34). Some TIL can be isolated and demonstrate antitumor activity in vitro but later fail to grow to adequate numbers for cell transfer. Furthermore, not all patients have easily resectable melanoma tumors, and patients with widely metastatic disease must remain healthy and eligible during the 4 to 6 week cell growth period. The ability to introduce genes that code for TCRs specific for tumor antigens into PBL using gamma-retroviruses or lentiviruses provides a means by which some of the limitations of autologous TIL can be overcome. This process begins with the identification of a few cells with antitumor activity from which TCR genes can be isolated and cloned for incorporation into a retroviral vector. Gene transfer of a TCR increases the applicability of ACT not only in the melanoma patient population but also in other types of cancer.

The process of creating a successful genetically engineered TCR begins with selecting the method of TCR gene transfer. The selected method must have high transduction efficiency and be reproducible on a large clinical scale. RNA electroporation has been found to yield higher levels of gene transfer compared with DNA electroporation, but given the short half-life of RNA expression, this method has limitations for use on a clinical scale (35). Several small improvements in retroviral design and transfection methodology have allowed this route of genetic engineering to consistently and durably alter human lymphocytes with 50% to 80% efficiency.

A conventional TCR is composed of an alpha and a beta chain. For effective transduction, the amount of each chain should equally be expressed. Placing the coding regions for both the alpha and beta chains, separated by a picornavirus ribosomal skip peptide in the retroviral vector, has proven the most effective method (36). Activity of the TCR is maximized when the introduced alpha and beta chains selectively bind one another and mispairing with the endogenous TCR chains is minimized. The introduction of murine residues into human constant regions on the TCR increases specific pairing between transduced chains (37,38). The introduction of cysteines to form disulfide bonds has also improved the desired pairing. In addition to improving the overall TCR activity, facilitation of specific pairing decreases potentially dangerous self-reactivity of T cells, which has resulted from TCR mispairing in murine models (39).

Although the advances in the construction of active and stable TCRs have been substantial, the choice of target antigen is most critical for success of ACT with gene-engineered lymphocytes. The first successful use of genetically engineered lymphocytes modified to express a TCR was reported by Morgan et al. in 2006 (40). In this series, the MART-1 reactive TCR, DMF-4, was genetically cloned from a melanoma patient and transduced into the PBL of 17 metastatic melanoma patients through a gamma-retroviral vector. MART-1 is a tumor antigen that is known to be expressed on not only melanoma tumor cells but also normal melanocytes of the skin, eye, and inner ear. The modified T cells of all the patients showed in vitro biologic reactivity in coculture with MART-1 positive melanoma cell lines as measured by specific secretion of INF-γ. The cells were delivered similar to the TIL protocols, which included a lymphodepleting, nonmyeloablative chemotherapy regimen followed by cell transfusion and administration of high dose IL-2. Two of the 17 patients receiving anti-MART-1 TCR cells demonstrated objective clinical regression of disease. The 2 patients who responded were found to have sustained high levels of circulating gene-transduced cells at 1 year postinfusion. No cell-related toxicities were observed. Given the responses seen with the DMF4 TCR, which was characterized as a TCR of low avidity, a more reactive TCR was sought, in the hopes of a higher clinical response rate.

Johnson et al. (41) isolated a high-avidity TCR (referred to by this group as DMF5) from a human T cell that recognized the same MART-1 epitope as DMF4. A highly expressed epitope from the gp-100 melanoma–melanocyte antigen was also identified as a potential target; however, attempts to generate a high-avidity TCR against this antigen from patients were unsuccessful. Ultimately, the researchers were able to generate a highly avid TCR to this gp-100 epitope using HLA-A2 transgenic mice. In short, HLA transgenic mice were immunized with human tumor antigens, which differed slightly from the homologous sequences found in the mouse, thus circumventing thymic tolerance to these human proteins. These high-avidity murine TCR were not only restricted by the transgenic HLA so that they could recognize human target cells but also functioned when introduced into human PBL without modification (42). Thirty-six metastatic melanoma patients were treated, 20 of whom received cells with the human anti-MART-1 DMF5 TCR and 16 received cells with the murine anti-gp-100 TCR. Similar to the previous study, the cells were administered after lymphodepletion, and high-dose IL-2 was given after TCR-cell infusion. Six of the 20 DMF5 TCR patients and 3 of the 16 patients treated with gp-100 experienced objective tumor responses by RECIST criteria. Regression was seen in multiple organs, including brain, lung, liver, lymph nodes, and subcutaneous disease. The presence of the transferred cells was monitored in these patients, and all were found to have detectable levels at 1 month posttreatment, with varying levels of activity. Responding patients were all found to have high levels of active cells based on INF-γ and IL-2 assays; however, this was also the case for some of the non-responders. This suggested that persistent cell activity may be necessary but not sufficient for response. Furthermore, there was no difference between the persistence of human-derived DMF5 TCR cells and the murine gp-100 TCR containing cells, suggesting that immune reactions against mouse TCR sequences was not a limiting factor.

There were several differences in the clinical course of the patients in this study compared with the experience with the DMF4 TCR. The mean peak INF-γ serum levels, markers of transferred cell activity, were notably higher in the DMF5 and gp-100 patients than in the DMF4 patients. During the INF-γ peaks, the DMF5 and the gp-100 patients exhibited a diffuse erythematous rash, which, when biopsied, showed destruction of epidermal melanocytes. These rashes resolved within several days of onset, but some patients subsequently had diffuse vitiligo in the affected areas. Some patients also experienced toxicities involving the melanocytic cells of the eye and ear, including anterior uveitis, hearing loss, and vestibulitis (43). These on-target toxicities were effectively treated with local steroids, and all patients reverted to normal, with the exception of 1 patient who had mild residual hearing loss. These observed toxicities highlight the importance of carefully selecting the targeted tumor antigen. Melanoma–melanocyte antigens, such as MART-1 and gp-100, represent target antigens overexpressed on tumor tissue in comparison with normal tissues. Other antigens in this category include tyrosinase, tyrosinase-related protein-1 (TRP-1), and tyrosinase-related protein-2 (TRP-2), and toxicity related to normal melanocyte destruction may also limit their utility.

Cancer testis antigens are another group of tumor associated antigens (TAAs) found to be expressed in fetal development and on the surface of common epithelial cancers (44,45) but are sparsely expressed in normal adult tissues, with the exception of the testes, which are protected from immune attack by the lack of MHC antigen expression. In a recent trial using the NY-ESO-1 cancer testis antigen as a target for genetically engineered T cells, objective cancer regressions were observed in melanoma and synovial cell sarcoma patients whose tumors were confirmed to have expression of the NY-ESO-1 protein. PBL of the patients were genetically modified in the manner previously described to express a TCR that recognized an

HLA-A2 restricted epitope of NY-ESO-1. All patients had failed standard of care therapies and, in most of the patients with synovial cell sarcoma, second-line agents as well. Five of the 11 patients with metastatic melanoma and 4 of the 6 patients with synovial cell sarcoma experienced objective tumor responses by RECIST criteria. At the time of publication, 2 of the melanoma patients had complete responses ongoing at 22 and 20 months. A tumor response in this protocol is shown in Figure 4. Unlike the MART-1 and gp-100 trials, there was no association between the persistence of cells and response. There were also no on-target toxicities observed in patients treated with this anti-NY-ESO-1 TCR. Given the numerous cancer testis antigens described, ACT using cells that were gene modified

to target this family of antigens holds huge potential for the treatment of patients with common epithelial cancers, and these studies are actively being pursued (8,46).

■ ADOPTIVE CELL TRANSFER USING CHIMERIC ANTIGEN T-CELL RECEPTORS

Recognition of an antigen by a TCR requires that the antigen is presented by specific MHC molecules. This restricts the use of TCR therapy to patients who express that particular HLA type. Some tumors can also evade the immune system by downregulation of HLA. These limitations of a conventional TCR can be overcome by chimeric antigen

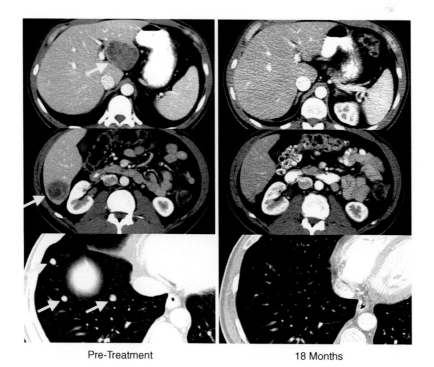

Pre-Treatment   18 Months

FIGURE 4

Objective tumor regression in a patient with metastatic melanoma involving the liver and lungs who was treated with adoptive cell transfer using T cells transduced with an anti-NY-ESO-1 T cell receptor.

receptors (CARs), which confer non–HLA restricted antigen specificity to T cells by using part of a monoclonal antibody to engage the tumor antigen (47,48). First reported by Eshhar and colleagues in 1989 (48), a CAR is constructed by fusing the variable region of the heavy and light chains of a single-chain monoclonal antibody (coupled by a peptide linker to form 1 polypeptide chain) with the intracellular signaling domains of a TCR. The CAR construct is retrovirally inserted into normal circulating T lymphocytes obtained from peripheral blood lymphopheresis, thereby eliminating the need for tumor resection.

The design of the CAR hybrid protein has evolved with time to improve T-cell function and persistence in vivo. The first-generation CARs used the CD3ζ intracellular signaling domain, which allowed the T cell to secrete cytokines and mediate cell lysis upon activation. The second-generation CARs added a second intracellular domain, often a T-cell costimulatory molecule, such as CD28, to increase cell activation and proliferation. Additional signaling domains, such as 41BB and OX40, are now used in third-generation CARs to enhance effector function and T-cell survival in vivo (49).

The clinical efficacy of cells expressing this hybrid receptor has been best shown in the targeting of the CD19 antigen on B cell malignancies (47–51). CD19 is expressed on the cell surface of almost all B-lineage cells, including normal mature B cells, malignant B cells, B cell precursors, and some plasma cells (52). In murine models, 1 infusion of anti-CD19-CAR-transduced T cells after lymphodepletion by irradiation completely eliminated intraperitoneally injected lymphoma cells and large subcutaneous lymphoma masses (52). The result was superior to that seen in mice treated with anti-CD19

monoclonal antibody alone. Success in the murine models led to a clinical trial in which 8 patients with treatment-refractory B cell lymphoma or chronic lymphocytic leukemia received the Cy-Flu preparative regimen, followed by the infusion of anti-CD19-CAR-transduced T cells and IL-2 (720,000 IU/kg every 8 hours) (53). One patient died 18 days post–cell infusion as a result of culture-proven influenza A pneumonia. Of the remaining 7 patients, 6 achieved objective remission with 1 complete response (ongoing at 18 months) (53). Four of the 7 patients developed long-term depletion of normal B cells treated with occasional intravenous immunoglobulin infusions for hypogammaglobulinemia. Additional toxicities seen on the study included fever, hypotension, fatigue, reversible renal failure, and obtundation. These toxicities seemed to correlate with the peak of IFN-γ and tumor necrosis factor (TNF) production within the first 8 days of cell transfer and completely resolved with time.

Because CAR-transduced T cells rely on antibody recognition of a tumor antigen for T-cell activation, they may only be targeted against cell-surface antigens (unlike conventional TCRs, which can recognize both intracellular and extracellular processed peptides). However, the antibody recognition of a CAR allows it to recognize non–protein surface molecules such as carbohydrates and glycolipids, which may be expressed on the surface of tumor cells. The number of antitumor antibodies currently available for engineering CARs exceeds the number of known antitumor TCRs, giving CAR-transduced T cells potential to extend the application of adoptive immunotherapy. Preclinical studies using a CAR directed against the high molecular weight melanoma-associated antigen (HMW-MAA), a cell-surface protein expressed on a majority of melanomas but with restricted expression in normal tissue, have shown promising results (54).

■ FUTURE EFFORTS WITH GENE-ENGINEERED T-CELLS

Reengineering T cells is not only limited to retargeting their specificity but can also be used to reprogram the function of tumor-specific T cells. Genes that encode cytokines can be introduced into antitumor T cells to enable them to produce their own growth factors in an autocrine fashion or provide local paracrine stimulation to enhance tumor killing. Both IL-2 and IL-15 have been tried in murine models of autocrine growth support. In the latter instance, Hsu et al. (55) transduced PBLs with a retroviral vector encoding IL-15. These T cells demonstrated prolonged survival and resistance to apoptosis in the absence of exogenous IL-2 support. Perhaps even more promising is the example of engineering paracrine secretion of IL-12 by T cells to enhance the antitumor effects in the tumor microenvironment. IL-12 is a cytokine known to augment the function of CD4+, CD8+, NK, and dendritic cells. Animal studies have shown IL-12 to have potent antiangiogenic and immune-stimulatory effects. This was initially demonstrated by administering recombinant IL-12 in murine models and later in clinical studies (56). The greatest limiting factor in more widespread applications of IL-12 was the dose-limiting toxicities associated with systemic delivery. This prompted clinical trials designed around delivery of the cytokine at the tumor site. In 1 animal study, a very small number of tumor antigen-specific T cells that were engineered to produce IL-12 led to regression of large tumors (57). The T cells secreted IL-12 only when encountering their nominal antigen in the tumor microenvironment,

because the IL-12 transgene was driven by an NFAT-sensitive promoter. This not only limited the systemic toxicity of IL-12 in vivo but also reduced its antiproliferative effects during in vitro T cell culture. Improved tumor infiltration with the IL-12 tumor-specific cells was also demonstrated compared with the tumor-specific cells alone. Clinical trials with TIL engineered to express IL-12 upon tumor recognition are currently under way, with promising early results.

The experience, so far, of ACT with autologous TIL from melanoma has proved how powerful and effective T cells can be in the treatment of melanoma. Similar to most effective immunotherapies that can induce major tumor regressions, complete responses from ACT seem to have the potential to cure patients of widespread metastatic disease. Unlike those other immunotherapies, the ability to achieve complete regressions may not be such an infrequent accomplishment. The ability to retarget T cells through gene modification enhances and extends T-cell efficacy in the treatment of melanoma and opens possibilities for treating other refractory cancer types. Nevertheless, the broader promise of ACT may lie in the modification of T-cell function through genetic redesign to create the exact T cell one might want to affect tumor destruction and control toxicity. The current challenge is to better understand what that T cell should look like.

■ REFERENCES

1. Smith FO, Downey SG, Klapper JA, et al. Treatment of metastatic melanoma using interleukin-2 alone or in conjunction with vaccines. *Clin Cancer Res.* 2008;14(17):5610–5618.
2. Rosenberg SA, Dudley ME. Adoptive cell therapy for the treatment of patients with metastatic melanoma. *Curr Opin Immunol.* 2009;21(2):233–240.

3. Topalian SL, Hodi FS, Brahmer JR, et al. Safety, activity, and immune correlates of anti-PD-1 antibody in cancer. *N Engl J Med.* 2012;366(26):2443–2454.

4. Ridgway D. The first 1000 dendritic cell vaccinees. *Cancer Invest.* 2003;21(6):873–886.

5. Rosenberg SA, Yang JC, Restifo NP. Cancer immunotherapy: moving beyond current vaccines. *Nat Med.* 2004;10(9):909–915.

6. Rosenberg SA, Yang JC, Sherry RM, et al. Durable complete responses in heavily pre-treated patients with metastatic melanoma using T-cell transfer immunotherapy. *Clin Cancer Res.* 2011;17(13):4550–4557.

7. Rosenberg SA. Cell transfer immunotherapy for metastatic solid cancer–what clinicians need to know. *Nat Rev Clin Oncol.* 2011;8(10):577–585.

8. Rosenberg SA. Cell transfer immunotherapy for metastatic solid cancer–what clinicians need to know. *Nat Rev Clin Oncol.* 2011;8(10):577–585.

9. Morgan DA, Ruscetti FW, Gallo R. Selective *in vitro* growth of T lymphocytes from normal human bone marrows. *Science.* 1976;193(4257):1007–1008.

10. Rosenberg SA, Grimm EA, McGrogan M, et al. Biological activity of recombinant human interleukin-2 produced in Escherichia coli. *Science.* 1984;223(4643):1412–1414.

11. Yron I, Wood TA Jr, Spiess PJ, Rosenberg SA. *In vitro* growth of murine T cells. V. The isolation and growth of lymphoid cells infiltrating syngeneic solid tumors. *J Immunol.* 1980;125(1):238–245.

12. Rosenstein M, Yron I, Kaufmann Y, Rosenberg SA. Lymphokine-activated killer cells: lysis of fresh syngeneic natural killer-resistant murine tumor cells by lymphocytes cultured in interleukin 2. *Cancer Res.* 1984;44(5):1946–1953.

13. Mazumder A, Rosenberg SA. Successful immunotherapy of natural killer-resistant established pulmonary melanoma metastases by the intravenous adoptive transfer of syngeneic lymphocytes activated *in vitro* by interleukin 2. *J Exp Med.* 1984;159(2):495–507.

14. Lotze MT, Line BR, Mathisen DJ, Rosenberg SA. The *in vivo* distribution of autologous human and murine lymphoid cells grown in T cell growth factor (TCGF): implications for the adoptive immunotherapy of tumors. *J Immunol.* 1980;125(4):1487–1493.

15. Rosenberg SA. Immunotherapy of cancer by systemic administration of lymphoid cells plus interleukin-2. *J Biol Response Mod.* 1984;3(5):501–511.

16. Rosenberg SA, Lotze MT, Yang JC, et al. Prospective randomized trial of high-dose interleukin-2 alone or in conjunction with lymphokine-activated killer cells for the treatment of patients with advanced cancer. *J Natl Cancer Inst.* 1993;85(8):622–632.

17. Rosenberg SA, Spiess P, Lafreniere R. A new approach to the adoptive immunotherapy of cancer with tumor-infiltrating lymphocytes. *Science.* 1986;233(4770):1318–1321.

18. Spiess PJ, Yang JC, Rosenberg SA. *In vivo* anti-tumor activity of tumor-infiltrating lymphocytes expanded in recombinant interleukin-2. *J Natl Cancer Inst.* 1987;79(5):1067–1075.

19. Muul LM, Spiess PJ, Director EP, Rosenberg SA. Identification of specific cytolytic immune responses against autologous tumor in humans bearing malignant melanoma. *J Immunol.* 1987;138(3):989–995.

20. Schwartzentruber DJ, Topalian SL, Mancini M, Rosenberg SA. Specific release of granulocyte-macrophage colony-stimulating factor, tumor necrosis factor-alpha, and IFN-gamma by human tumor-infiltrating lymphocytes after autologous tumor stimulation. *J Immunol.* 1991;146(10):3674–3681.

21. Topalian SL, Solomon D, Rosenberg SA. Tumor-specific cytolysis by lymphocytes infiltrating human melanomas. *J Immunol.* 1989;142(10):3714–3725.

22. Hom SS, Schwartzentruber DJ, Rosenberg SA, Topalian SL. Specific release of cytokines by lymphocytes infiltrating human melanomas in response to shared melanoma antigens. *J Immunother Emphasis Tumor Immunol.* 1993;13(1):18–30.

23. Hom SS, Topalian SL, Simonis T, Mancini M, Rosenberg SA. Common expression of melanoma tumor-associated antigens recognized by human tumor infiltrating lymphocytes: analysis by human lymphocyte antigen restriction. *J Immunother.* 1991;10(3):153–164.

24. Aebersold P, Hyatt C, Johnson S, et al. Lysis of autologous melanoma cells by tumor-infiltrating lymphocytes: association with clinical response. *J Natl Cancer Inst.* 1991;83(13):932–937.

25. Rosenberg SA, Packard BS, Aebersold PM, et al. Use of tumor-infiltrating lymphocytes and interleukin-2 in the immunotherapy of patients with metastatic melanoma. A preliminary report. *N Engl J Med.* 1988;319(25):1676–1680.

26. Rosenberg SA, Yannelli JR, Yang JC, et al. Treatment of patients with metastatic melanoma with autologous tumor-infiltrating lymphocytes and interleukin 2. *J Natl Cancer Inst.* 1994;86(15):1159–1166.

27. Wrzesinski C, Paulos CM, Kaiser A, et al. Increased intensity lymphodepletion enhances tumor treatment efficacy of adoptively transferred tumor-specific T cells. *J Immunother.* 2010;33(1):1–7.

28. Gattinoni L, Powell DJ Jr, Rosenberg SA, Restifo NP. Adoptive immunotherapy for cancer: building on success. *Nat Rev Immunol.* 2006;6(5):383–393.

29. Dudley ME, Gross CA, Langhan MM, et al. CD8+ enriched "young" tumor infiltrating lymphocytes can mediate regression of metastatic melanoma. *Clin Cancer Res.* 2010;16(24):6122–6131.

30. Goff SL, Smith FO, Klapper JA, et al. Tumor infiltrating lymphocyte therapy for metastatic melanoma: analysis of tumors resected for TIL. *J Immunother.* 2010;33(8):840–847.

31. Zhou J, Shen X, Huang J, Hodes RJ, Rosenberg SA, Robbins PF. Telomere length of transferred lymphocytes correlates with *in vivo* persistence and tumor regression in melanoma patients receiving cell transfer therapy. *J Immunol.* 2005;175(10):7046–7052.

32. Huang J, Khong HT, Dudley ME, et al. Survival, persistence, and progressive differentiation of adoptively transferred tumor-reactive T cells associated with tumor regression. *J Immunother.* 2005;28(3):258–267.

33. Besser MJ, Shapira-Frommer R, Treves AJ, et al. Clinical responses in a phase II study using adoptive transfer of short-term cultured tumor infiltration lymphocytes in metastatic melanoma patients. *Clin Cancer Res.* 2010;16(9):2646–2655.

34. Dudley ME, Wunderlich JR, Shelton TE, Even J, Rosenberg SA. Generation of tumor-infiltrating lymphocyte cultures for use in adoptive transfer therapy for melanoma patients. *J Immunother.* 2003; 26(4):332–342.

35. Morgan RA, Dudley ME, Rosenberg SA. Adoptive cell therapy: genetic modification to redirect effector cell specificity. *Cancer J.* 2010;16(4):336–341.

36. Wargo JA, Robbins PF, Li Y, et al. Recognition of NY-ESO-1+ tumor cells by engineered lymphocytes is enhanced by improved vector design and epigenetic modulation of tumor antigen expression. *Cancer Immunol Immunother.* 2009;58(3):383–394.

37. Bialer G, Horovitz-Fried M, Ya'acobi S, Morgan RA, Cohen CJ. Selected murine residues endow human TCR with enhanced tumor recognition. *J Immunol.* 2010; 184(11):6232–6241.

38. Sommermeyer D, Uckert W. Minimal amino acid exchange in human TCR constant regions fosters improved function of TCR gene-modified T cells. *J Immunol.* 2010; 184(11):6223–6231.

39. Bendle GM, Linnemann C, Hooijkaas AI, et al. Lethal graft-versus-host disease in mouse models of T cell receptor gene therapy. *Nat Med.* 2010;16(5):565–70, 1p following 570.

40. Morgan RA, Dudley ME, Wunderlich JR, et al. Cancer regression in patients after transfer of genetically engineered lymphocytes. *Science.* 2006;314(5796):126–129.

41. Johnson LA, Morgan RA, Dudley ME, et al. Gene therapy with human and mouse T-cell receptors mediates cancer regression and targets normal tissues expressing cognate antigen. *Blood.* 2009;114(3):535–546.

42. Cohen CJ, Zheng Z, Bray R, et al. Recognition of fresh human tumor by human peripheral blood lymphocytes transduced with a bicistronic retroviral vector encoding a murine anti-p53 TCR. *J Immunol.* 2005;175(9):5799–5808.

43. Seaman BJ, Guardiani EA, Brewer CC, et al. Audiovestibular dysfunction associated with adoptive cell immunotherapy for melanoma. *Otolaryngol Head Neck Surg.* 2012;147(4):744–749.

44. Scanlan MJ, Gure AO, Jungbluth AA, Old LJ, Chen YT. Cancer/testis antigens: an expanding family of targets for cancer immunotherapy. *Immunol Rev.* 2002;188:22–32.

45. Simpson AJ, Caballero OL, Jungbluth A, Chen YT, Old LJ. Cancer/testis antigens, gametogenesis and cancer. *Nat Rev Cancer.* 2005;5(8):615–625.

46. Robbins PF, Morgan RA, Feldman SA, et al. Tumor regression in patients with metastatic synovial cell sarcoma and melanoma using genetically engineered lymphocytes reactive with NY-ESO-1. *J Clin Oncol.* 2011;29(7):917–924.

47. Kochenderfer JN, Wilson WH, Janik JE, et al. Eradication of B-lineage cells and regression of lymphoma in a patient treated with autologous T cells genetically

engineered to recognize CD19. *Blood.* 2010; 116(20):4099–4102.

48. Eshhar Z, Waks T, Gross G, Schindler DG. Specific activation and targeting of cytotoxic lymphocytes through chimeric single chains consisting of antibody-binding domains and the gamma or zeta subunits of the immunoglobulin and T-cell receptors. *Proc Natl Acad Sci USA.* 1993;90(2):720–724.

49. Park TS, Rosenberg SA, Morgan RA. Treating cancer with genetically engineered T cells. *Trends Biotechnol.* 2011;29(11):550–557.

50. Cooper LJ, Topp MS, Serrano LM, et al. T-cell clones can be rendered specific for CD19: toward the selective augmentation of the graft-versus-B-lineage leukemia effect. *Blood.* 2003;101(4):1637–1644.

51. Kowolik CM, Topp MS, Gonzalez S, et al. CD28 costimulation provided through a CD19-specific chimeric antigen receptor enhances *in vivo* persistence and antitumor efficacy of adoptively transferred T cells. *Cancer Res.* 2006;66(22):10995–11004.

52. Kochenderfer JN, Yu Z, Frasheri D, Restifo NP, Rosenberg SA. Adoptive transfer of syngeneic T cells transduced with a chimeric antigen receptor that recognizes murine CD19 can eradicate lymphoma and normal B cells. *Blood.* 2010;116(19):3875–3886.

53. Kochenderfer JN, Dudley ME, Feldman SA, et al. B-cell depletion and remissions of malignancy along with cytokine-associated toxicity in a clinical trial of anti-CD19 chimeric-antigen-receptor-transduced T cells. *Blood.* 2012;119(12):2709–2720.

54. Burns WR, Zhao Y, Frankel TL, et al. A high molecular weight melanoma-associated antigen-specific chimeric antigen receptor redirects lymphocytes to target human melanomas. *Cancer Res.* 2010;70(8):3027–3033.

55. Hsu C, Jones SA, Cohen CJ, et al. Cytokine-independent growth and clonal expansion of a primary human CD8+ T-cell clone following retroviral transduction with the IL-15 gene. *Blood.* 2007;109(12):5168–5177.

56. Del Vecchio M, Bajetta E, Canova S, et al. Interleukin-12: biological properties and clinical application. *Clin Cancer Res.* 2007; 13(16):4677–4685.

57. Kerkar SP, Muranski P, Kaiser A, et al. Tumor-specific CD8+ T cells expressing interleukin-12 eradicate established cancers in lymphodepleted hosts. *Cancer Res.* 2010;70(17):6725–6734.

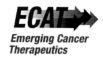

Immunotherapies for Metastatic Melanoma

Kevin Conlon*

Metabolism Branch, Center for Cancer Research, National Cancer Institute, Bethesda, MD

■ ABSTRACT

During the last several years, a number of promising new immunotherapeutic agents for the treatment of advanced or metastatic melanoma have emerged. Continuing the seeming momentum generated by the positive phase III registration trials for ipilimumab and vemurafenib, publication of the results of several phase I trials evaluating antibodies directed at programmed death 1 (anti-PD-1) or 1 of its physiologic ligands, PD ligand 1 (PD-L1), demonstrated striking efficacy in the early clinical trials. Treatment with recombinant human (rh) Interleukin 21 (IL-21) has shown response rates (RRs) as high as 24% for melanoma patients in early phase I/II single-agent trials. Recently, the first-in-human (FIH) clinical trials with rhIL-15 have been initiated, and there are clinical trials currently assessing the reformulated glycosylated rhIL-7, which is now produced in mammalian cell lines. Results from clinical trials evaluating these 2 promising cytokines with potential activity are eagerly awaited. After a period when interest immunotherapeutic strategies had plateaued and new cytokines were not as efficacious in human cancer patients as the preclinical animal models indicated, a palpable enthusiasm is evident for the clinical evaluation of these promising new agents and in combination with the active cellular therapies or immunotherapy drugs.

Keywords: interleukin-7, interleukin-21, interleukin-15, class I cytokines, common γ chain cytokines, anti-PD-1, anti-PD-L1

*Corresponding author, Metabolism Branch, Center for Cancer Research, National Cancer Institute, Bldg. 10, CRC, Room 4E-5322, 9000 Rockville Pike, Bethesda, MD
  E-mail address: conlonkc@mail.nih.gov

Emerging Cancer Therapeutics 3:3 (2012) 547–582.
DOI: 10.5003/2151–4194.3.3.547

■ INTRODUCTION

This chapter will review the current pre-clinical data and important clinical trial results and briefly discuss the implications of this information with regard to newly opened or clinical trials and strategies in development for the common gamma (γ) chain cytokines interleukin-21 (IL-21), interleukin-15 (IL-15), interleukin-7 (IL-7), and monoclonal antibodies (1) directed at the immune checkpoint inhibitor pro-grammed-death receptor 1 (PD-1) or the PD-1 ligands 1 and 2 (PD-L1, PD-L2) (2,3). Published results from clinical trials examining rhIL-21 and rhIL-7 have reported immune activation and, in certain cases, encouraging preliminary clinical activity (4,5). Recombinant human IL-15 (RhIL-15) was identified as a highly desirable immunotherapy candidate by the 2007 National Cancer Institute (NCI) Immunotherapy Agent Workshop and has finally entered the clinical arena with the initiation of the FIH clinical trials at the NCI, Ipilimumab is clearly an effective treatment for advanced or metastatic melanoma and the evolving data suggest that inhibition of other "immune checkpoint" molecules is an extremely viable treatment strategy (6,7). In addition, with the very promising early results from anti-PD-1 or anti-PD-L1 monoclonal antibodies clinical trials (MoAbs) (3,8), there is a sense of positive expectation for the anticipated next round of clinical trial presentations from the studies evaluating the PD-1/PD-L1 agents. Presentations at the recent clinical or scientific meetings and formal publication of results from recent clinical trials have validated these strategies or agents and suggest that the dramatic improvement in clinical activity long sought from the immunotherapy of melanoma may be nearer at hand. Better understanding of the basic immune cellular processes and the prospects of combining these new active agents with existing cellular therapies, other immune cytokines, chemotherapies, and vaccine approaches suggests a wealth of rationale treatment strategies to be assessed in melanoma patients.

■ PROGRESS IN THE TREATMENT OF ADVANCED MELANOMA

In the last 3 years, melanoma treatment has welcomed 2 new therapeutic entities with clear clinical benefit to patients with metastatic melanoma: ipilimumab (6,7) (anti-cytoxic T-lymphocyte antigen-4 [anti-CTLA-4] antibody) and the serine-threonine B-Raf kinase (BRAF) inhibitor vemurafenib (9). Both agents were granted U.S. Food and Drug Administration (FDA) approval soon after the review of the pivotal licensing trial data. Although vemurafenib is not an immunologic agent, better understanding of the molecular aberrations in melanoma has increased our ability to combine immunologic and molecular therapies. The effort to define new more effective treatments has further been energized by the recent publications of long-anticipated investigational trial results with MoAbs targeting PD-1 or PD-L1. Provocative indications of clinical benefit from anti-PD-1 treatment had been published with the initial phase I report (10) for this agent almost 2 years ago, and continued by rumors of a substantial single-agent response rated were generated by patient's testimonials. Ongoing refinements, novel combination treatments, or molecular manipulations of tumor-infiltrating lymphocytes (TILs), chimeric antigen receptor (CAR) cells (11), and ipilimumab (6,7), which will be discussed in another section in this chapter, have also contributed to the improvement in the treatment of melanoma. Reinitiated evaluation of the reformulated rhIL-7 now glycosylated because of production in a mammalian cell, continued investigations with rhIL-21, and the initiation of the FIH rhIL-15 trials have caused much anticipation for melanoma immunotherapy that has been dormant for nearly 20 years, when rh cytokines first became widely available for clinical use and produced the first wave of positive clinical data.

■ BACKGROUND PD-1, PD-L1 AND PD-L2

The effector cell molecule, now called PD-1, was initially described as a unique member of the immunoglobulin gene superfamily or cluster of differentiation molecule 28-B7 (CD28-B7) family (12,13), which was upregulated on the surface of activated T-cell lines and murine thymocytes undergoing programmed cell death, hence the designation. Subtractive hybridization was used to isolate a gene now called Pdcd1, encoding a 288 amino acid (aa) single-chain molecule with an extracellular and cytoplasmic domain (14, 15), which was shown to inhibit lymphocyte activation when it engaged by its ligands at the same time the T- or B-cell receptors (TCR or BCR) are stimulated by a cognate antigen (Ag). As shown in Figure 1, when PD-1 and the TCR are stimulated, simultaneous critical tyrosines residues, particularly the N-terminal tyrosine, which is located in an immunoreceptor tyrosine-based inhibitory motif (ITIM) in the cytoplasmic portion of the molecule, bind the Src homology region phosphatases (SHP) 2 and, to a lesser degree, SHP-1, leading to the dephosphorylation of critical tyrosines that are normally phosphorylated during the TCR activation cascade (16,17). This dephosphorylation of CD3 ζ chain and ζ chain—associated protein kinase 70 (CD3ζ ZAP70) and protein kinase theta (PKCθ) reduce the phosphatidylinositol-3-OH kinase (PI3k) signal, subsequently reducing the phosphorylation of

the serine/threonine protein kinase Akt and other distal activation pathways (18).

Similar in structure to PD-1, the PD-Ls are single-chain transmembrane proteins that are also members of the immunoglobulin super gene or CD28-B7 family. PD-L1 is constitutively expressed on T cells, B cells, dendritic cells (DCs), macrophages, mesenchymal stem cells, and bone marrow (BM)-derived mast cells. It is also important to note that PD-L1 has been demonstrated to be present on multiple human tumors (melanoma, breast, colorectal [CRC], ovarian, other gastrointestinal [GI] mucosal cells, thyroid, thymic, and H&N) cells (19–22). PD-L1 has also been shown to be upregulated when T cells, B cell, macrophages, and DCs are activated (23,24). In contrast with the wide expression of PD-L1, PD-L2 expression is restricted to activated macrophages and DCs. Initially, there were reports indicating that these ligands functioned as stimulators of T-cell activation similar to other members of the CD28 family, but it subsequently became very clear that they functioned as antagonists for the developing immune response.

■ IMMUNOBIOLOGY OF PD-1, PD-L1, PD-L2 AND CANCER IMMUNOTHERAPY

After a molecule or functional pathway has been identified as a "druggable" target, a key part of the preclinical evaluation of therapeutic potential of the target is to assess the effect of inhibiting or augmenting its function on the cell, host, or disease. Early in the preclinical evaluation of PD-1 and the PD-1 ligands, it became clear that antibodies that blocked the immunosuppressive signal through PD-1 had significant potential as an immunotherapeutic strategy. Evaluation of anti-PD-1 antibodies alone or in combination

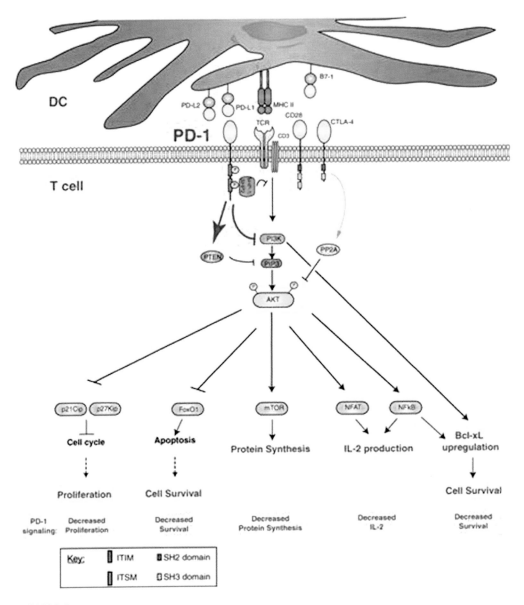

FIGURE 1

PD-1, PD-L1, and PD-L2 immune checkpoint blockade and immunotherapy.

PD-1 is expressed not only on T cells, B cells, and myeloid cells. PD-L1 and, to a lesser extent, PD-L2, which are expressed on some tumor cells, but also on antigen presenting cells (APCs), T cells, B cells, macrophages, mesenchymal stem cells, and bone marrow–derived mast cells that are or can be present in tumor deposits transmits a negative signal through PD-1. When PD-1 and the TCR are stimulated simultaneous critical tyrosines residues, especially the N-terminal tyrosine that is located in an immunoreceptor tyrosine-based inhibitory motif (ITIM) in the cytoplasmic portion of the molecule bind the Src homology region phosphatases (SHP) 2 and to a lesser degree SHP-1 leading to the dephosphorylation of critical tyrosines that are normally phosphorylated during the TCR activation cascade.

Reproduced with permission from Immunol Rev. 2010; 236:219–42. The PD-1 pathway in tolerance and auto-immunity. Francisco LM, Sage PT, Sharpe AH.

with other therapeutic components that included cytokine-secreting tumors and adoptive cellular therapies to treat a wide spectrum of malignancies in multiple animal model systems of breast cancer (mammary carcinoma cell lines 4T1, EMT6), melanomas (B16), and CRC cancers (CT26, murine colorectal cell lines MC38) showed that anti-PD-1 produced or augmented the antitumor response in these models (25–27). In another immunotherapeutic strategy, coimmunization with adenoviruses containing the human papilloma virus 16 (HPV16) E7 DNA and another DNA construct that encoded for soluble PD-1 (sPD-1) improved the immune response against E7 expressing tumors. It is important to note that, given the expected effects for human immunotherapy, the sPD-1 increased Ag-specific total CD8$^+$ and memory subset cellular responses by decreasing activation-induced apoptosis through the upregulation of Bcl-xL expression (28). The sPD-1 also augmented DC maturation as measured by the upregulation of major histocompatibility class II (MHCII) expression in these Ag-presenting cells (APCs), both indicating potential application for anti-PD-1 treatment in tumor vaccine efforts.

In addition to the functional data from tumor model systems, there is substantial information indicating a central role of these immune checkpoint molecules in shaping the immune response to viral pathogens. Blockade of PD-1 blockade with a murine antihuman PD-1 shifted the immune response to superantigen (*Staphylococcus* *(aureus)* enterotoxin BSEB) and tetanus toxoid (TT) away from the T helper 2 (Th2) ($\downarrow$IL5, IL13) profile toward Th1- and Th17-like cytokine responses ($\uparrow$ interferon gamma [IFNγ], IL2, tumor necrosis factor alpha [TNFα], IL6, and IL7) (29). There are multiple reports demonstrating that PD-1 expression is high in chronic viral infections and contributes to the immune evasion or

exhaustion, which prevents clearance of these viral pathogens. PD-L1 has also been shown to be upregulated on circulating monocytes and myeloid DCs (MyDCs) in chronic hepatitis B (CHB) infected animals (30) and CD14$^+$ monocytes and T cells in the human immunodeficiency virus (HIV) patients (31). This possibly represents another facet of the defective immune system present in HIV infection patients. As such, it is very provocative that the CD8$^+$ cells of long-term HIV infected nonprogressors have been shown to have low PD-1 expression (31).

Data from PD-1 and PD-ligand knockout (KO) mice (C57BL/6-Pdcd1$^{-/-}$ and BALB/c-Pdcd1$^{-/-}$) have provided additional insight into the importance of this pathway on cellular or immune processes (32). C57BL/6-Pdcd1$^{-/-}$ mice develop a systemic lupus-like glomerulonephritis and arthritis. BALB/c-Pdcd1$^{-/-}$ have a dilated cardiomyopathy marked by high titers of circulating IgG autoantibodies and diffuse cardiac deposition of antibodies specific for a particular cardiomyocyte protein (33). Other autoimmune dysfunctions in receptor-deficient mice are further indication of a central role for PD-1, PD-L1, and PD-L2 in modulating the immune response (34,35).

Additional data from the analyses of cancer patients have demonstrated that the understanding gained from these studies of cell lines and animal models applies to the human situation. Several groups have reported the correlation of higher PD-1 expression on effector cells and PD-L1 on tumor cells or other leukocytes in the tumor deposits, with poor prognosis in patients with prostate cancer, melanoma, breast cancer, and metastatic renal cell carcinoma (mRCC) (36–38). Freshly harvested TILs from patients with non–small cell lung cancer (NSCLC), melanoma, and mRCC are known to be anergic in a unique way and have depressed activity pathways compared with peripheral blood leukocytes (PBLs) obtained from normal healthy donors (39). Again not surprisingly, analysis of freshly harvested TILs from 50 patients showed strong expression PD-1 in >90% of the TIL specimens. This finding may in part identify why initially inactive TILs become effective in cellular therapies. Analysis of TILs after 2 days of ex vivo culturing produced a 4-fold reduction PD-1 expression on the TILs, and this change coincided with functional recovery in terms of calcium (CA^{++}) flux and tyrosine phosphorylation of kinases in the activation pathways. It is important to note that stimulation of these TILs with anti-CD3 MoAb maintained PD-1 expression in the activated TILs, unlike the TILs that were cultured without stimulation. It has previously been shown that PD-1/PD-L1 inhibitory effects can also be overcome by the addition of exogenous IL-2 or anti-CD3/ anti-CD28 stimulation. Both these observation are interesting, given the shift in many clinical trials from the older long-term TILs cultured only with rhIL-2 toward "young TILs" that are generally expanded over a shorter time frame with the addition of anti-CD3 activation Comparative analysis of lymphocytes from nontumor sites for the same patients or benign tissue specimens has also shown lower expression of PD-1. Similar analyses of PD-L1 expression on tumor cells has been shown to be variable, depending on the tumor type: 40% melanoma (N = 15), 35% NSCLC (N = 15), 18% mRCC (N =12). it is also interesting to note that PD-L2 expression on tumor cells was much lower (< 5% melanoma and NSCLC; ≈ 10% RCC) compared with PD-L1 (39). Analysis of PD-L1 and PD-L2 expression on non–malignant myeloid cells obtained from the tumor harvest showed slightly higher expression of PD-L1 than was noted on the tumor cells and much higher (35%–40%) expression on the myeloid cells than

was noted on the tumor cells. It is not clear if the PD-L1 and PD-L2 on malignant cells tumor have a different effect than the intratumoral myeloid cells on the TILs (40,41).

The critical role of $CD4^+$ $CD25^{high}$ T regulatory cells (Tregs) in suppressing the immune response and, probably, contributing to the immune evasion of cancers is now much clearer. Consistent with this role, the recent data demonstrating differential expression of PD-1 and PD-L1 on Tregs and nonsuppressor $CD4^+$ and $CD8^+$ cells suggests an additional way PD-1 and PD-L1 may contribute to the immunosuppressive microenvironment in tumor deposits (42). Analysis of changes in PD-L1 expression on "conventional" $CD4^+$ (C-CD4) cells and Tregs and expansion of $CD4^+$ subsets and $CD8^+$ cells in cancer patients receiving immunotherapy with agonist anti-CD40 antibody and Inlerleukin-2 (IL-2) showed that total $CD4^+$ cell numbers remained stable, but the numbers of Tregs were seen to increase, whereas C-CD4 cells decreased. This was correlated with the finding that stimulated C-CD4 cells but not Tregs upregulated PD-1 expression and decrease of the C-CD4 numbers was directly correlated with PD-L1 expression. Although the total number of $CD8^+$ cells initially increased, the secondary $CD8^+$ responses become impaired after initial productive stimulation.

■ CLINICAL TRIALS RESULTS

CA209001

The initial clinical report (10) that generated significant interest was from a relatively small multicenter standard phase I dose escalation trial with humanized monoclonal antibody (MoAb) MDX-1106 (ONO-4538) that enrolled a mixed group of 39 patients with CRC, castrate resistant prostate cancer (CRPC), NSCLC, melanoma, and mRCC. This was presented at the American Society of Clinical Oncology (ASCO) meetings in 2008 and 2009 and formally reported in a peer-review journal in 2010. The initial plan was to enroll 6 patient cohorts for treatment at dose levels of 0.3, 1, 3, and 10 mg/kg of MDX-1106 given as a 1 hour infusion with patient assessment each week for 8 weeks. The assessment was to include clinical safety evaluation and radiographic restaging response at weeks 8 and 12 using Response Evaluation Criteria in Solid Tumors (RECIST) 1.0 criteria. Then, an expanded cohort of 15 patients was to be treated at the maximum tolerated dose (MTD) or maximum administered dose. The expanded cohort was treated at the 10 mg/kg dose level, and limited retreatment of radiographically stable or improved patients who did not experience significant ($\geq$ grade 3) adverse events without dose-limiting toxicities (DLTs) was later allowed.

Safety

The safety profile was good, with 1 metastatic ocular melanoma patient who received multiple doses over an 8 month period developing an immune-related adverse event (irAE) grade 3 colitis that required IV corticosteroids and infliximab to control. One of the 2 patients who developed an elevated thyroid stimulating hormone (TSH) progressed to frank hypothyroidism requiring thyroid replacement. Two other patients developed (grade 2) polyarthropathies that may have been related to prior underlying diagnoses (Lyme arthritis and polymylagia rheumatica with pretreatment antinuclear antibodies titer > 1:1,000) that required oral corticosteroids and discontinuation of their treatment. Mild fatigue and musculoskeletal complaints were reported in a small percentage of the patients.

Laboratory Analyses

Changes in routine clinical labs included an almost immediate decrease in the absolute lymphocytes count (ALCs), reflected equally in both CD4$^+$ and CD8$^+$ cells. The ALCs gradually recovered back toward the pretreatment baseline level over the next 30 days, which ultimately resulted in a modest decrease ($\approx$ 10%) in ALCs over the 3 months of observation in the 17 patients with detailed information. No consistent change in the percentage of either CD4$^+$ or CD8$^+$ with memory phenotype (CD45RO$^+$) or activated (CD25$^+$ and HLA-DR$^+$) T-cells. Serial biopsies of a regressing-tumor-involved lymph node from 1 of the melanoma patients developed an infiltration of CD8$^+$ cells, and 2 responding patients showed diffuse expression of PD-L1 (B7-H1). It is important to note that no patient demonstrated the production of anti-MDX-1106 antibodies or changes in their delayed-type hypersensitivity responses against standard recall Ags. Pharmacokinetic (PK) and pharmacodynamic (PD) analyses showed some variability for the in vivo PD-1 receptor occupancy data, but the maximum concentration (C_{max}) and the area under the curve (AUC) were dose proportional. These analyses demonstrated a prolonged half life for the MDX-1106 antibody of 12 to 20 days and greater than 70% occupancy of PD-1 on circulating T-cells for more than 2 months, which indicated that every other week dosing was appropriate for future clinical studies.

Clinical Efficacy

A complete response (CR) in a CRC patient that was ongoing for greater than 21 months at the time of the report and partial responses (PRs) in a metastatic melanoma and RCC patients, as well as less significant regressions (2), resulted in 12 patients with tumor shrinkage or stabilization.

CA209003

The early reports of clinical activity and relative absence of irAEs had led to a heightened sense of expectation with regard to the subsequent clinical trial reports with MDX-1106 that had been redesignated BMS-936558. The presentations at the 2012 ASCO Meeting and the related publication (3) of the results of a larger multicenter phase I dose escalation trial in 296 patients with the same 5 metastatic diseases (CRC. CRPC, NSCLC, melanoma and RCC) did not disappoint. Although the same dose levels were again examined, repeat dosing every 2 weeks was used from the start of the protocol, and patients could continue treatment for up to 2 years in the absence of unacceptable side effects or disease progression. Patients with SD, PR, or CR with their initial (up to 2 years of) treatment were eligible for retreatment at progression.

The majority of the patients enrolled in the trail had melanoma (104) or NSCLC (122), but there were adequate numbers of RCC (34), CRPC (17), and CRC (19) entered who were included in the 236 patients analyzable for efficacy to evaluate the response rate to BMS-936558 in these histologies. In addition to respective histologies, the patients enrolled in the study represented a good cross section of good performance status (>96% were Eastern Cooperative Oncology Group [ECOG] 0 or 1) metastatic patients in terms of their treatment histories, with 49% of the efficacy population having >3 prior systemic therapies, >80% surgical resection of their diseases, nearly half with prior radiation therapy, and 50% having received appropriate hormonal or immunologic treatments. In addition, the patients did not represent a select group of better prognosis patients; a substantial percentage had bone or visceral (liver) metastases (Table 1).

Safety

The overall result was, again, good in this trial, with only 15 patients (5%) discontinuing the treatment for AEs considered related to the study drug. Nearly all patients (97%) experienced an AE while on treatment, with the most common events being fatigue (49%), decreased appetite (31%), diarrhea (28%), cough (25%), dyspnea (22%), constipation (22%), vomiting (22%), rash (20%), fever (18%), and headache (18%). The most common AEs assessed as related to BMS-936558 treatment were fatigue (24%), rash (12%), diarrhea (11%), pruritis (10%), decreased appetite (8%), and nausea (8%). Grade 3 or 4 treatment-related AEs occurred in 41 of the 296 patients (14%), without any evidence of dose relationship with the AEs, any significantly more common individual AE, or the severity of these events. The irAEs that are now designated as "drug-related adverse events of special interest" included pneumonitis (3%), vitiligo (3%), colitis, hepatitis, hypophysitis, and thyroiditis (all <1%). This spectrum of auto-immune-type phenomena or AEs of special interest seen in smaller-sized data base that includes nonmelanoma patients seems similar but possibly superior to the safety profile of ipilimumab. In the randomized 3 arm phase III ipilimumab licensing trial, the rate of colitis any-grade, or grades 3 to 5, colitis (8% and 5%, respectively) must be seen as higher compared with anecdotal cases of lower-grade colitis in the anti-PD-1 trial. Although there are some commonalities in the irAEs for either treatment, the frequency of particular irAEs indicates difference in the side-effect profile most notably for pneumonitis with BMS-936558.

As seen in Table 2, comparison of irAEs or AEs of special interest from the BMS-936558 phase I trial that includes a substantial number of nonmelanoma patients to the ipilimumab phase III trial

TABLE 1 Patient profile phase I protocol CA209003

Disease	NSCLC N = 122 (%)	Melanoma N = 104 (%)	RCC N = 34 (%)
Number of prior therapies			
1	18 (15)	41 (39)	10 (29)
2	31 (25)	36 (35)	9 (26)
3	27 (22)	18 (17)	5 (15)
≥4	40 (33)	9 (9)	10 (29)
Not reported	6 (5)		
Systemic therapies			
Chemotherapy (platinum containing regimen)	115 (94)		
Tyrosine kinase or angiogenesis inhibitor	41 (34)		25 (74)
Immunotherapy		67 (64)	32 (94)
BRAF inhibitor		8 (8)	
Sites of disease			
Lung	107 (88)	63 (6)1	(30) 88
Liver	24 (20)	37 (36)	(9) 26
Bone	21 (17)	13 (13)	(10) 29
Lymph Node	81 (66)	69 (66)	(28) 82
Other	46 (38)	64 (62)	(20) 59

Source: Adapted from Topalian et al. (3).

data is informative, but it must be recognized that the NSCLC patients would be receiving cytotoxic chemotherapeutics and radiation therapy, which might have some effect on some of these events, most notably pneumonitis, where 2 of the cases in this trial were NSCLC patients. Pruritus was seen in the BMS-936558 patients but less commonly than for the ipilimumab patients. Hypothyroidism and hepatitis, including higher-grade AEs, were uncommon and occurred at a similar frequency in both groups of patients. Colitis, including severe cases (≥grade 3), occurred at a much higher rate in the ipilimumab patients and was so rare in the BMS-936558 patients that it seems it was an anecdotal event. No events of hypopituitarism or hypophysitis were reported in the anti-PD-1 trial, but hypophysitis has been seen in patients treated with BMS-936558. Conversely, pneumonitis was not seen in the ipilimumab phase III trial but is known to occur in patients receiving this treatment and was notably seen in the antiPD-1 trial including three grade 5 events. Any patients experiencing pneumonitis were treated aggressively with discontinuation of the BMS-936558, initiation of IV corticosteroids, and, in 3 cases of treatment, the addition of infliximab and mycophenolate to terminate the event (Table 2).

Laboratory Analyses

Roughly 10% of the patients had elevations of their aspartate aminotransferase (AST) or alanine aminotransferase (ALT), with 1% of these AEs being grade 3 or 4 events. The PK parameters for BMS-936558 measured in this trial was very similar to the data from the previously published smaller dose

TABLE 2 Comparison of adverse events of special interest ipilimumab phase III trials and CA209003

Treatment	Ipilimumab N = 131		Ipilimumab plus gp100 N = 380		BMS-936558 N = 296	
AE of Special Interest	All	Grade ≥ 3	All	Grade ≥ 3	All	Grade ≥ 3
Pruritis	24.4%	0	17.6%	0.3%	10%	0.3%
Colitis	7.6%	5.3%	5.3%	2.9%	<1%	–
Hypothyroidism	1.6%	0.3%	1.5%	0	1%	0.3%
Hypopituitarism	2.3%	0.8%	0.8%	0.5%	–	–
Hypophysitis	1.5%	1.5%	0.5%	0.5%	–	–
Hepatitis	0.8%	0	0.5%	0.3%	1%	0.3%
Pneumonitis	–	–	–	–	3%	1%

Source: Adapted from Topalian et al. (3, 6 and 7)

escalation phase I trial. The Cmax and AUC were proportional for the dose range examined in this trial (0.1–10 mg/kg), and the in vivo PD-1 receptor occupancy analysis ranged from approximately 65% for the 0.1 mg/kg dose to 70% for the 10 mg/kg dose. One important result that had been less well studied in the prior trial correlative studies was the effect of PD-L1 expression on the surface of the tumor cells with the response to BMS-936558 treatment. In the 42 patients (61 specimens) with pretreatment tumor deposit material amenable to immunohistochemical (IHC) analysis for PD-L1 expression with the murine anti-human PD-L1 MoAb by 2 pathologists, 25 patients demonstrated PD-L1 expression. Nine of these 25 patients (36%) responded to anti-PD-1 treatment. It is important to note that none of the 17 patients who were PD-L1 negative responded to treatment and this indicates a potential important predictor of the lack of efficacy to this treatment, which needs to prospectively be examined in a larger sample group to fully verify this observation.

Clinical Efficacy

As seen in Table 3, the response rates for all doses in the 3 largest disease cohorts were 18% (14/76) for NSCLC, 28% (26/94) for melanoma, and 27% (9/33) for RCC. Even with the size of the melanoma patient cohort, this single-agent response rate must be regarded as impressive. The melanoma-specific response rates were not that different across the dose range, but the 3 and 10 mcg/kg dose levels would have to be considered the best choice for future trials.

CA210001

As the physiologic interactions between PD-1, PD-L1 and PD-L2 become clearer, it would be predicted that an antagonist MoAb directed toward PD-L1 would have similar results as a MoAb directed at PD-1 (8). Nevertheless, the results of similar phase I dose escalation trial examining the safety and efficacy of the humanized IgG4 directed against PD-L1 are impressive, with evidence of clinical benefit in the treatment of patients with metastatic melanoma, NSCLC, and mRCC. Because the trials were conducted by the same industry

TABLE 3 Objective response rate, duration of response and progression-free survival melanoma patients

Dose	Objective Response Rate		Duration of Response (Months)	Stable Disease ≥24 Weeks		Progression-Free Survival Rate at 24 Weeks
0.1	4/14	29%	7.5+, 5.6+, 5.6, 5.6	1/14	7%	40%
0.3	3/16	19%	3.8+, 2.1+, 1.9+	1/16	6%	31%
1	8/27	30%	24.9+, 22.9, 20.3+, 19.3+, 18.4+, 7.6+, 5.6+, 5.3+	3/27	11%	45%
3	7/17	41%	22.4+, 18.3+, 15.2+, 12.9, 11.1, 9.3, 9.2+	1/17	6%	55%
10	4/20	20%	24.6+, 23.9+, 18.0+, 17.0	0/20	0	30%
All doses	26/94	28%		6/94	6%	41%

Source: Adapted from Topalian et al. (3).

sponsor, it is not surprising that there were many similarities for the patient selection, dosing, schedule, design, and eligibility for these 2 trials. The trial enrolled 207 patients, with the most common tumor types being NSCLC (75), melanoma (55), CRC (18), and mRCC (17), and patients with ovarian, pancreatic, gastric, and breast cancer. The patient characteristics in this trial, summarized in Table 4, were remarkably similar in terms of performance status, prior local treatments, and the number and types of systemic therapies. With the exception of the relatively low number of melanoma patients who were treated with a BRAF inhibitor, the systemic therapies reflect the consensus standards of care for these cancers. This phase I dose escalation trial evaluated cohorts patients treated with BMS-639559 treated at dose levels of 0.3, 1, 3, and 10 mg/kg administered once every 14 days for the 6 week treatment cycle, with the potential to receive up to a total of 16 cycles (96 weeks) of treatment. After the MTD had been defined, the trial planned to enroll 5 disease-specific expansion cohorts of 16 patients, each to better assess clinical activity of BMS-639559.

Safety

Sixty-one percent of the patients (121/207) experienced an AE, 19 of which were grade 3 or 4 events. The most common study-drug-related AEs were fatigue (16%), infusion reactions (10%), diarrhea (9%), rash (9%), arthralgias (7%), nausea (6%), pruritus (6%), and headache (4%). There seemed to be no relationship between the number or the severity of the AEs and the dose of BMS-639559, and again, no MTD was defined in this study. Grade 3 or 4 AEs occurred in 9% of the patients; 23/207 (11%) stopped treatment because of an adverse event, and 12 (6%) were considered related to treatment Rx. Common AEs were fatigue, infusion reaction (10% most common at 10 mg/kg dose), diarrhea, arthralgias, rash, nausea, pruritis, and HA. Rx-related AEs of special interest seen in 81 of the 237 patients (39%) included not only rash, hypothyroidism, and hepatitis but also sarcoidosis, endopthalmitis, DM, and myasthenia; 9 patients required corticosteroids. There were 11 SAEs; in addition to common GI toxicities, 1 patient had pancreatitis.

TABLE 4 Patient profile phase I protocol CA210001

Disease	NSCLC N = 75 (%)	Melanoma N = 55 (%)	RCC N = 17 (%)
ECOG Performance status			
0	21 (28)	33 (60)	7 (41)
1	50 (67)	22 (40)	10 (59)
2	3 (4)	0	0
Surgery	43 (57)	–	16 *(94)
Radiation Therapy	24 (32)	–	–
Systemic therapies			
Chemotherapy (platinum containing regimen)	71 (95)	–	–
Tyrosine kinase or angiogenesis inhibitor	31 (41)	–	14 (82)
Immunotherapy	–	31 (56)	7 (41)
BRAF inhibitor	–	5 (9)	–
Sites of disease			
Lung	64 (85)	36 (65)	11 (65)
Liver	18 (24)	13 (24)	7 (41)
Bone	15 (20)	3 (5)	5 (29)
Lymph Node	46 (61)	28 (51)	7 (41)
Other	35 (47)	38 (69)	10 (59)

* nephrectomy

Source: Adapted from Brahmer et al. (8).

There was 1 case of adrenal insufficiency and 1 case of grade 1 myocarditis.

Laboratory Results

PK was dose proportional, t ½ is approximately 15 days, and receptor occupancy exceeded 65% for all groups. Hyperglycemia (all grades) was seen in 11% of the patients, and in 2% of the patients, it was ≥grade 3. Anemia occurred in 16% of the patients, and in 4% of the patients, it was ≥grade 3.

Clinical Efficacy

The median duration of Rx was 12 weeks. In the melanoma patients treated with BMS-936559, the disease control rate (DCR) was slightly lower (18%), but the CR rate of 6% (3/52) was higher than the rate seen in the comparable anti-PD-1 trial.

The progression-free survival rate at 24 weeks in a relatively modest-sized cohort of melanoma patients was 42%, which is again remarkably similar to the rate seen in the anti-PD-1 trial.

Comparison of Immune Checkpoint Inhibitors

The comparison of efficacy data assessment from the phase III ipilimumab and for the melanoma patients in the phase I BMS-936558 and 936559 trials, summarized in Table 5, demonstrates some provocative results. Although the CR rates (all 1% or less) for the 3 treatments (both ipilimumab arms are being considered together here) are not impressive, the 27% PR rate (25/94) for BMS-936558 is approximately 3 times the rate observed in the ipilimumab monotherapy arm and

TABLE 5 Comparison of efficacy for immune checkpoint inhibitors

Treatment	Ipilimumab N = 137	Ipilimumab plus gp100 N = 403	BMS-936558 N = 94	BMS-936559 N = 52
Complete response	1.5%	0.2%	1%	6%
Partial response	9.5%	5.5%	27%	12%
Stable disease	17.5%	14.4%	6%	24%
Disease control rate	28.5%	20.1%	33%	18%
Progression-free survival	12%*	7%*	41%#	42%#

* @ 12 weeks for ipilimumab trial

@ 24 weeks for BMS-936558 and 936559 trials

Source: Adapted from Topalian et al. (3, 6, 7 and 8)

still higher than vaccine/ipilimumab arm. The rate of stable disease (SD) reported in the BMS-936558 trial is certainly lower than for both ipilimumab treated cohorts and results in fairly similar DCRs for the 3 treatment groups, suggesting that the long-term outcome for either treatment is similar. Nevertheless, the progression-free survival percentage at 2 observation intervals for BMS-936558 (24 weeks) compared with ipilimumab (12 weeks) is another indicator of the efficacy potential for anti-PD-1 therapy in the treatment of metastatic melanoma. The precise role of treatment sequence, results of the combination trials, and longer-term follow-up will greatly inform as to how these agents will be used in the future.

CT-011

BMS-936558 is not the only anti-PD-1 that is currently in clinical trials evaluating the efficacy of blocking signals through PD-1 as a treatment for advanced malignancies. A phase I dose escalation protocol with CT-011, humanized IgG1 MoAb, was performed in refractory or relapsed patients having the hematologic malignancies of acute myeloid leukemia (AML), chronic lymphocytic leukemia (CLL), Hodgkin's disease (HD), non-Hodgkin's lymphoma (NHL), and multiple myeloma (MM) (43). The 17 patients enrolled included many high-risk patients, with 5 patients who had undergone a stem cell transplant (SCT; 4 allogeneic and 1 autologous) and several patients with ECOG PS 2, 1 each ECOG PS 3 and 4. Patients received a single 5 hour infusion of CT-011 at doses of 0.2, 0.6, 1.5, 3, and 6 mg/kg.

Safety

Eleven of the 18 patients (61%) enrolled reported an adverse event in a pattern that did not suggest relationship to the dose of CT-011. The most common adverse events were diarrhea (2) and pain (2), and there was 1 event each of rash, shortness of breath (SOB), weakness, flushing, blurred vision, pressure (ulcer) wound, and urinary tract infection (UTI). The events of weakness and flushing that occurred in the same CLL patient were considered possibly related to the CT-011 treatment. The MTD was not defined in this study, and although no treatment related toxicities were seen, 4 SAEs was observed, all in AML patients, and eventually resulted in the death of these patients over the 21 day study period. One of the deaths as a result of resistant acute myeolmonocytic (M4) AML and grade 4 graft versus host disease (GVHD) occurred in a patient who, 8 weeks before entering this trial, had undergone an SCT with an unmanipulated peripheral stem cell harvest from an HLA-matched unrelated donor had evidence of early grazed 1 GVHD (rash) that progressed to grade 4 GI tract GVHD after receiving the lowest dose (0.2 mg/kg) given in this study. The time course of the events and the progression of the patient's skin GVHD are not clear from the report, but the events were assessed as not related to the study drug by the study physicians. Two patients died during treatment, and 2 other patients withdrew from the protocol. In the first case, the patient was unable to travel to the research center for routine evaluations because of poor general condition, and the second patient underwent an allogeneic SCT. Details with regard to the time course for the emerging GVHD were not provided, making it difficult to evaluate the relationship of CT-011 treatment and this SAE.

Laboratory Analyses

With the exception of 1 AML patient, none of the AML patients demonstrated any reduction in their peripheral blast count nor did the nonleukemic patients demonstrate reduction of their disease burden as assessed by radiographic or laboratory measurements. Limited assessment of CT-011 PKs performed at 24 and 48 hours, days 7, 14, and 21 postinfusion showed dose-proportional increases in CT-011 levels across the dose range evaluated, with some variability in the median t ½, which ranged from 217 to 410 hours, with some suggestion of a longer t ½ for

the 6 patients felt to have clinical benefit. In contrast with the decreases in ALC, CD4+, and CD8+ cells for the BMS-936558 patients, the patients receiving CT-011 demonstrated an early increase in the median number of CD4+ cells, which was somewhat sustained throughout the 21 day evaluation, but no consistent change in the median number of CD8+ cells or activated CD69+ lymphocytes was noted.

Clinical Efficacy

Clinical benefit was felt to be seen in 5 patients, with prolonged disease stabilization seen in 2 CLL patients (>17 and 8 months), 1 post auto-SCT HD patient (8 months), 1 MM patient (>13 months), a "minimal" response in an AML patient (transfusion independent for 9 months), and a CR in a follicular NHL patient with bulky lymphadenopathy above and below the diaphragm. The clinical end-point assessment is difficult here because of the nature of the patient population, their substantial comorbities, and the absence of improvements in their laboratory or radiographic assessments to support the apparent benefits of treatment.

MK-3475

Preliminary results of a phase I dose escalation trial with another commercial sponsor's antibody against PD-1 were presented at the 2012 ASCO meeting (44). The MoAb is also an IgG4; doses evaluated to date were 1, 3, and 10 mg/kg, initially given as a 1 time dose. After an initial observation period for safety assessment, patients were allowed to receive repeat dosing every other week. At the time of the report, 9 patients (3 NSCLC, 2 melanoma, 2 rectal cancer, 1 sarcoma, 1 carcinoid) had been enrolled.

Safety

The most common drug-related AEs were fatigue (33%), nausea (22%), and diarrhea, dysgeusia, breast pain, and pruritus (11% each). All events, except for pruritus (grade 2), were grade 1 AEs.

Laboratory Analyses

Very early PK analysis indicated a t ½ of between 13 and 22 days.

Clinical Efficacy

One of the melanoma patients had an ongoing PR at the time of the report, and 3 patients had SD.

■ ANTI-PD-1 AND PD-L1 SUMMARY COMMENTS

Although the clinical data and experience with agents targeting the PD-1 and PD-L1 interaction is not extensive, a number of observations about anti-PD-1 and anti-PD-L1 therapies seem appropriate:

- There was impressive single-agent (BMS-936558 and BMS-936559) clinical activity in early clinical trials in several solid tumors, including a malignancy (NSCLC) not normally sensitive to immunotherapy.
- Awaiting additional clinical data from CT-011 and MK-3475 in solid tumor patients.
- Half life of approximately 2 weeks suitable for every other week dosing.
- Rate of AEs and spectrum of toxicities are not problematic.
- Patients with PD-L1 negative tumors do not respond to anti-PD-1 treatments.
- The rate of irAEs or drug-related adverse events of special interest is low and better than ipilimumab.

- Results of combination anti-PD-1 and ipilimumab trial awaited.
- Very limited information on the potential risk for autoimmune toxicities because of sequential or concordant use of 2 immune checkpoint inhibitors.
- Initiation of trials with anti-PD-1 or PD-L1 agents and other standard immunotherapeutics (adoptive cellular, vaccine, cytokine) are anticipated.
- Other new candidate drugs targeting these immune checkpoint molecules are expected to be available or more widely available for clinical investigations.

■ COMMON γ CHAIN CYTOKINES

After a significant period of time where candidate cytokines with promising preclinical data proved to be a disappointment in human clinical trials, several new stimulatory cytokines are beginning or extending encouraging early data in new clinical investigations (Figure 2). RhIL-21 has been tested in a number of phase I and II trials, and reports from several of these trials have demonstrated highly encouraging activity in early IL-21 clinical trials. IL-21 a class I cytokine (45,46) initially described in 2000 is grouped in light of a γ chain common to the cytokines IL-2, 3, 4, 6, 11, 12, 15, 18, 21. Activated $CD4^+$ cells are the primary producer of IL-21, but natural killer T (NK-T) cells are also a source. IL-21, often synergistically with IL-7 and IL-15, has been shown to stimulate other T-cells and act on B-cells to have a major effect on Ig production. These common γ chain cytokine also promote the maturation of NK cells by increasing

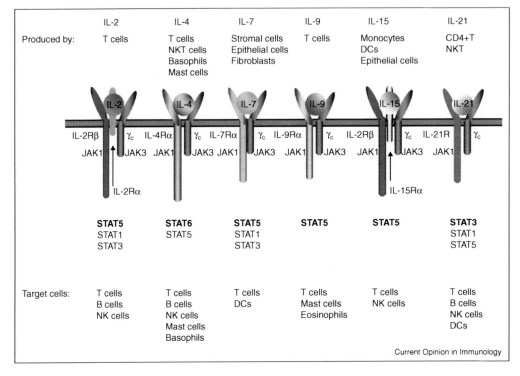

FIGURE 2

Common γ chain cytokines, receptors, and signaling molecules.

γc-family cytokines. Shown are the receptors for IL-2, IL-4, IL-7, IL-9, IL-15, and IL-21. These cytokines each activate STAT proteins through phosphorylation of JAK1 and JAK3. The principal STAT protein activated by each cytokine is in bold. DC, dendritic cell; NK cell, natural killer cell; NKT cell, natural killer T cell. STAT5 refers collectively to STAT5A and STAT5B, which are closely related tandem head-to-head genes.

Reproduced with permission from: *Current Opinion in Immunology*, 2011, 23:598–604 IL-2. Family cytokines: new insights into the complex roles of IL-2 as a broad regulator of T helper cell differentiation Wei Liao, Jian-Xin Lin and Warren J. Leonard.

their cytotoxicity and obviously play an important role in the innate immune response against viruses (47). IL-21's primary signaling pathway is through Janus kinase 1 (JAK1) and 3, which transmits the activation signal through STAT 3 and, to a lesser extent, through STAT1 and STAT 3. Analysis immune response from patients treated with IL-21 shows a pattern of cytokine secretion that is difficult to assign as a Th1-, Th2- or Th17-like pattern, but IL-10, IL-18, TNFα, and the chemokine monocytes chemotactic protein-1 (MCP-1) showed the greatest increase above pretreatment levels (48).

Most prominently, IL-21 does not significantly stimulate T Regs and has been reported to reverse the effects of these immunosuppressive cells (49). In addition to these effects on different T-cell sets, IL-21 is an important regulator or stimulator of NK Cell responses (50).

Open-Label 2 Arm Phase I rhIL-21

An older report of an open-label 2 arm phase I trial enrolled 29 patients with melanoma evaluated similar IV infusion regimens of IL-21 at dose levels of 1 to 100 mcg/kg but does not present clinical information remains pertinent when discussing IL-21 (51). Patients were either treated with the now common daily × 5, followed by 9 days of rest (5 +9) schedule or tiw for 6 consecutive weeks. Although this trial did not establish the daily × 5 regimen to be evaluated in future trial, the similarity in terms of tolerance (AEs), laboratory abnormalities, immune activation, and clinical efficacy are interesting and helped define 30 mcg/kg as the recommended phase II dose (RPh2D) but not the MTD after review of the AEs for 4 patients treated at the 50 mcg/kg dose level and 2 patients treated at the 100 mcg/kg dose level.

Safety

The 14 patients treated at the 1, 3, and 10 mcg/kg dose levels tolerated either treatment arm well, but 3 of the 7 patients treated with the tiw regimen at the 30 mcg/kg dose level had DLTs, including late elevation of ALT, grade 3 neutropenia, fevers, and rigors for the third patient. The daily × 5 patients at this junction had a better safety profile; enrollment to tiw arm was discontinued, and all patients were enrolled in the daily × 5 arm as the dose escalation continued. When both patients at the 100 mcg/kg dose level experience DLTs, a new intermediate dose of 50 mcg/kg was added, and eventually, 4 patients were treated, with 1 patient having DLT of grade 3 thrombocytopenia and fatigue. With this finding, additional dosing of more than 30 mcg/kg was ceased, and the 30 mcg/kg was assigned as the MTD. All the patients had at least 1 AE, and approximately half (14 of 29) of the patients had a grade ≥3 AE. The most common AEs were fatigue (55%), fever and nausea (52%), and HA (45%), followed by rash, myalgias, vomiting (31%), and pruritus, anorexia, and influenza-like syndrome (28%). The initial differential in AEs based on the treatment regimen, in retrospect, was not valid, and ultimately, the authors concluded that the safety profile for the 2 regimens were really very comparable. Thirteen patients had an SAE (30 events), most notably elevated ALT, fever, fatigue, nausea, and neutropenia, and there was 1 on study death; a myocardial infarction in a patient with ischemic heart, abdominal aortic aneurism, and hypertension not considered related to IL-21.

Laboratory Analysis

The laboratory data from this trial was reported in 2 different publications with somewhat different slants. Besides the laboratory information contained in the clinical trial report, the publication presented a more detailed analysis of changes in molecular signaling, absolute lymphocyte, and phenotypes of lymphocyte subsets. PK analysis showed the expected dose-dependent increase in AUC for IL-21, which was linear across the dose levels, but the t ½ was also seen to increase from 1.1 hours for the 1 mcg/kg dose level to 4.2 hours for the 100 mcg/kg dose level. The authors felt that the t ½ was underestimated for the lower dose cohorts, because IL-21 level had fallen below the lower limit of detection in the assay measuring the drug concentration. In addition to the laboratory abnormalities cited in the Safety section, grade 3 increases in LFTs (γ glutamyl transferase, ALT, AST) were seen (5 patients), and decreases in fibrinogen (3 patients) and increases in alkaline phosphatase, total bilirubin, and uric acid (1 patient each) were observed. Increased levels of sIL-2R were measured during the times the patients were receiving IL-21; therefore, the patients being treated with the tiw regimen had a more consistent elevation modestly above baseline for the 1 and 10 mcg/kg patients, 5- to 10-fold above baseline for the 30 mcg/kg patients, and, interestingly, very high for one 3 mcg/kg patient, with evidence of a cumulative increase in this activation parameter for this particular patient. In the patients treated with the "5 + 9" schedule, there was a peak valley effect with high levels of sIL-2 receptor at levels comparable or slightly above the equivalent tid dose level results during the daily treatment period and a return to baseline levels during the 9 day break. The "5 + 9"patients treated at the 50 and 100 mcg/kg dose levels had the maximum concentrations of sIL-2R. Five- to 10-fold increases in perforin-1 and granzyme B mRNA were measured in CD8+ cells on day 5 of treatment, most apparent at the patients dosed more than 30 mcg/kg.

More extensive evaluation the total number of lymphocytes, CD4+, CD8+, and NK cells during the initial 5 day treatment again demonstrated an early decline in T and NK cells, which trended back up toward the baseline levels, and, possibly, a slight expansion in the ALC measured by day 12 for the 2 highest dose levels of IL-21 during the first 2 cycles. Increases in the percentage of chemokine receptor type 7 (CCR7+), CD62 ligand (CD62L+), and, possibly, naive CD45RA+ lymphocytes were also seen, with dose-related increase possibly present for the 1 to 30 mcg/kg dose cohorts but apparently lower for the 50 and 100 mcg/kg cohorts, which may be more related to the smaller number of patients analyzed. A significant, consistent, and comparable increase in STAT3 phosphorylation in CD3+ cells was seen at all dose levels. Analyses of NK (CD56+) and CD8+ cells showed increases in granzyme B and perforin mRNA and increases for NK cells in vitro cytotoxicity toward K562 cells from a number of the patients without any evidence of a treatment dose or schedule-related effect. Increases in IFNγ, granzyme A, and CXCR3 mRNA were also seen in the analysis of CD8+, with

some evidence of a dose-related effect on IFNγ mRNA levels. No patient developed antibodies directed against IL-21.

Clinical Efficacy

There was 1 PR in the 21 patients evaluable for response who was subsequently converted to a CR surgically, and another 9 patients had SD at the week 8 response evaluation time point and received additional IL-21 treatment. There was no evidence that either regimen was superior in terms of activity.

Phase I Trial in Metastatic Melanoma and Renal Cell Cancer

The clinical evaluation of Rh IL-21 has been under way for a number of years, and the results of some the early trials have been reported. Although reports have been encouraging in certain cases, the development of this immunomodulator has not rapidly proceeded. One of the early clinical efforts in melanoma and mRCC patients was a phase I dose escalation trial of intravenous bolus (IVB) administration daily × 5 weeks 1 and 3 (d1–5, 15–19) given at doses of 3, 10, 30, and 100 mcg/kg with plans for treatment of an expanded cohort at MTD (52). One patient was also treated at an intermediate dose level after the only 2 patients at the 100 mcg/kg dose level experienced DLTs. Forty-three patients were eventually enrolled (24 melanoma, 19 RCC); 34 of the patients were treated at the MTD of 30 mcg/kg, and additional treatment cycles were later allowed for patients with evidence of clinical benefit.

Safety

The side-effect profile are similar to most cytokine treatments, with the most common AEs being flu-like symptoms: fevers (91%), fatigue (82%), chills (68%), HA

(56%), nausea (47%), pruritis (47%), myalgias (41%), anorexia/arthralgias/constipation (29%), and rash (24%). These toxicities were generally lower grade, but 3 patients had grade 3 events (abdominal pain, thrombocytopenia, and hypophosphatemia). One patient had significant hepatotoxicity (grade 4) during his second course with ALT/AST > 100 × the upper limit of normal (ULN) for a time, a total bilirubin of 188 mcmol/L, and a prolonged PT A biopsy confirmed hepatic necrosis, and the patient required a longer time to recover than the other patients with less severe events did. There was no clear indication that repeat treatment was associated with an increase of toxicity.

Laboratory Analyses

At the 30 mcg/kg dose level, 1 of the 6 patients had transient grade 3 ALT elevation, but both patients treated at the 100 mcg/kg dose level had DLTs. In 1 case, there was grade 3 hyponatremia, and the other patient had multiple AEs grade 3 platelets, leucopenia, hyperbilirubinemia, hypophosphatemia, and grade 4 lymphopenia. The 1 patient treated at the added 50 mcg/kg dose level had grade 3 neutropenia without fever or infection. In all cases, the DLTs were rapidly reversible, with the exception of the patient with the grade 4 hepatotoxicity. The AUC for IL-21 was dose proportional, and the terminal t ½ of IL-21 (≈ 3 hours) was similar for the dose levels, with the possible exception of the 3 mcg/kg dose level. Most patients had initial lymphopenia that nadired at approximately 50% of the starting ALC and rose to nearly 50% above the baseline in the week after treatment. It is important to note that, for cytokine produced in *Escherichia coli* that is not glycosylated like a natural IL21, 6 of the 43 patients developed anti IL-21 antibodies. All 6 patients were treated at the 30 mcg/kg dose level; 5 patients converted to being antibody positive after retreatment, and in 3 cases the antibodies were neutralizing.

Clinical Efficacy

One CR and 11 patients with SD was seen in the 24 melanoma patients (4% RR and 50% disease control rate [DCR]), and 4 PRs and 13 SDs were noted in the 19 mRCC patients (21% RR and 90% DCR).

Treatment-Naive Metastatic Melanoma Phase IIa trial

A subsequent phase II trial using the established daily × 5 IVB schedule (days 1–5, 15–19, and 29–33 and then 2 week rest before the next cycle) using the Simon 2 stage phase II design enrolled a total of 24 patients (14 stage 1; 10 stage 2) (53). Although the protocol required good performance status (ECOG 0 or1) for entry and adequate physiologic parameters, more than half of the patients had advanced visceral metastases (M1a 20%, M1b 25%, and M1c 54%). Patients were eligible for additional 8 week cycles of treatment in the absence of symptomatic disease progression.

Safety

On the basisof the prior experience with IL-21 given as a daily IVB, tolerance of the treatment was considered good, with no grade 4 or 5 AEs. There were still a substantial number of AEs observed during the treatment (282), of which 75% (212) were considered treatment related, but these AEs were mostly grade 1 (73%) or grade 2 (23%). Minor decreases in blood pressure (BP), concordant increases in heart rate (HR), and fevers were observed during treatment, but these changes quickly returned to baseline levels after treatment has been completed. The most common

AEs were rash (63%), fever, fatigue (58%), and HA, nausea, and influenza symptoms (46%), with only common cytokine side effects seen in 1/3 or less of the patients. Nine patients had grade 3 laboratory AEs most prominently low ALC (17 events), hyponatremia (5 events), elevated ALT and AST (4 events), elevated INR (2 events), and 1 episode of hyperkalemia. Many patients experienced lower grade laboratory AE such as low ALC (100%), hypoalbuminemia (92%), thrombocytopenia (75%), anemia (58%), decreased serum bicarbonate (79%), hyponatremia (75%), elevated ALT, and AST (67%). Thirteen SAEs were noted during the protocol treatment period. Eight of the events (hypersensitivity, fever, sinus tachycardia, myalgias/arthralgias, chills, and hepatitis) that occurred in 4 of the patients were considered, probably or definitely related to the IL-21 treatment. With the exception of the patients with the hypersensitivity SAE (discontinued treatment) and hepatitis (dose reduced), no patients had their IL-21 dosing changed because of their AEs.

Laboratory Analysis

This particular trial provided the best picture of IL-21 effects on immune cells demonstrated a prompt reduction in the total number of CD4$^+$, CD8$^{+,}$ and NK cells during the initial 5 day treatment and a substantial increase in monocytes at the day 4 immune assessment. Similar evaluation on day 29 of the cycle 3 "baseline" showed a modest increase in the total number of CD8$^+$ (approaching 150% of initial pretreatment level) without substantial increases in the number of CD4$^+$ and NK cells. The end of treatment assessment on day 32 again demonstrated decreased numbers of CD4$^+$, CD8$^+$, and NK cells, with an even more profound monocytosis now almost 2.5 times the starting number

of cells. Despite the decreases in the number of lymphocytes, there was still ample evidence of immune activation measured as increases in the mRNA for lytic or effector molecules (granzyme B, perforin and IFNγ) in CD8$^+$ and NK cells, sustained increases in the percentage of CD4$^+$, CD8$^+$, and NK cells that were CD25$^+$ (IL-2R) or the activation marker CD69, monocytes with increased expression or density of FC receptor CD16 (FcγRIII) or CD64 (FcγRI) and an initial increase in the percentage of CD62L$^+$ chemokine receptor 7 positive (CCR7$^+$) most indicative of central memory cells during the initial 5 day treatment, which later declined. The development of anti-IL-21 antibodies was detected in 1 patient. The results of the flow cytometry or technically fluorescence-activated cell sorting (FACS) analysis for changes in the immunophenotype of lymphocytes were very similar to the results of another phase I trial evaluating IL-21 treatment in melanoma and mRCC patients.

Clinical Efficacy

One patient in the first stage group had a short lived CR (11 weeks), and 1 patient in the second stage group had a PR. Another patient had a CR in baseline marker lesions but was found to have new brain lesions at restaging and was not considered a responder, and the overall RR was 8.3%,

Phase I Trial Dose Escalation Subcutaneous rhIL-21 in Melanoma and Renal Cell Carcinoma

The specific effects and toxicity profile related to a new route of administration or schedule for an untested cytokine cannot reliably be predicted, even when in vivo human data are available and still require testing in human subjects. SC dosing offers PK advantages, theoretical immunologic advantages, and clear logistical advantages in terms of outpatient or self-administered treatment. Many cellular immunotherapy trials evaluating subcutaneous (SC) cytokine administration have reported clinical efficacy, but SC treatment regimens are still generally considered inferior to IV regimens. A phase I dose escalation trial enrolling 26 patients with melanoma and mRCC evaluating SC rhIL-21 given at dose levels of 3, 10, 30, 100, 200, and 300 mcg/kg 3 times a week (tiw) for 8 to 16 weeks (54). Patients were restaged with CT scans after 8 and 16 weeks.

Safety

The AE profile was similar to the IVB trial; headaches (81%), fatigue (65%), fever (62%), injection site reaction (58%), nausea (50%), myalgias (42%), arthralgias/pruritus/vomiting, rash, and anemia (<25%), with the majority of the event being grade 1 or 2. The MTD was 200 mcg/kg, and 15 of the 26 patients had ≥grade 3 AEs, most often hematologic laboratories, and these AEs resulted in 3 patients withdrawing from the trial.

Laboratory Analyses

The AUC of IL-21 was dose proportional across the IL-21 dose levels. As expected, the t ½ of IL-21 administered by the SC route was slightly longer (mean 3.6–5.2 hours) than the 3.1 hours seen in the 30 mcg/kg dosing cohort evaluated in the rhIL-21 IVB trial. Again, acute decreases in the number of NK, CD8+, and CD4+ lymphocytes, and B-cells were noted in the peripheral blood (PB), and these cell counts remained below the normal range or pretreatment levels for the patients for the treatment period. There was evidence of immune activation as measured increases in soluble IL-2 receptor (sIL-2R) and in the mRNA for IFNγ, perforin, and granzyme B in the patient's

PBLs. Analysis of sIL-2R levels demonstrated minimal increase in sIL-2R at doses of 3 to 30 mcg/kg, but much higher levels measured at 100, 200, and 300 mcg/kg with a rapid return to pretreatment levels when the rhIL-21 was interrupted for the week 8 radiographic evaluation.

Clinical Efficacy

Three patients were classified as having PRs (1 melanoma, 2 mRCC) in the 25 patients evaluable for response, 5 patients were early progressive disease, and 3 later developed new sites of disease. The melanoma patient called a PR was really an unconfirmed CR, and 15 patients had SD for an RR of 12% and a DCR of 69%.

A Phase IIa Trial of Intravenous rhIL-21 in Treatment-Naive Metastatic Melanoma

A phase II trial that has been reported in abstract form only evaluated IL-21 IVB given on the standard "5 + 9" schedule to 40 previously untreated metastatic melanoma patients evaluated to different dose levels and essentially different lengths of treatment, which resulted in 3 different treatment cohorts (55). All patient were again treated weeks 1 and 3 but cohort 3 did not receive treatment week 5. Cohorts 1 and 3 were dosed at 50 mcg/kg/day, and cohort 2 patients received 30 mcg/kg/day; the treatments were given as follows: cohort 1, 50 mcg/kg/day weeks 1, 3, and 5 every 8 weeks; cohort 2, 30 mcg/kg/day weeks 1, 3, and 5 every 8 weeks; and cohort 3, 50 mcg/kg/day weeks 1 and 3 every 6 weeks. Treatment at 50 mcg/kg every other week × 3 proved too difficult to administer, and this cohort was terminated after 3 patients have been treated. In contrast, the cohort receiving rhIL-21 at 50 mcg/kg only weeks 1 and 3 every 6 weeks proved tolerable, and a total of 7 patients were treated with this schedule. The vast majority of the patients were treated with the now standard IL-21 regimen of three 5 day cycles every other week with a 2 week rest afterward. Patients had good performance status (all ECOG 0 or 1) but had significant disease burden, with 45% having ≥3 sites of metastatic disease.

Safety

Two of the 3 patients in cohort 1 and 4 of the 7 patients in cohort 3 had DLTs. The most common AEs were fatigue, rash, fever, myalgias, anorexia, chills, and nausea. It is interesting to note that 40% of the patients receiving the 50 mcg/kg dose had grade 3 rash. Four (infection with grade 4 neutropenia, 2 patients with grade liver function test (4 LFT) abnormalities and a second malignancy [AML]) of the total of 9 SAEs were probably or definitely related to the IL-21 treatment.

Laboratory Analyses

More detailed analysis of biologically important molecules that included IL-21R, Bcl-2 expression (immunohistochemistry), presence of BRAF (V600E) mutation, ulceration of primary, serum vascular endothelial growth factor (VEGF), or CD25 levels were not seen to correlate with clinical activity.

Clinical Activity

PRs were seen in 9 of the 37 patients (24%) evaluable for response, 16 patients had SD (40%) with a median duration of 5.3 months, and 14 patients had progressive disease at their initial evaluation. The median progression-free survival of 4.3 months was felt to be favorable to the median 1.58 months predicted by the 2008 Korn meta-analysis of progression and overall survival benchmarks for metastatic melanoma.

Laboratory Analysis of Patients Treated With Intravenous rhIL-21

Another report has detailed laboratory information but does not present clinical data for 72 patients treated with rhIL-21 in 2 earlier phase I trials in Australia using similar but not identical IV infusion regimens at dose levels between 100 mcg/kg (56). Patients were either treated with the now common daily × 5 followed by 9 days of rest (5 +9) schedule or tiw for 6 consecutive weeks.

Laboratory Analysis

This particular publication provided the best picture of rhIL-21 effects on immune cells demonstrated a prompt reduction in the total number of CD4+, CD8+, and NK cells during the initial 5 day treatment and a substantial increase in monocytes at day 4 of immune assessment. Similar evaluation on day 29 of the cycle 3 "baseline" showed a modest increase in the total number of CD8+ (approaching 150% of initial pretreatment level) without substantial increases in the number of CD4+ and NK cells. The end of treatment assessment on day 32 again demonstrated decreased numbers of CD4+, CD8+, and NK cells, with an even more profound monocytosis now almost 2.5 times the starting number of cells. Despite the decreases in the number of lymphocytes, there was still ample evidence of immune activation measured as increases in the mRNA for lytic or effector molecules (granzyme B, perforin and IFNγ) in CD8+ and NK cells, sustained increases in the percentage of CD4+, CD8+, and NK cells that were CD25+ (IL-2R) or the activation marker CD69, monocytes with increased expression or density of FC receptor CD16 (FcγRIII) or CD64 (FcγRI) and an initial increase in the percentage of CD62L+ chemokine receptor 7 positive (CCR7+) most indicative of central memory cells during the initial 5 day treatment, which later declined. The development of anti-IL-21 antibodies was detected in 1 patient.

RhIL-21 Summary

There have been some encouraging results from the early clinical trials with rhIL-21, but definitive clinical trials must be performed. Still a number of conclusions can be made about rhIL-21:

- RhIL-21 has a good safety profile, with constitutional, musculoskeletal, and GI AEs being the predominant side effects with rare severe hepatotoxicity.
- The daily × 5 IV regimen given every other week has become the most widely used regimen.
- Immune activation clearly occurs, but lymphocyte counts remain slightly depressed during treatment.
- Important stimulator of CD8$^+$ and NK cells but not Tregs.
- Clinical efficacy in melanoma patients has been demonstrated in several trials, but response rates are highly variable.

Background for rhIL-7

IL-7 is another common γ chain (CD132) cytokine with a number of important biologic functions and potential as an oncology immunotherapeutic agent (57). The prospective therapeutic role for IL-7 is not limited to the treatment of advanced solid tumors, because IL-7 has an important contribution in the development of thymic (T cell) lymphocytes or reconstitution of the T-cell repertoire after hematopoietic stem cell transplantation (58). IL-7 is produced by nonhematopoietic stromal or epithelial cells, BM stromal cells, MHC II$^+$ thymic epithelial cells, liver and intestinal

epithelial cells, keratinocytes, follicular DCs, smooth muscle cells, and, sometimes, DCs and macrophages. Given the diverse and widely available tissue sources of IL-7, it is not surprising that nearly all PB T cells express the IL-7 receptor (IL-7R), and both findings indicate the important physiologic role for this cytokine. Similar to the IL-21 receptor (IL-21R), only IL-7R has the common γ chain, and IL-7 has a specific alpha chain (IL-7Rα or CD127) that is distinct from the trimeric IL-15R. After IL-7 has engaged IL-7R, it transmits the activation signal through JAK 1 and JAK3, primarily through STAT5 and the common RAS/RAF/PI3K pathways. CD132 expression is constitutive or constant, but CD127 expression is most common early in thymopoieses, "naive" (CD45RA$^+$) and, importantly, on effector T cells that upregulate the receptor during the contraction phase of an immune response on the cells that ultimately become "central memory" cells (59). Type I IFNs, Fms-like tyrosine kinase 3 ligand (FLT3 ligand), TNFα, and corticosteroids increase the expression of CD127 and stimuli normally associated with T-cell activation such as IL-2 or IL-15 diminish CD127 transcription and translation as evidenced by the low expression of CD127 on "memory" (CD45RO$^+$) or chronically activated T-cells and importantly TRegs.

Preclinical Tumor Models

Because the focus of this chapter is on the immunotherapy of metastatic melanoma, this section will not discuss preclinical data that support the post SCT immune reconstitution strategies. The translation of positive preclinical results into the efficacy in patients can be difficult, but sometimes, delineation of precise conditions in the preclinical models are very informative. As might be predicted by the immunologic role of IL-7, coadministration during the contraction phase of the immune response after vaccinia virus or DNA vaccination increased the number of lymphocytic choriomeningitis virus (LCMV) Ag-specific CD8+ effector cells, thereby producing an improved recall response and viral control (60,61). The stimulatory effects of IL-7 have been examined in a murine renal cell cancer (RCC-26) allogeneic transfected with genes for IL-7, IL-2, and B7.1 (CD80). Comparison of IFNγ production from renal cell cancer–specific TILs (TIL26) by ELISPOT showed comparable levels of when these cells were incubated with RCC-26 cells cotransfected with IL-7/CD80 or IL-2/CD80 (62). Comparison of effects of adjuvant rhIL-2, rhIL-7, and rhIL-15 when mice were immunized against specific (male HY) Ag showed that IL-7 and IL-15 increased the number of specific effector cells against the dominant and subdominant Ags, but IL-2 did not. Both the rhIL-7 and rhIL-15 treated mice showed sustained survival of long-term specific memory cells and indicated that IL-7 and IL-15 had greater potential as immune adjuvants for vaccines. In a murine preclinical model for adoptive immunotherapy of melanoma (Pmel) with CD8+effector cells, mice treated with IL-7 had an antitumor immune response that was as effective as mice receiving IL-2, IL-15 or IL-21 (63,64). Treatment with rhIL-7 has been shown to augment the immune response generated by in GM-CSF transfected B16F10 and CT26 tumors. Increased numbers of lymphocytes in the draining lymph nodes, increased numbers of tumor specific effector cells, and improved survival were observed in the animals treated with the cytokine (65).

Given the biologic and immunologic functions of IL-7, therapeutic administration of this cytokine has also been shown to promote antiviral immune responses in preclinical models for the HIV infection and other viral diseases. Despite the differences in the 2 disease groups (cancer and HIV infections), there are similarities in terms of immune function and dysfunction that make preclinical and clinical trial data from HIV studies informative (66–68).

NCI Phase I Clinical Trials

Two phase I dose escalation trials have been conducted at the NCI. The initial trial was an FIH dose escalation trial administering SC rhIL-7 at doses of 3, 10, 30, and 60 mcg/kg every third day (0, 3, 6, 9, 12, 15, 18 and 21) for 8 doses in conjunction with 2 well characterized 9 mer melanoma peptides, gp100: 209–217 (210M) and MART-1: 26–35 (27L) emulsified in incomplete Freund adjuvant on days 7, 14, and 21. Five of the 12 patients (11 melanoma and 1 sarcoma) enrolled in the trial were treatment naive and had undergone surgical resection of their disease. Extensive PK, immunologic, FACS analyses, BM, and molecular analyses were performed as part of this study (69).

Safety

The treatments were well tolerated, with fevers and injection site reactions being the most common AEs. Three patients had more notable grade 3 events, 1 patient had transient hypocalcemia soon after the protocol prescribed leukopheresis that was probably related to citrate anticoagulant, and 2 patients had grade 3 elevations of their LFTs during the treatment period that the promptly resolved after IL-7 was stopped.

Laboratory Analyses

Analysis of IL-7 showed linear PK at the 24 hour postdose assessment for 3 highest dose levels, but no IL-7 could be measured in the serum of the 3 patients treated at the 3 mcg/kg dose level. Although all 3 60 mcg/kg patients had detectable IL-7 at the 48 hour time point and had consistent t ½ for IL-7 of approximately 12 hours, only 1 patient from the 30 mcg/kg cohort had measurable levels of IL-7 on day 2. Only minor changes in absolute neutrophil count (ANC), ALC, absolute CD4$^+$, CD8$^+$, and FoxP3$^+$ Treg counts were seen in the patients treated with 3 mcg/kg over the 4 week study assessment period. Beginning at the 10 mcg/kg dose level, moderate and then more notable increases in ALC, absolute CD4$^+$and CD8$^+$ (≈ 3 times baseline for 30 mcg/kg dose) up to 6 to 7 times baseline numbers for the patient receiving the highest dose of IL-7. This lymphocytosis persisted sometimes through the day 28 time point. In contrast, all the patients treated at the 60 mcg/kg dose level showed decreases in the absolute FoxP3$^+$ Treg counts as measured by semiquantitative polymerase chain reaction (PCR)assessment of FoxP3 mRNA (normalized to β actin) on day 28, which ranged from 29% to 73% below their baseline Treg assessment. Although there was no consistent change in the percentage of T cells expressing CD25 (IL-2 receptor) or HLA-DR, there was evidence of a shift in the percentage of CD45RA$^+$ cells toward CD45RO$^+$ cells.

Although none of the patients entered had evidence of anti-IL-7 antibodies pretreatment, 5 of the 6 patients treated at the 30 and 60 mcg/kg dose levels developed anti-IL-7 neutralizing antibodies by the day 28 analyses with titers of 1:50 to 1:200, which did not meet the protocol-defined level for a significant antibody titer.

Clinical Efficacy

None of the patients had an objective clinical response.

The most recent trial (70) enrolled 16 patients with incurable nonhematologic malignancies were treated with doses of rhIL-7 at doses of 3, 10, 30, and 60 mcg/kg given as a SC injection every other day for 2 weeks. Approximately half of the patients had melanoma (N = 5) or mRCC (N = 2), which are considered immunologically responsive diseases, with 3 patients having sarcomas (osteogenic, rhabdomyosarcoma, synovial cell), 2 having GI primaries (colon, duodenal), and the other patients having various solid tumors (hemangiopericytoma, cancer unknown primary, pheochromocytoma, and ovarian) that are not usually treated with immunotherapies. The 6 patients treated at the 3 and 10 mcg/kg dose levels tolerated the treatment with minimal side effects. The 30 mcg/kg dose level was defined as the MTD after 2 of the 4 patients enrolled at the 60 mcg/kg dose level had DLTs.

Safety

Beginning with the patients treated at the 10 mcg/kg dose level, mild generalized lower grade constitutional symptoms and local injection site reactions (erythema, pruritus, and induration) were consistently noted approximately 6 to 8 hours after IL-7 treatment. All 3 of the 10 mcg/kg patients had grade 2 injection site reactions and grade 1 constitutional symptoms, and 1 patient had a slight elevation in ALT. Injection site reaction (grade 1 or 2) were noted in 3 of the 4 patients treated with 30 mcg/kg, and all had low-grade constitutional complaints, with 1 patient having a grade 3 elevation of their AST, which constituted a DLT. Only 1 of the 60 mcg/kg patients tolerated their treatment well. In addition to the injection site reaction and the constitutional symptoms, another patient with the diagnosis of pheochromocytoma had a grade 3 cardiac event (chest pains, hypertension, and elevated troponins without EKG changes) several hours after their third 60 mcg/kg dose. This event was assessed as a cardiac DLT, but the authors considered that the event was not unexpected for a patient with pheochromocytoma diagnosis and concluded that this "DLT" was not applicable to the MTD determination for the trial. The other AEs seen at this dose level included grade 2 shortness of breath, grade 1 thrombocytopenia, elevated LFTs in all 4 patients, and >50% increase in mean spleen size at day 14 as measured with CT scan.

Laboratory Analysis

First clearly seen at the 10 mcg/kg dose level and above, patients showed a prompt decline of approximately 50% in ALC after their first dose, followed by a gradual increase in the count, which was maximal at day 21 or 28 most often. In the 3 mcg/kg cohort, the ALC never really returned to baseline levels, and the 10 mcg/kg cohort increase peaked at approximately 120% of the baseline ALC. The 30 and 60 mcg/kg cohorts showed dose-dependent increases in ALC up to 3 times the starting ALC. The ALC remained elevated for these groups through the last evaluation performed at day 56. This lymphocytosis was equally seen, for the most part, in CD4$^+$ and CD8$^+$ cells, but not in CD3$^-$ NK or B-cells. Transient increases in the percentage of IL-2R$^+$ (CD25$^+$) CD8$^+$ and non–Treg CD4$^+$ were noted during the treatment period in a limited analysis of the patients receiving the higher IL-7 doses. Transient drops in platelet counts were seen during the treatment period with some possible relationship to dose, but recovered without any clinical bleeding events. Hemoglobin showed a modest decreased without a clear dose relationship during the active treatment period. In contrast, for the 2 highest dose levels, absolute eosinophil and 3 highest dose level neutrophil counts substantially

increased above the baseline, but the numbers of monocytes did not increase as consistently.

Compared with other recombinant human cytokines synthesized in E. coli, the IL-7 used in the protocol was not glycosylated similar to a mammalian or human cytokine and was potentially immunogenic (71). Analysis for the development of anti-IL-7 antibodies during treatment showed 1 of the 6 patients in the 3 and 10 mcg/kg dose levels who was treated with a different lot of drug-developed antibodies (1/1600 titer), and another patient developed a low measurable level (1/100 titer) that was considered negative. However 5 of the 9 patients assessed for antibodies from the 30 and 100 mcg/kg cohorts developed antibodies with titers ranging from 1/400 to 1/1200. Of the remaining 4 patients, 1 was not evaluated, 1 had no measurable antibodies (0), and the other 2 were negative with titers measured at 1/100, which was below the 1/200 cut for positive result. In no case were these antibodies able to neutralize IL-7.

Clinical Efficacy

No clinical responses were seen, and with the exception of the hemangiopericytoma patient who had nonsignificant shrinkage (20%) of his metastatic abdominal mass, all other patients had progressive disease.

RhIL-7 Summary

Very important clinical results from trials with the reformulated rhIL-7 are still not available and the current data leads to these conclusion about rhIL-7:

- RhIL-7 has a good safety profile, with mild side effects.
- Support immune reconstitution contributes to the production of effector

memory, central memory, and naive T cells and is potentially inhibitory for Tregs.

- Initial human clinical trials showed a substantial number of patients who developed anti-IL-7 antibodies Although considered nonneutralizing, it was of concern, because the clinical product was E. coli derived and nonglycosylated.

- New formulation produced in the mammalian (CHO) cell line has now entered clinical trials and lessens the issues with repeat cycles of treatment.

Background for rhIL-15

The cytokine that is now called interleukin-15 was initially reported nearly simultaneously by 2 different research groups, 1 at the NCI and the other at Immunex Corporation (72,73). Interleukin-15 is produced not only by APCs such as DCs but also by other mononuclear cells after encounters with double-stranded RNA, viral, bacterial, and fungal pathogens and also type 1 interferons (IFNs). IL-15 is normally not secreted as a free cytokine in vivo but, most often, with IL-15Rα on the cell surface of APCs and presented in trans to nearby effector T and NK cells (74,75). Interleukin-15 has a heterotrimeric receptor (IL-15R) composed of a unique alpha subunit (IL-15Rα chain), a beta subunit that it shares with IL-2 (IL-2R/IL-15Rβ chain), and the previously discussed common gamma-chain (γc). In contrast with IL-2, IL-15 does not cause activation-induced cell death (AICD) and seemingly has greater capacity to maintain high-avidity CD8+ memory T-cell responses to invading pathogens by supporting the survival of these T-cells (76,77). In addition to promoting the global CD8+ response, IL-15 preferentially expands the most

active CD8+, CD95+, CCR7−, and CD28− effector memory cells and increases their T-cell receptor avidity by inducing higher expression of CD8αβ, which, as expected, augments these cells' functional capacity (78). Administration of IL-15 has also been shown to upregulate IL-15Rα expression, which allows the effector cells to respond to lower local concentrations of IL-15, which resulted in increased production of secondary stimulatory cytokines such as IFNγ and tumor necrosis factor alpha (TNFα) and increased production of lytic molecules such as perforin (79,80). It is important to note that, similar to IL-21, IL-15 was initially described as inhibiting T regs but is now understood to provide limited stimulation of these immunosuppressive cells in contrast with the effects of IL-2.

Preclinical Tumor Models

Preclinical experiments indicate that IL-15 is superior to IL-2 in the maintenance of NK cells, NK-T cells, intraepithelial lymphocytes, and memory phenotype CD8+ T-cells (81). The antitumor effect of IL-2 probably results from its ability to expand lymphocyte populations in vivo and to increase the effector functions of these cells, thereby inhibiting tumor growth. Attempts to prevent tumor growth in mice by administration of IL-15 have proven effective (81–83) in multiple tumor types: CRC (MC38 and CT-26), melanoma (Pmel and B16), and other tumors alone or in combination with other cytokines, cellular therapies, or vaccines.

Results From Nonhuman Primate Toxicology Studies

A toxicology study with 24 adult rhesus macaques nonhuman primate (NHP) performed to support the FIH clinical protocol

(84,85) evaluated treatment with recombinant human interleukin-15 (rhIL-15) given at doses of 10, 20, 50, or 200 mcg/kg as a 30 minute daily infusion (IVB) for 12 days. Animals treated with the 200 and 50 mcg/kg doses exhibited lethargy, a disheveled appearance, diarrhea, and dehydration that, in some cases, required IV fluids. Laboratory results from this time period showed transient grade 3 or 4 granulocytopenia in the rhesus macaques receiving rhIL-15 at a dose of 50 mcg/kg/day, but no consistent changes in platelet counts or hemoglobin. Concurrent BM samples showed a hypercellular marrow containing all elements of the granulocytes, and none of the animals had any evidence of an infection Histologic examination of the macaques' livers demonstrated granulocytes and other leukocytes in the sinusoids adjacent to normal appearing hepatocytes, suggesting that redistribution to the tissues is a contributing factor in the apparent neutropenia. No significant changes in BUN, creatinine, transaminases, bilirubin, or albumin were seen in the macaques treated at doses of 50 mcg/kg or less. Normal or elevated granulocyte counts were restored within 48 to 72 hours of discontinuation of the rhIL-15 dosing. No antibodies directed against rhIL-15 were detected in the animals, and no animals developed antinuclear antibodies. At necropsy, the only gross or microscopic abnormalities were loss of adiposities in the hyperplastic marrows and the presence of neutrophils and other white blood cells (WBCs) in the liver sinusoids. No animal deaths occurred on this study.

NCI Phase I Dose Escalation Study in Patients with Metastatic Melanoma and mRCC

Phase I trial of daily IVB administration of rhIL-15 given for a single 12 day cycle to patients with metastatic malignant melanoma and metastatic renal cell cancer was begun in 2010 (86). The trial was initially planned with ascending doses beginning at 3 mcg/kg/day to be followed with doses at 7, 10, 15, 20, and 25 mcg/kg/day. Dose levels at 0.3 and 1 mcg/kg/day were added after the first patient has experienced a dose-DLT. The first 5 patients were treated with 3 mcg/kg/day, 4 patients were treated at the 1.0 mcg/kg/day dose level after DLTs, and all 6 subsequent patients have been treated with 0.3 mcg/kg. Table 6 summarizes the experience of the patients treated to date in the initial phase 1 rhIL-15 trial.

Safety

The first patient treated (83 year old woman with melanoma) at the 3 mcg/kg dose level developed symptomatic hypotension (grade 3) with her first rhIL-15dose. The fifth patient developed dose-limiting thrombocytopenia (platelet count nadir of 35,000) after 6 doses, in part because of preprotocol radiation therapy to his right hemipelvis administered just before starting rhIL-15. Because the initial dose level exceeded the MTD, and the next cohort of patients was treated at the 1 mcg/kg dose level. Adverse events that have been observed include the development of fevers, chills, and, at the highest dose level, rigors beginning 2 to 2.5 hours and peaking approximately 3.5 hours after the rhIL-15 infusions. Several of the patients treated at the 3 mcg/kg dose level experienced transient asymptomatic decreases in their BP in the period 3 to 6 hours after the infusions, which was addressed by increases in the rate of normal saline infusions.

The first and, recently, the fourth patients treated at the 1 mcg/kg dose level also had dose-limiting grade 3 aspartate

TABLE 6 Summary of the first 13 patients treated in the NCI FIH trial

Diagnosis/Age	Prior treatment	Doses	Discontinuation
3 µg/kg Patients			
Melanoma/83 F	None	1	DLT grade 3 hypotension
Ocular melanoma/43 M	None ineligible for HD IL-2	12	Completed treatment
Melanoma/53 M	HD IL-2, Ipilimumab, TILs with LD IL-2, AZD-6244, XRT	10	Non-DLT hypotension, pleural effusion
Ocular melanoma/57 F	Anti-CD137, Ipilimumab, CR011 Immunotoxin, XL-184	12	Completed treatment
Melanoma/34 M	HD IL-2, TILs with HD IL-2, young TILs with HD IL-2, Ipilimumab, XRT	6	DLT grade 3 thrombocytopenia
1 µg/kg Patients			
Renal Cell/57 M*	IMRT to jaw, XRT to pelvis, TroVax vaccine with sunitinib, pazopanib, everolimus	4	DLT persistent grade 3 AST/ALT abnormalities
Renal Cell/67 M	Sunitinib, axitinib, sorafenib with LBH589, everolimus	12	Completed treatment
Melanoma/21 F	Young TILs with HD IL-2, Ipilimumab, IL-12 transduced TILs	12	Completed treatment
Mucosal melanoma/50 M	None	4	DLT persistent grade 3 AST/ALT abnormalities
0.3 µg/kg Patients			
Melanoma/68F**	Mod Neck dissection + XRT, Ipilimumab (stopped with colitis) temozolomide, Taxol plus IGF inhibitor	12	Completed treatment
Melanoma/66 F**	HD IL-2, Ipilimumab, CDDP Plus ALT08 vaccine, Ipilimumab with NY-ESO-1 CD8 cells	12	Completed treatment
Renal cell/71M	Sunitinib X 4, pazopanib, everolimus, Rexin-G (intratumoral retroviral GM-CSF), photodynamic therapy	12	Completed treatment
Renal cell/43M	HDIL-2 X 3, anti-PD-1, sunitinib	12	Completed treatment
Renal cell/47M	anti-PD-1, sunitinib	12	Completed treatment

aminotransferase or alanine aminotransferase (AST/ALT) elevations, which halted both their treatments after 4 doses, but all the 1 mcg/kg patients had significant less BP changes, rigors, and constitutional symptoms and required less supportive care. The 6 patients entered when all these AEs have been treated at the 0.3 mcg/kg dose level without any remarkable side effects. All 0.3 mcg/kg patients have received the prescribed 12 doses with incident, and the protocol has recently been amended to allow repeat treatments for patients with evidence of responsive disease.

Laboratory Analyses

Although only 2 of the patients treated with the 3 mcg/kg dose of rhIL-15 had elevations of their transaminases (mild grade 2 elevations of their AST returned to baseline levels within 2 to 4 days), both DLTs at the 1 mcg/kg were grade 3 ALT elevation (5 and 11 × the ULN). One of these patients had a history of idiopathic steatohepatitis (fatty liver), but the other patient was ECOG performance status 0 with no identified liver abnormality. In addition, several of the 0.3 mcg/kg patients developed mild grade 2 elevations of either AST or ALT, and another patient had transient grade 3 transaminases. All patients have demonstrated an increase in the ALC with maximum expansion ranging from 4.2 to 1.5 times their baseline value. This lymphocytosis is most apparent with increases NK cells, but $CD8^+ CD45RO^+$ cells have also substantially increased, and the expansion in cell numbers persists for at least 1 week sometime 2 weeks after completion of treatment. In the limited number of repeat rhIL-15 courses given to date, there is no evidence of differences in laboratory results. Laboratory and immunologic assessments have shown considerable immune activation. Preliminary analyses of 2 immunologic end points (50% increase in the pretreatment number of $CD8^+ CD45RO^+$ memory cell and $\geq 50\%$ increase in pretreatment absolute number of NK cells maintained for at least 1 week) shows that these end points have been met by nearly all patients. Consistent with the clinical events, analysis of inflammatory cytokines in the patients showed maximum concentrations in the serum at 4 hours, including marked increases of IL-6, IFNγ, and IL-1β and lesser increases of TNFα. There was no obvious correlation between rhIL-15 dose or the degree of lymphocytosis and cytokine production for the patients treated to date. The preliminary rhIL-15 PK analysis shows the Cmax and AUC for rhIL-15 to be dose proportional with a serum t ½ of approximately 1 hour (data not shown), and PKs after the 12th infusion did not appreciably change compared with day 1 results. It is important to note that serial assessments for anti-IL-15 antibodies in the patients have not demonstrated antibody formation in any of the 15 patients treated to date.

Clinical Efficacy

No clinical responses by RECIST criteria have been observed, but nonsignificant decreases in the sum of the marker lesions and stabilization for more than the 3 month study period have been observed in patients who had active disease before rhIL-15 treatment.

Additional Active or Soon-to-be-Open rhIL-15 Trials

Two other rhIL-15 clinical trials have been initiated at the NCI. The Surgery

Branch has begun a phase I dose escalation trial administering rhIL-15 with TILs. The Metabolism Branch has also initiated a phase I trial administering rhIL-15 as a 10 day (120 hour) continuous intravenous (CIV) infusion based on toxicology study performed in rhesus macaques, which showed a dramatically higher lymphocytosis that was primarily seen in the CD8$^+$ and CD45RO$^+$ T cell subsets. Another phase I dose escalation trial assessing the therapeutic potential of NK cell stimulation at the University of Minnesota has treated 5 patients. Finally, the NCI Cancer Therapy Evaluation Program through the newly established Cancer Immunotherapy Trials Network (CITN), which will essentially function as an Immunotherapy Cooperative group, will initiate their first rhIL-15 trial on the third quarter of 2012, with anticipation of additional trials to follow soon after.

RhIL-15 Summary

The clinical experience with rhIL-15 is still very limited, but some preliminary conclusions can be made about this agent:

- RhIL-15 has a good safety profile with mild side effects.
- Sporadic Liver function test abnormalities which do not seem dose related.
- Stimulates T-cells and NK cells.
- Moderate sustained lymphocytosis in patients more NK mediated with the IVB regimen.
- Preclinical NHP data indicate that continuous intravenous regimen is better for expansion of (CD8) T cells.
- Additional clinical trials that include combination treatments have or soon will open.

■ FUTURE DIRECTIONS IN THE TREATMENT OF ADVANCE MELANOMA: 2012

As discussed in the Introduction, there have been a number of very positive clinical trial reports indicating significant activity in new investigational agents. In addition, there have been a large number of publications that have provided important preclinical or translational information not discussed in detail in this chapter that have broadened our understanding of the human immune system. These data have clarified how the now well-recognized counterregulatory forces such as CTLA-4, PD-1 and Tregs act to inhibit the in vivo activation expected to occur with our immunotherapeutic efforts. Greater understanding of the functional role of the different lymphocyte effector cell subsets has elucidated how the newer rh cytokines now available for clinical use can provide superior activation or support of in situ or infused tumor specific effector cells. Application of our growing ability to modulate immune checkpoint molecules and more precise use of stimulatory cytokines in combination with established adoptive cellular therapies or vaccine strategies has led to renewed expectations that immunotherapy can now be the powerful therapeutic modality predicted many years ago when the anticancer role of the human immune system was initially recognized. Therefore, we await, with great anticipation, the results of newly active or planned immunotherapy trials evaluating anti-PD-1, anti-PD-L1, rhIL-21, rhIL-7, and rhIL-15.

■ REFERENCES

1. Liao W, Lin JX, Leonard WJ. IL-2 family cytokines: new insights into the complex roles of IL-2 as a broad regulator of T helper

cell differentiation. *Curr Opin Immunol.* 2011;23(5):598–604.

2. Topalian SL, Drake CG, Pardoll DM. Targeting the PD-1/B7-H1(PD-L1) pathway to activate anti-tumor immunity. *Curr Opin Immunol.* 2012;24(2):207–212.

3. Topalian SL, Hodi FS, Brahmer JR, et al. Safety, activity, and immune correlates of anti-PD-1 antibody in cancer. *N Engl J Med.* 2012;366(26):2443–2454.

4. Davis ID, Skrumsager BK, Cebon J, et al. An open-label, two-arm, phase I trial of recombinant human interleukin-21 in patients with metastatic melanoma. *Clin Cancer Res.* 2007;13(12):3630–3636.

5. Rosenberg SA, Sportès C, Ahmadzadeh M, et al. IL-7 administration to humans leads to expansion of CD8+ and CD4+ cells but a relative decrease of CD4+ T-regulatory cells. *J Immunother.* 2006;29(3):313–319.

6. Robert C, Thomas L, Bondarenko I, et al. Ipilimumab plus dacarbazine for previously untreated metastatic melanoma. *N Engl J Med.* 2011;364(26):2517–2526.

7. Hodi FS, O'Day SJ, McDermott DF, et al. Improved survival with ipilimumab in patients with metastatic melanoma. *N Engl J Med.* 2010;363(8):711–723.

8. Brahmer JR, Tykodi SS, Chow LQ, et al. Safety and activity of anti-PD-L1 antibody in patients with advanced cancer. *N Engl J Med.* 2012;366(26):2455–2465.

9. Chapman PB, Hauschild A, Robert C, et al.; BRIM-3 Study Group. Improved survival with vemurafenib in melanoma with BRAF V600E mutation. *N Engl J Med.* 2011;364(26):2507–2516.

10. Brahmer JR, Drake CG, Wollner I, et al. Phase I study of single-agent anti-programmed death-1 (MDX-1106) in refractory solid tumors: safety, clinical activity, pharmacodynamics, and immunologic correlates. *J Clin Oncol.* 2010;28(19):3167–3175.

11. Rosenberg SA, Dudley ME. Adoptive cell therapy for the treatment of patients with metastatic melanoma. *Curr Opin Immunol.* 2009;21(2):233–240.

12. Sharpe AH, Freeman GJ. The B7-CD28 superfamily. *Nat Rev Immunol.* 2002;2(2):116–126.

13. Nishimura H, Honjo T. PD-1: an inhibitory immunoreceptor involved in peripheral tolerance. *Trends Immunol.* 2001;22:265–268.

14. Finger LR, Pu J, Wasserman R, et al. The human PD-1 gene: complete cDNA, genomic organization, and developmentally regulated expression in B cell progenitors. *Gene.* 1997;197(1–2):177–187.

15. Jeffrey Weber Immune Checkpoint Proteins. A new therapeutic paradigm for cancer—preclinical background: CTLA-4 and PD-1 blockade. *Semin Oncol.* 2010;37:430–439.

16. Zanin-Zhorov A, Dustin ML, Blazar BR. PKC-? function at the immunological synapse: prospects for therapeutic targeting. *Trends Immunol.* 2011;32(8):358–363.

17. Sherman E, Barr V, Manley S, et al. Functional nanoscale organization of signaling molecules downstream of the T cell antigen receptor. *Immunity.* 2011;35(5):705–720.

18. Fischer A, Picard C, Chemin K, Dogniaux S, le Deist F, Hivroz C. ZAP70: a master regulator of adaptive immunity. *Semin Immunopathol.* 2010;32(2):107–116.

19. Chen J, Feng Y, Lu L, et al. Interferon-?-induced PD-L1 surface expression on human oral squamous carcinoma via PKD2 signal pathway. *Immunobiology.* 2012;217(4):385–393.

20. Krönig H, Julia Falchner K, Odendahl M, et al. PD-1 expression on Melan-A-reactive T cells increases during progression to metastatic disease. *Int J Cancer.* 2012;130(10):2327–2336.

21. Iwai Y, Ishida M, Tanaka Y, Okazaki T, Honjo T, Minato N. Involvement of PD-L1 on tumor cells in the escape from host immune system and tumor immunotherapy by PD-L1 blockade. *Proc Natl Acad Sci USA.* 2002;99(19):12293–12297.

22. Gao Q, Wang XY, Qiu SJ, et al. Overexpression of PD-L1 significantly associates with tumor aggressiveness and postoperative recurrence in human hepatocellular carcinoma. *Clin Cancer Res.* 2009;15(3):971–979.

23. Latchman Y, Wood CR, Chernova T, et al. P D-L2 is a second ligand for PD-1 and inhibits T cell activation. *Nat Immunol.* 2001 Mar;2(3):261–268.

24. Mendoza-Coronel E, Camacho-Sandoval R, Bonifaz LC, López-Vidal Y. PD-L2 induction on dendritic cells exposed to Mycobacterium avium downregulates BCG-specific T cell response. *Tuberculosis (Edinb).* 2011;91(1):36–46.

25. Chemnitz JM, Parry RV, Nichols KE, June CH, Riley JL. SHP-1 and SHP-2 associate with immunoreceptor tyrosine-based switch motif of programmed death 1 upon primary human T cell stimulation, but only receptor ligation prevents T cell activation. *J Immunol.* 2004;173(2):945–954.

26. Hirano F, Kaneko K, Tamura H, et al. Blockade of B7-H1 and PD-1 by monoclonal antibodies potentiates cancer therapeutic immunity. *Cancer Res.* 2005;65(3):1089–1096.

27. Li B, VanRoey M, Wang C, Chen TH, Korman A, Jooss K. Anti-programmed death-1 synergizes with granulocyte macrophage colony-stimulating factor–secreting tumor cell immunotherapy providing therapeutic benefit to mice with established tumors. *Clin Cancer Res.* 2009;15(5):1623–1634.

28. Song MY, Park SH, Nam HJ, Choi DH, Sung YC. Enhancement of vaccine-induced primary and memory CD8(+) T-cell responses by soluble PD-1. *J Immunother.* 2011;34(3):297–306.

29. Dulos J, Carven GJ, van Boxtel SJ, et al. PD-1 blockade augments Th1 and Th17 and suppresses Th2 responses in peripheral blood from patients with prostate and advanced melanoma cancer. *J Immunother.* 2012;35(2):169–178.

30. Tzeng HT, Tsai HF, Liao HJ, et al. PD-1 blockage reverses immune dysfunction and hepatitis B viral persistence in a mouse animal model. *PLoS ONE.* 2012;7(6):e39179.

31. Wang X, Zhang Z, Zhang S, et al. B7-H1 up-regulation impairs myeloid DC and correlates with disease progression in chronic HIV-1 infection. *Eur J Immunol.* 2008;38(11):3226–3236.

32. Nishimura H, Nose M, Hiai H, Minato N, Honjo T. Development of lupus-like autoimmune diseases by disruption of the PD-1 gene encoding an ITIM motif-carrying immunoreceptor. *Immunity.* 1999;11(2):141–151.

33. Tarrio ML, Grabie N, Bu DX, Sharpe AH, Lichtman AH. PD-1 protects against inflammation and myocyte damage in T cell-mediated myocarditis. *J Immunol.* 2012;188(10):4876–4884.

34. Nishimura H, Minato N, Nakano T, Honjo T. Immunological studies on PD-1 deficient mice: implication of PD-1 as a negative regulator for B cell responses. *Int Immunol.* 1998;10(10):1563–1572.

35. Menke J, Lucas JA, Zeller GC, et al. Programmed death 1 ligand (PD-L) 1 and PD-L2 limit autoimmune kidney disease: distinct roles. *J Immunol.* 2007;179(11):7466–7477.

36. Nakanishi J, Wada Y, Matsumoto K, Azuma M, Kikuchi K, Ueda S. Overexpression of B7-H1 (PD-L1) significantly associates with tumor grade and postoperative prognosis in human urothelial cancers. *Cancer Immunol Immunother.* 2007;56(8):1173–1182.

37. Konishi J, Yamazaki K, Azuma M, Kinoshita I, Dosaka-Akita H, Nishimura M. B7-H1 expression on non-small cell lung cancer cells and its relationship with tumor-infiltrating lymphocytes and their PD-1 expression. *Clin Cancer Res.* 2004;10(15):5094–5100.

38. Wu C, Zhu Y, Jiang J, Zhao J, Zhang XG, Xu N. Immunohistochemical localization of programmed death-1 ligand-1 (PD-L1) in gastric carcinoma and its clinical significance. *Acta Histochem.* 2006;108(1):19–24.

39. Wang SF, Fouquet S, Chapon M, et al. Early T cell signalling is reversibly altered in PD-1+ T lymphocytes infiltrating human tumors. *PLoS ONE.* 2011;6(3):e17621.

40. Dong H, Strome SE, Salomao DR, et al. Tumor-associated B7-H1 promotes T-cell apoptosis: a potential mechanism of immune evasion. *Nat Med.* 2002;8(8):793–800.

41. Latchman Y, Wood CR, Chernova T, et al. PD-L2 is a second ligand for PD-1 and inhibits T cell activation. *Nat Immunol.* 2001;2(3):261–268.

42. Alderson KL, Zhou Q, Berner V, et al. Regulatory and conventional CD4+ T cells show differential effects correlating with PD-1 and B7-H1 expression after immunotherapy. *J Immunol.* 2008;180(5):2981–2988.

43. Berger R, Rotem-Yehudar R, Slama G, et al. Phase I safety and pharmacokinetic study of CT-011, a humanized antibody interacting with PD-1, in patients with advanced hematologic malignancies. *Clin Cancer Res.* 2008;14(10):3044–3051.

44. Patnaik A, Kang SP, Tolcher AW, et al. Phase I study of MK-3475 (anti-PD-1 monoclonal antibody) in patients with advanced solid tumors. *Proc ASCO.* 2012; Abstract 2512.

45. Ozaki K, Kikly K, Michalovich D, Young PR, Leonard WJ. Cloning of a type I cytokine receptor most related to the IL-2 receptor beta chain. *Proc Natl Acad Sci USA.* 2000;97(21):11439–11444.

46. Meazza R, Azzarone B, Orengo AM, Ferrini S. Role of common-gamma chain cytokines in NK cell development and function: perspectives for immunotherapy. *J Biomed Biotechnol.* 2011;2011:861920.

47. Parrish-Novak J, Dillon SR, Nelson A, et al. Interleukin 21 and its receptor are involved in NK cell expansion and regulation of lymphocyte function. *Nature.* 2000;408(6808):57–63.

48. Dodds MG, Frederiksen KS, Skak K, et al. Immune activation in advanced cancer patients treated with recombinant IL-21: multianalyte profiling of serum proteins. *Cancer Immunol Immunother.* 2009; 58(6):843–854.

49. Peluso I, Fantini MC, Fina D, et al. IL-21 counteracts the regulatory T cell-mediated suppression of human CD4+ T lymphocytes. *J Immunol.* 2007;178(2):732–739.

50. Watanabe M, Kono K, Kawaguchi Y, et al. Interleukin-21 can efficiently restore impaired antibody-dependent cell-mediated cytotoxicity in patients with oesophageal squamous cell carcinoma. *Br J Cancer.* 2010;102(3):520–529.

51. Davis ID, Skrumsager BK, Cebon J, et al. An open-label, two-arm, phase I trial of recombinant human interleukin-21 in patients with metastatic melanoma. *Clin Cancer Res.* 2007;13:3630–3636.

52. Thompson JA, Curti BD, Redman BG, et al. Phase I study of recombinant interleukin-21 in patients with metastatic melanoma and renal cell carcinoma. *J Clin Oncol.* 2008;26(12):2034–2039.

53. Davis ID, Brady B, Kefford RF, et al. Clinical and biological efficacy of recombinant human interleukin-21 in patients with stage IV malignant melanoma without prior treatment: a phase IIa trial. *Clin Cancer Res.* 2009;15(6):2123–2129.

54. Schmidt H, Brown J, Mouritzen U, et al. Safety and clinical effect of subcutaneous human interleukin-21 in patients with metastatic melanoma or renal cell carcinoma: a phase I trial. *Clin Cancer Res.* 2010;16(21):5312–5319.

55. Petrella TM, Tozer R, Belanger K, et al. Interleukin-21 (IL-21) activity in patients (pts) with metastatic melanoma (MM). *Proc ASCO.* 2010; Abstract 8507.

56. Frederiksen KS, Lundsgaard D, Freeman JA, et al. IL-21 induces *in vivo* immune activation of NK cells and CD8(+) T cells in patients with metastatic melanoma and renal cell carcinoma. *Cancer Immunol Immunother.* 2008;57(10):1439–1449.

57. Mackall CL, Fry TJ, Gress RE. Harnessing the biology of IL-7 for therapeutic application. *Nat Rev Immunol.* 2011;11(5):330–342.

58. Capitini CM, Chisti AA, Mackall CL. Modulating T-cell homeostasis with IL-7: preclinical and clinical studies. *J Intern Med.* 2009;266(2):141–153.

59. Ramanathan S, Gagnon J, Dubois S, Forand-Boulerice M, Richter MV, Ilangumaran S. Cytokine synergy in antigen-independent activation and priming of naive CD8+ T lymphocytes. *Crit Rev Immunol.* 2009;29(3):219–239.

60. Nanjappa SG, Walent JH, Morre M, Suresh M. Effects of IL-7 on memory CD8 T cell homeostasis are influenced by the timing of therapy in mice. *J Clin Invest.* 2008;118(3):1027–1039.

61. Pellegrini M, Calzascia T, Elford AR, et al. Adjuvant IL-7 antagonizes multiple cellular and molecular inhibitory networks to enhance immunotherapies. *Nat Med.* 2009;15(5):528–536.

62. Frankenberger B, Pohla H, Noessner E, et al. Influence of CD80, interleukin-2, and interleukin-7 expression in human renal cell carcinoma on the expansion, function, and survival of tumor-specific CTLs. *Clin Cancer Res.* 2005;11(5):1733–1742.

63. Klebanoff CA, Gattinoni L, Palmer DC, et al. Determinants of successful CD8+ T-cell adoptive immunotherapy for large established tumors in mice. *Clin Cancer Res.* 2011;17(16):5343–5352.

64. Markley JC, Sadelain M. IL-7 and IL-21 are superior to IL-2 and IL-15 in promoting human T cell-mediated rejection of systemic lymphoma in immunodeficient mice. *Blood.* 2010;115(17):3508–3519.

65. Li B, VanRoey MJ, Jooss K. Recombinant IL-7 enhances the potency of GM-CSF-secreting tumor cell immunotherapy. *Clin Immunol.* 2007;123(2):155–165.

66. Lévy Y, Sereti I, Tambussi G, et al. Effects of recombinant human interleukin 7 on T-cell recovery and thymic output in HIV-infected patients receiving antiretroviral therapy: results of a phase I/IIa randomized, placebo-controlled, multicenter study. *Clin Infect Dis.* 2012;55(2):291–300.

67. Leone A, Rohankhedkar M, Okoye A, et al. Increased CD4+ T cell levels during IL-7 administration of antiretroviral therapy-treated simian immunodeficiency virus-positive macaques are not dependent on strong proliferative responses. *J Immunol.* 2010;185(3):1650–1659.

68. Beq S, Rozlan S, Gautier D, et al. Injection of glycosylated recombinant simian IL-7 provokes rapid and massive T-cell homing in rhesus macaques. *Blood.* 2009;114(4):816–825.

69. Rosenberg SA, Sportès C, Ahmadzadeh M, et al. IL-7 administration to humans leads to expansion of CD8+ and CD4+ cells but a relative decrease of CD4+ T-regulatory cells. *J Immunother.* 2006;29:313–319.

70. Sportès C, Babb RR, Krumlauf MC, et al. Phase I study of recombinant human interleukin-7 administration in subjects with refractory malignancy. *Clin Cancer Res.* 2010;16(2):727–735.

71. Morre M, Beq S. Interleukin-7 and immune reconstitution in cancer patients: a new paradigm for dramatically increasing overall survival. *Target Oncol.* 2012;7(1):55–68.

72. Grabstein KH, Eisenman J, Shanebeck K, et al. Cloning of a T cell growth factor that interacts with the 1P chain of the interleukin-2 receptor. *Science.* 1994;264:965–968.

73. Bamford RN, Grant AJ, Burton JD, et al. The interleukin (IL) 2 receptor beta chain is shared by IL-2 and a cytokine, provisionally designated IL-T, that stimulates T-cell proliferation and the induction of lymphokine-activated killer cells. *Proc Natl Acad Sci USA.* 1994;91(11):4940–4944.

74. Lucas M, Schachterle W, Oberle K, Aichele P, Diefenbach A. Dendritic cells prime natural killer cells by trans-presenting interleukin 15. *Immunity.* 2007;26(4):503–517.

75. Dubois S, Patel HJ, Zhang M, Waldmann TA, Müller JR. Preassociation of IL-15 with IL-15R alpha-IgG1-Fc enhances its activity on proliferation of NK and CD8+/CD44high T cells and its antitumor action. *J Immunol.* 2008;180(4):2099–2106.

76. Oh S, Perera LP, Terabe M, Ni L, Waldmann TA, Berzofsky JA. IL-15 as a mediator of CD4+ help for CD8+ T cell longevity and avoidance of TRAIL-mediated apoptosis. *Proc Natl Acad Sci USA.* 2008;105(13):5201–5206.

77. Lu J, Giuntoli RL, Omisa R, et al. Interleukin 15 promotes antigen independent in vitro expansion and long term survival of antitumor cytotoxic T lymphocytes. *Clin Cancer Res.* 2002;8:3877–3884.

78. Oh S, Perera LP, Burke DS, Waldmann TA, Berzofsky JA. IL-15/IL-15Ralpha-mediated avidity maturation of memory CD8+ T cells. *Proc Natl Acad Sci USA.* 2004;101(42):15154–15159.

79. Ozdemir O, Ravindranath Y, Savasan S. Mechanisms of superior anti-tumor cytotoxic response of interleukin 15-induced lymphokine-activated killer cells. *J Immunother.* 2005;28(1):44–52.

80. King JW, Thomas S, Corsi F, et al. IL15 can reverse the unresponsiveness of Wilms' tumor antigen-specific CTL in patients with prostate cancer. *Clin Cancer Res.* 2009;15(4):1145–1154.

81. Waldmann TA. The biology of interleukin-2 and interleukin-15: implications for cancer therapy and vaccine design. *Nat Rev Immunol.* 2006;6(8):595–601.

82. Lu J, Giuntoli RL 2nd, Omiya R, Kobayashi H, Kennedy R, Celis E. Interleukin 15 promotes antigen-independent *in vitro* expansion and long-term survival of antitumor cytotoxic T lymphocytes. *Clin Cancer Res.* 2002;8(12):3877–3884.

83. Tagaya Y, Bamford RN, DeFilippis AP, Waldmann TA. IL-15: a pleiotropic cytokine with diverse receptor/signaling pathways whose expression is controlled at multiple levels. *Immunity.* 1996;4(4):329–336.

84. Lugli E, Goldman CK, Perera LP, et al. Transient and persistent effects of IL-15 on lymphocyte homeostasis in nonhuman primates. *Blood.* 2010;116(17):3238–3248.

85. Waldmann TA, Lugli E, Roederer M, et al. Safety (toxicity), pharmacokinetics, immunogenicity, and impact on elements of the normal immune system of recombinant human IL-15 in rhesus macaques. *Blood.* 2011;117(18):4787–4795.

86. Conlon K, Morris JC, Janik, et al. Phase I study of intravenous recombinant human interleukin-15 (rh IL-15) in adults with metastatic malignant melanoma and renal cell carcinoma. *Proc SITC.* 2011.

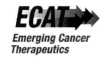

ECAT
Emerging Cancer Therapeutics

Updated Approach to the Patient With Metastatic Melanoma

Rodabe N. Amaria[1] and Rene Gonzalez[*,2]

[1]*Department of Medicine, University of Colorado, Aurora, CO;*

[2]*Cutaneous Oncology Program, University of Colorado, Aurora, CO*

■ ABSTRACT

Melanoma has traditionally been a devastating malignancy in advanced stages as a result of the paucity of effective therapies. In 2011, two drugs have been approved for the management of advanced melanoma: the immune system stimulator ipilimumab and the targeted agent vemurafenib. We will review the management of advanced melanoma with specific emphasis on targeted therapies against *BRAF, NRAS,* and *C-KIT,* as well as immunotherapy options. We will also discuss the management of oligometastatic disease, central nervous system disease, and in-transit metastases. Although ipilimumab and vemurafenib have dramatically altered the management of advanced melanoma, there is much work to be done in developing additional agents, and we will discuss ongoing and eagerly awaited research.

Keywords: melanoma, ipilimumab, vemurafenib, dabrafenib, trametinib, anti-PD-1/PD-L1 antibody

*Corresponding author, Anschutz Cancer Pavillon, 1665 Aurora Court, Suite 3070, Mail Stop F703, Aurora, CO
   E-mail address: Rene.gonzalez@ucdenver.edu

Emerging Cancer Therapeutics 3:3 (2012) 583–602.
DOI: 10.5003/2151–4194.3.3.583
demosmedpub.com/ecat

■ INTRODUCTION

The incidence of melanoma is increasing faster than any other cancer, with approximately 68,000 new cases diagnosed yearly in the United States (1). Melanoma is the fifth most common newly diagnosed malignancy in males and seventh most common in females (2). Because melanoma tends to affect people at younger ages than most cancers do, it is the leading cancer in terms of years of life lost (3). When diagnosed early and appropriately excised, melanoma is a curable malignancy. However, mortality is high for patients with advanced disease because of the lack of effective treatment options. The only commonly used drugs that were approved by the Food and Drug Administration (FDA) for treatment of advanced melanoma before 2011 were high-dose interleukin 2 (IL-2) and dacarbazine, which both have response rates of 5% to 15% (4,5). Until recently, none of the agents used for treating melanoma demonstrated an improvement in the overall survival (OS), thus emphasizing the urgent need for new therapies. This chapter will focus on recent progress in the treatment of advanced melanoma, with specific focus on molecularly targeted therapies and immunotherapies.

■ MOLECULAR CHARACTERIZATION OF MELANOMA

Advances in understanding the biology of melanoma have helped elucidate the varied molecular mechanisms that drive tumorigenesis. As our understanding of the molecular heterogeneity of malignancy evolves, our ability to generate targeted therapies that are more efficacious and less toxic than traditional chemotherapy improves. Melanoma oncologists have embraced the idea of molecularly therapies, and at present, melanoma is an example of a malignancy with a variety of effective targeted therapeutic options.

In 2002, a landmark showed that approximately 50% of melanomas harbor a mutation in the *BRAF* gene (6). BRAF is a serine-threonine kinase that plays a role in the mitogen-activated protein kinase (MAPK) pathway. The mutant BRAF kinase allows for unregulated signaling through the MAPK pathway and therefore leads to unregulated cancer cell growth and tumor proliferation (Figure 1). Of the entire cohort of melanomas with mutated *BRAF*, approximately 80% have a specific amino acid substitution of valine to glutamic acid at position 600 (V600E). Of the 20% of non-V600E mutations, the most common variant is V600K, although a variety of different mutations have been reported (V600R, V600D) (7).

The natural history of melanoma in patients that harbor *BRAF* mutations differs from those with wild-type disease. In a prospective analysis of consecutive melanoma patients with stage IIIc or IV disease evaluated at a single institution in Australia, it was found that patients with *BRAF*-mutated disease tend to be, on the average, 10 years younger than wild-type patients are. Primary tumors of patients with *BRAF*-mutated disease are more often the superficial spreading and nodular subtypes of melanoma in contrast with acral-lentiginous or desmoplastic histopathologies. Primary *BRAF*-mutated tumors tend to develop in areas without chronic sun damage (CSD), such as the trunk, and tend to be more mitotically active. There was no statistically significant difference in the depth of the primary tumor at diagnosis, no gender preference, and no difference in the rates of ulcerated primary tumors based on *BRAF* mutational status (7).

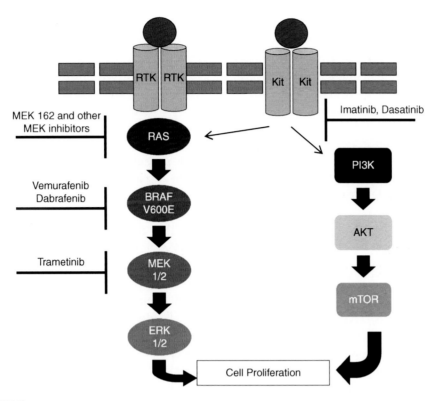

FIGURE 1

Schematic of the MAPK and PI3K pathways depicting molecular targets for current and emerging small molecule inhibitors.

Modified from Anthony Ribas with permission.

Although *BRAF* mutations are the most common molecular driver in non-CSD skin, *NRAS* mutations are also found in approximately 15% to 20% of patients with cutaneous lesions arising in non–sun damaged skin (8). In a recent prospective analysis of 249 consecutive patients with cutaneous melanoma treated at a single institution, *NRAS* mutations were found in approximately 14% of the analyzed tumor samples. There was shorter melanoma-specific survival in the patients with *NRAS* mutations compared with those patients with *BRAF* mutations (hazard ratio [HR] 2.51; P = .05). *NRAS*-mutated tumors were found to be thicker at the time of diagnosis and were more likely to have greater than 1 mitosis/mm^2 of tumor than *BRAF*-mutated or wild-type tumors do (9).

Although *BRAF* and *NRAS* mutations are mostly found in patients with melanomas arising from non-CSD skin, they can be seen in a minority (5%–15%) of patients with melanomas in CSD skin or in acral or mucosal distributions. Acral and mucosal melanomas tend to predominantly have increased copy number or activating mutations in *Kit*, as seen in approximately 15% to 20% of patients. *Kit* is a transmembrane receptor tyrosine kinase (RTK) and, when active, can initiate downstream signaling either through the MAPK or phosphati-dyl-inosital-3-OH kinase (PI3K) pathways to activate transcription (Figure 1) (10). It is unknown if *Kit* activation in melanoma worsens prognosis.

Our practice is to obtain *BRAF* mutational analysis on all patients with stage

III and IV melanoma. *Kit* mutational analysis should also be done in patients with primary acral and mucosal tumors. *NRAS* mutational analysis should also be implemented, because of emerging data on agents specifically targeting the mutated NRAS kinase.

■ TARGETED THERAPIES IN ADVANCED MELANOMA

BRAF Inhibition

Vemurafenib

Previous attempts at targeting the MAPK pathway for antimelanoma effects have shown limited efficacy using the drug sorafenib (Nexavar, Bayer/Onyx Pharmaceuticals) (11). The promiscuity of sorafenib with its multikinase inhibitory effects was thought to be the reason for its poor efficacy in melanoma; therefore, further attempts at targeting the MAPK pathway were directed at specifically targeting the mutated BRAF kinase. The scaffold-based drug design approach, in which the mutated BRAF kinase domain was crystallized to generate a compound with specificity for only the mutated BRAF, yielded the drug vemurafenib in 2006 (Zelboraf, Genentech/Roche; also known as PLX4032/RG7204) (12).

Preclinical data showed that vemurafenib is effective in preferentially destroying melanoma cell lines harboring *BRAF* V600E mutations, with minimal effect on cell lines without oncogenic BRAF (13). Therefore, vemurafenib clinical trials were ultimately designed only for patients with documentation of *BRAF* V600 mutations. The extension cohort/phase II portion of the initial phase I/II vemurafenib trial enrolled 32 patients with unresectable stage IIIc or IV disease treated at 960 mg twice daily until disease progression or unacceptable toxicity. Out of the 32 total

patients, 26 had a favorable response, with 2 patients having a complete response (CR) and the rest with partial response (PR), leading to an unconfirmed response rate of 81%. The duration of response ranged from 2 months to more than 18 months. In addition, vemurafenib was shown to exert antimelanoma effects very rapidly, and patients with symptomatic disease such as pain or fatigue had significant improvement in their symptoms within 2 weeks of initiating treatment (14).

The BRAF inhibitor in melanoma (BRIM-2) trial is a phase II study that enrolled 132 patients with previously treated advanced melanoma harboring a *BRAF* V600 mutation (Table 1). The confirmed overall response rate was 53%, with only 15% of patients showing primary resistance. The median progression-free survival (PFS) was 6.8 months. With a median of 12.9 months of follow-up, the OS was 15.9 months (15).

A randomized phase III study of vemurafenib versus dacarbazine (BRIM-3) enrolled 675 treatment-naive patients with locally advanced or metastatic melanoma harboring a BRAF V600E mutation. Patients were randomized either to vemurafenib at 960 mg orally twice daily or dacarbazine dosed at 1000 mg/m^2 intravenously every 3 weeks until disease progression or intolerable toxicity. At the study's first interim analysis, the independent data safety and monitoring board concluded that the study met its coprimary end points, with significant improvements in both OS and PFS in the vemurafenib-treated patients, and allowed for crossover from dacarbazine to vemurafenib (16). A recent update of the data with a median of 10 months of follow-up showed an OS of 13.2 months with a hazard ratio (HR) for death of 0.62 in favor of the vemurafenib-treated patients (17).

Vemurafenib side effects are generally mild and easily tolerated. Arthralgia and fatigue are commonly reported, and asymptomatic elevations in liver function test can also be seen. Cutaneous effects are the most common group of adverse effects (AEs), including rash, photosensitivity, pruritis, hand/foot tenderness, keratoacanthomas, and cutaneous squamous cell cancers in approximately 20% to 30% of vemurafenib-treated patients. A detailed DNA analysis of 35 squamous cell carcinoma (SCC) samples induced by vemurafenib revealed the presence of concurrent RAS mutations (specifically HRAS) in approximately 60% of the tested samples. Thus, it is likely that patients who are prone to develop SCCs are those with preexisting RAS mutations. Vemurafenib itself does not seem to be carcinogenic but can potentiate the effects of preexisting mutations (18). There is no evidence that vemurafenib has induced any cancers other than cutaneous SCCs. The vast majority of keratoacanthomas and SCCs can be treated with surgical excision alone and rarely lead to the need for vemurafenib discontinuation or dose reduction.

On the basis of the aforementioned data, vemurafenib was FDA approved in August 2011 for treatment of unresectable stage IIIc or IV disease in patients with the presence of *BRAF* V600E–mutated disease. The COBAS® assay is the companion diagnostic test FDA approved along with vemurafenib to verify the presence of *BRAF* V600–mutated disease.

Dabrafenib

Dabrafenib (GSK2118436) is a selective BRAF inhibitor manufactured by GlaxoSmithKline. In an initial phase III trial, 250 patients with previously untreated stage IIIc/IV *BRAF* V600E–mutated melanoma were randomized in a 3:1 ratio to dabrafenib at 150 mg orally twice daily versus dacarbazine. Crossover was allowed in the dacarbazine-treated patients experiencing

progression. The HR for PFS was 0.3 (*P* < .0001), with a median PFS of 5.1 months on dabrafenib versus 2.7 months for the dacarbazine-treated patients. The confirmed response rate (RR) to dabrafenib was 53%, and survival data were not yet mature at the time of data presentation (19). These data essentially mimic the responses seen with vemurafenib therapy. The side-effect profile of dabrafenib, however, is slightly different from vemurafenib, with the most common AEs being pyrexia, arthralgias, skin hyperkeratosis, and papillomas. Only approximately 6% of patients treated with dabrafenib developed cutaneous SCCs (19).

MEK Inhibition

Trametinib

Similar to inhibition of BRAF, inhibition of the mitogen-activated protein kinase (MEK) is also an attractive target for drug development, in particular because the only substrates for MEK1/2 are ERK 1/2. Because MEK is downstream of BRAF, it can be reasoned that MEK inhibition would be most effective when BRAF is mutated and constitutively activated. This hypothesis has been validated in preclinical studies, indicating that inhibition of MEK was more effective in *BRAF*-mutated melanoma cell lines compared with *BRAF* wild-type or *RAS*-mutated cell lines (20).

Trametinib (GSK1120212) is a reversible highly selective allosteric inhibitor of MEK1/2. In preclinical models, trametinib produced tumor regression and showed success in early phase clinical trials in patients with *BRAF* mutations. A phase III study enrolled 322 patients with stage IIIc and IV melanoma with *BRAF* V660E– or V600K– mutated disease in a 2:1 ratio to trametinib 2 mg oral daily versus intravenous dacarbazine or paclitaxel. Crossover to trametinib was allowed for patients who progressed on the intravenous chemotherapy. The PFS was 4.8 months on trametinib versus 1.5 months in the chemotherapy arm based on investigator and independent review. The hazard ratio for progression was 0.45. The overall response rate (ORR) was 24% for trametinib treated patients compared with 7% in the chemotherapy treated patients. The 6 month OS was 81% versus 67% (21).

Trametinib is generally well tolerated, with acneiform rash, diarrhea, fatigue, and peripheral edema being the most common AEs. Rarely, ocular effects such as blurred vision or reversible chorioretinopathy have been observed. Reversible left ventricular ejection fraction depression has also been attributed to trametinib. No cutaneous SCCs have been observed in patients treated with trametinib.

Combined BRAF and MEK Inhibition

Dabrafenib and Trametinib

The development of resistance to single-agent vemurafenib occurs almost universally, as evidenced by the median PFS of approximately 7 months. Although only a minority of patients are primarily resistant to vemurafenib, most patients will develop secondary resistance mechanisms. A variety of resistance mechanisms were hypothesized, and research into preventing resistance is ongoing. The hypotheses with the most supporting data include bypassing the signaling of BRAF by the upregulation of NRAS and CRAF and of alternative signaling pathways such as the phosphatidyl-inosital-3 kinase (PI3K) pathways (Figure 1) (22,23). These data provide rationale for using BRAF-inhibiting drugs in combination with other targeted agents within the MAPK or PI3K pathways.

A phase I/II study enrolled 247 patients with BRAF V600 mutated advanced melanoma. All doses of dabrafenib and trametinib were well tolerated, including the highest dose cohort with patients receiving dabrafenib 150 mg twice daily and trametinib 2 mg daily. The median PFS was 9.4 months for patients treated with the dabrafenib and trametinib combination compared to 5.8 months for the dabrafenib only treated cohort. Use of the dabrafenib/trametinib combination seems to be better tolerated than using dabrafenib alone with pyrexia and fatigue being seen more commonly in the patients receiving combination therapy. In addition, the rate of cutaneous SCCs and other proliferative skin lesions was less in patients treated with combination therapy than those treated with dabrafenib (24).

Management of NRAS-Mutated Disease

As previously mentioned, NRAS-mutated disease tends to portend a worse prognosis (9). Previous attempts at targeting tumors with NRAS mutations have been challenging, with no positive trial results until recently. MEK162 is a potent MEK1/2 inhibitor with favorable preclinical data in BRAF- and NRAS-mutated melanoma. An open-label phase II study using MEK162 enrolled 24 patients with NRAS-mutated disease. Of the 13 patients with data available for analysis, 3 patients had PRs, and 4 patients had stable disease (SD) with acceptable toxicity, including rash and diarrhea (25). MEK162 is the first targeted agent to ever show activity in patients with NRAS-mutated disease. There are currently accruing trials using MEK162 in combination with either BEZ235 (PI3K/mTOR inhibitor) or BKM120 (PI3K inhibitor) in advanced solid tumors for patients with BRAF, KRAS, or NRAS mutations (NCT01337765/NCT01363232 from clinicaltrials.gov).

Management of Disease With C-KIT Gene Alterations

C-KIT gene amplification or gene activation can be seen in a variety of malignancies and has been seen in up to 25% of patients with acral or mucosal primary melanomas. Previous studies using imatinib in metastatic melanoma patients were unsuccessful, because an unselected patient population was used (26). More recent trials have mandated documentation of *KIT* gene alterations, which has led to increased clinical efficacy. In a recent multi-institution phase II trial, 43 patients with metastatic melanoma and documentation of *KIT* gene mutation or amplification were initiated on imatinib 400 mg orally daily. Ten patients (23%) had a PR, 13 patients had SD, and the PFS was 3.5 months. Increasing the dose of imatinib to 800 mg in patients with progressing disease on 400 mg of imatinib was largely unsuccessful in controlling disease (27). Of the 10 patients with PR, all had mutations in either exon 11 or 13 of *KIT*. There are ongoing clinical trials for patients with *KIT*-mutated disease, including the TEAM trial, which was initially designed as a randomized phase III trial between nilotinib and dacarbazine. However, accrual on this trial was poor, and a significant protocol amendment was approved such that it is now a single-arm phase II trial of nilotinib in patients with metastatic melanoma (NCT0102822).

■ IMMUNOTHERAPY IN THE MANAGEMENT OF ADVANCED MELANOMA

Ipilimumab

Cytotoxic T lymphocyte-associated antigen-4 (CTLA-4) is a T-cell surface receptor that works as an immune system checkpoint to regulate immune responses. The antigen is expressed when the immune system is stimulated and competes with CD28 for binding on antigen presenting cells (APCs), thus leading to blockade of costimulatory signals needed for T-cell activation (Figure 2). Blockade of CTLA-4 releases immune system inhibition, allowing for enhanced T-cell-mediated immunity and the ability to recognize cancer cells as foreign (28). Ipilimumab is a fully humanized monoclonal antibody directed against CTLA-4. Successful results in preclinical models led to the design of an initial phase III study that enrolled 676 patients with previously treated, unresectable stage III or IV melanoma randomized to receive ipilimumab at 3 mg/kg intravenously every 3 weeks with or without a glycoprotein-100 (gp100) vaccine versus gp100 alone (Table 2). Patients who were treated with ipilimumab and gp100 had an OS of 10 months compared with 6.4 months in the gp100 control group ($P < .001$). The best overall response rate was 10.9%, and the disease control rate, including CR, PR, and SD, was 28.5% in patients treated with ipilimumab. The PFS in patients treated with ipilimumab and gp100 compared with gp100 alone was not different (2.76 months), which highlights the latency period of approximately 3 months for the drug to take effect. The 1 and 2 year survival rates for patients treated with ipilimumab are 45.6% and 23.5%, respectively (29).

In a second phase 3 study, half of the patients received ipilimumab in conjunction with dacarbazine, and the other half received dacarbazine with placebo. The dose of ipilimumab used in this study was 10 mg/kg, and all patients had treatment-naive advanced melanoma. The best overall response rate was 15% for the ipilimumab with dacarbazine arm compared with 10% in the dacarbazine arm. The OS was statistically and significantly improved in the patients receiving ipilimumab by 2 months (30).

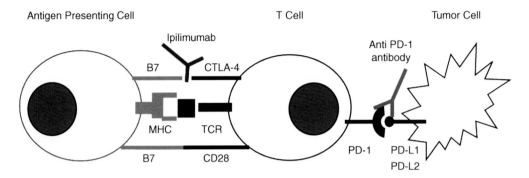

FIGURE 2
Immunologic interplay between antigen presenting cells (APCs), T cells, and tumor cells with areas of activity of ipilimumab and anti-PD-1 antibody.

Immune-related adverse events (IRAEs), including dermatitis, hepatitis, nephritis, hypophysitis, and, more commonly, diarrhea and enterocolitis, are seen with ipilimumab. In the phase III trials of ipilimumab, 60% of the patients experienced an IRAE, with 10% to 15% being grade 3 or 4. Most of these adverse events remit within 6 weeks of discontinuing ipilimumab. Approximately 2% of the patients treated with ipilimumab died as a result of complications of the study drug However, with close monitoring of patients for the development of potential AEs, ipilimumab is a safe and viable option to treat patients with advanced disease. (29). Diarrhea and enterocolitis are the most common IRAEs occurring in approximately 20% to 30% of treated patients, although grade 4 colitis is rare. Prompt initiation of treatment (including steroids) is effective in alleviating symptoms in the vast majority of patients within 2 weeks, although a small proportion of patients require treatment with infliximab, an antibody against tumor necrosis factor alpha (31).

High-Dose Interleukin 2

IL-2 was identified in the 1970s as a T-cell growth factor. A recombinant form of IL-2 was subsequently generated, and initial studies in murine tumor models led to the development of the high-dose IL-2 (HDIL2) regimen. In 1993, HDIL2 administered at a dose of 600,000 to 720,000 IU/kg intravenously every 8 hours for a maximum of 14 doses over 5 days was approved for treatment of metastatic renal cell carcinoma. The FDA approval of HDIL2 for melanoma came a few years later, after a meta-analysis of 270 patients with metastatic melanoma showed an overall response rate of 16%, with 6% of the patients having a CR and 10% having PR (5). Of the 6% of patients achieving a CR, these responses are generally durable over 5 years of follow-up. Toxicities of HDIL2 can be severe, including hypotension requiring the use of vasopressors, myelosuppression with risk for serious infection or transfusion support, renal failure, hepatitis, and pulmonary and peripheral edemas (5). However, HDIL2 toxicities are predictable and are easily managed in a setting with expertise using this therapy. Therefore, we recommend that this treatment is administered only in high-volume HDIL2 treatment centers with physicians and nurses who have the knowledge and experience required for safe administration of this agent. In addition, patients must be fit enough to tolerate the therapy, and we often require normal pulmonary function tests, nuclear cardiac stress testing, and normal blood counts, kidney and liver function in determining if a patient is fit enough to tolerate the expected toxicities of therapy.

Biochemotherapy

Biochemotherapy (BCT) is an aggressive treatment approach that combines IL-2 and interferon alpha immunotherapy with cisplatin, vinblastine, and dacarbazine (CVD) combination chemotherapy. BCT has shown success when neoadjuvantly or adjuvantly administered for patients with high risk for recurrence but can also be used in patients with metastatic disease. A recently presented Southwest Oncology Group (SWOG) analysis compared 1 year of high-dose interferon alpha (HDI) with BCT in the adjuvant setting for patients with resected stage IIIa to IIIc disease and found that the BCT-treated patients had improved a median relapse-free survival of 4 years compared with 1.9 years for the HDI-treated patients. There was no improvement in the OS, with 5 year survival rates of 56% for both groups (32).

The use of BCT in patients with metastatic disease is feasible in a small subset of patients with good functional status. In a randomized phase III study of BCT versus combination CVD chemotherapy, an overall response rate of 48% was seen in the BCT-treated patients compared with 25% for the CVD-treated group. Of the 91 patients treated with BCT, 6 had CR (33). A meta-analysis of 18 trials with more than 2,600 patients with metastatic melanoma showed statistically significant improvement in PRs, CRs, and ORR for patients treated with BCT (given at various doses and schedules) versus chemotherapy but no improvement in OS (34). The addition of IL2 and interferon to CVD significantly increases the number of grade 3 or 4 toxic events; however, BCT remains a viable option for young and fit patients with aggressive disease.

■ EMERGING IMMUNOTHERAPEUTIC AGENTS

Anti-PD-1 Antibody

Programmed death 1 (PD-1) is a protein that is upregulated on activated T cells during an immune system response. In the presence of tumor cells, PD-1 binds to its ligands, programmed death-ligand 1 (PD-L1) or PD-L2, on the surface of tumor cells, thereby producing T-cell anergy and dampening of immune system responses (Figure 2). BMS-936558 (Bristol Myers-Squibb) is a monoclonal antibody that blocks the binding of PD-1 to PD-L1/PD-L2 on tumor cells, thus allowing for T cells to remain stimulated and mount a widespread antitumor immune reaction. In a recent large phase I study, BMS-936558 was used in 296 patients with refractory solid tumors, including 104 patients with advanced melanoma. Four different dosing cohorts were used, and the drug was intravenously administered every 2 weeks for a total of 4 infusions. A response rate of 28% overall was seen in the melanoma cohort, and most of the responses were durable (>1 year) in patients who had been followed for more than 1 year. The response rate varied, depending on the dosing cohort, with 41% responders in the 3 mg/kg cohort. Severe IRAEs were not seen, and BMS-936558 seemed to be generally well tolerated, with mild fatigue, diarrhea, rash, and cough being the most common side effects (35). Thus, this preliminary study using BMS-936558 shows an increased response rate and less frequent IRAEs than what is observed with ipilimumab therapy. There are ongoing trials involving other anti-PD-1 antibodies, including Merck's MK-3475 (36), showing great promise in early stage clinical trials. A monoclonal antibody against PD-L1 (MPDL3280A/Genentech) is also in early phase clinical trials (NCT01375842).

Adoptive Cell Therapy

Adoptive cell therapy (ACT) refers to the process of isolating a patient's anticancer T cells, expanding them to great quantities in an ex vivo setting and then transferring these cells back into an immunodepleted host in conjunction with IL-2. This therapy has been championed by the National Institutes of Health, and a variety of different protocols have been generated over the years, with a large number of published phase I/II trials. One of the most recent and efficacious protocols published by Rosenberg and colleagues (37) required harvesting tumor-infiltrating lymphocytes (TILs) from a patient's melanoma. These TILs were grown ex vivo and expanded to more than 50 million cells. Before TIL infusion, patients received a lymphodepleting conditioning regimen consisting of fludarabine and cyclophosphamide alone or in conjunction with 2 different doses of total body irradiation. TIL infusion was accompanied by HDIL2 to help augment the number and activity of the transferred cells. The overall response rate was 56% for the entire cohort but was 72% with 40% CRs in the patients receiving fludarabine and cyclophosphamide and the higher total body irradiation dosing (37).

There is a variety of ongoing research and debates in ACT, and much work remains to be done to determine the optimal regimen. However, ACT does have great potential, and it does represent a viable option for select patients who can sustain the rigors of therapy. In addition, the current ACT protocols require at least 3 weeks growing the transferred cells to sufficient quantities; thus, patients who are relatively asymptomatic and have slow enough growing disease are the ideal candidates for this therapy.

■ MANAGEMENT OF OLIGOMETASTATIC DISEASE

Surgical management for oligometastatic disease had long been the mainstay of therapy because of the lack of effective systemic therapies. Currently, the role of surgery for treatment of metastatic disease is under debate as the number of effective systemic therapies increases. Patient selection is a key factor as patients who are fit enough with limited comorbid conditions and with lower tumor doubling times being the preferred patient population for surgical resection of oligometastatic disease. The technical ability to perform a complete resection with adequate margins is another selection factor. With the correctly identified patient population, there does seem to be a survival benefit for resection of oligometastatic disease. A single-institution retrospective analysis was done on 4,426 consecutive patients with metastatic melanoma. Thirty-five percent (1,574) patients were eligible for resection of metastases, with approximately 56% of the resected cohort having a single site of metastatic disease. The 5 year survival rate was statistically and significantly improved in patients with a single site of resectable disease. Patients with skin or lymph node metastases had the best prognosis, with a median OS of 35 months (38). A recent meta-analysis analyzed pooled data from 33 retrospective studies on patients with resected or unresected metastases. The 2 year OS was 27% in patients with resected metastases versus 12% in the unresected group. Data from 7 specific studies reporting on resection of visceral metastases showed a 40% reduction in the risk of death for patients receiving palliative resections (39). Thus, patients with minimal sites of completely resectable disease with slow-growing tumors are the best candidates for resection as the data seem to confer a survival benefit for these select patients.

■ MANAGEMENT OF CENTRAL NERVOUS SYSTEM METASTASES

Central nervous system (CNS) metastasis in melanoma is common, with approximately 50% of patients with metastatic disease having CNS involvement during the course of their disease. Traditionally, patients with CNS metastases have a poor median survival of less than 6 months (40). Although surgery, whole brain radiotherapy (WBRT), and temozolomide have long been the mainstay of treatment of CNS disease, there is emerging data on the benefit of stereotactic radiosurgery (SRS) and systemic therapy such as ipilimumab and BRAF directed therapies.

Patients with symptomatic disease may require treatment with steroids to control cerebral edema and should be referred for craniotomy to resect symptomatic disease if possible. Patients with metastases less than 3 cm in size with asymptomatic or minimally symptomatic lesions should be considered for treatment with SRS. In a review of 333 consecutive melanoma patients with CNS metastases treated with gamma knife SRS, disease control rates were 47% at 6 months, 25% at 12 months, and 10% at 24 months after treatment. Sixty-seven percent of patients had multiple metastases treated in this series, with 13% of patients having more than 7 lesions treated (41).

In our opinion, WBRT should rarely, if ever, be done, with a potential exception being for palliative purposes to relieve symptoms in cases where surgery or SRS are contraindicated. Because melanoma is relatively radio resistant, the dose of radiation delivered during WBRT is often ineffective for adequate disease control and has been shown to contribute to neurocognitive decline (40). The use of WBRT in the adjuvant setting after surgical resection is highly controversial, because there have been no melanoma-specific studies of this approach, and data are extrapolated from series of solid tumors (40). We strongly discourage the use of WBRT in melanoma patients.

Systemic Therapies for CNS Metastases

Temozolomide

Temozolomide has long been the systemic agent of choice for treatment of patients with multiple CNS metastases because this agent can cross the blood brain barrier. An initial series of 151 melanoma patients with CNS metastases who were not treated with surgery or radiation showed a 7% response rate, with a median OS of 3 months (42). In a more recent series of 53 patients with melanoma CNS metastases treated with a dose-dense schedule of temozolomide (150 mg/m^2 orally daily on days 1–7 and 15–21 of either a 28 or 35 day cycle), 9% of patients had PR, and 23% had SD for a disease control rate (DCR) of 32% (43).

Ipilimumab

Ipilimumab has shown some efficacy in treating melanoma CNS metastases. A group of 72 patients were treated with ipilimumab at a dose of 10 mg/kg intravenously every 3 weeks for a total of 4 doses. In the group of 51 patients with asymptomatic CNS involvement, 24% of the patients achieved control of their CNS disease. In a group of 21 patients with symptomatic CNS metastases on stable doses of steroids, the disease control rate was 10% (44).

BRAF-Directed Therapies

There is emerging data that vemurafenib or its counterpart dabrafenib can penetrate the CNS to lead to disease control in patients with metastatic melanoma. An initial case report of a 16 year old girl with symptomatic, hemorrhagic CNS metastases progressed through prior SRS therapy had a dramatic CNS response to vemurafenib lasting more than 6 months (45). On the basis of this case and other similar observations, an open-label single-arm phase II trial testing the efficacy of vemurafenib in patients with metastatic melanoma with asymptomatic brain metastases is ongoing (NCT01378975). A recently presented phase I/II study of dabrafenib in 23 patients with melanoma and asymptomatic CNS metastases showed initial treatment responses in patients with either no prior CNS directed therapies or who had previously received radiation or surgery. Nineteen of the 23 patients went on to have progressive disease, with 5 of the 19 patients progressing intracranially, 6 of the 19 patients progressing systemically, and 8 of the 19 patients progressing at both sites (46).

■ MANAGEMENT OF IN-TRANSIT METASTASES

In-transit metastases are tumor deposits spreading from the primary tumor to the draining lymph node bed through the lymphatic system. Usually, surgical excision of an isolated metastasis is the treatment of choice; however, this can become technically challenging or not feasible when there are multiple metastases or multiple recurrences after surgery. In cases of locally unresectable in-transit metastases with or without lymph node–positive disease (stage IIIC by the American Joint Committee on Cancer [AJCC] staging system), patients can be candidates for systemic therapy. Patients with *BRAF*-mutated disease should be considered for BRAF-directed inhibition or immunotherapy with HDIL2 or ipilimumab, and patients who are *BRAF* wild type could consider immunotherapy. Hyperthermic limb perfusion or infusion therapy can be considered in selected cases. Hyperthermic limb perfusion/infusion therapy is a procedure in which the artery and vein are either surgically or percutaneously accessed or cannulated at the root of the affected limb. Heated melphalan is usually used to perfuse the affected limb, although there are emerging data with the use of tumor necrosis factor alpha (TNFα) alone or in conjunction with melphalan (47). A tourniquet is proximally placed to limit the melphalan exposure to the affected limb, which allows for up to 25-fold higher chemotherapy concentrations than what can systemically be delivered. The largest single-institution retrospective analysis from Duke University showed an overall response rate of 81%, with 55% complete responders lasting, on the average, 32 months with hyperthermic melphalan perfusion in 62 patients with melanoma in transit metastases (48). Local skin toxicities are expected to the treated limb, including swelling, skin erythema, and blistering, but compartment syndrome and limb necrosis can rarely develop, leading to limb amputation.

Areas of Debate

With the rapid pace of discovery in melanoma, a variety of debates are ongoing. One unresolved area of debate is with

TABLE 1 Key studies and results in BRAF-mutated disease

Trial	Phase	Number of Patients	ORR (%)	PFS (months)	OS (months)
BRIM-2: vemurafenib 960 mg twice a day	II	132	53	6.9	15.9
BRIM-3: vemurafenib 90 mg twice a day vs. dacarbazine	III	337 338	48 5	5.3 1.6	13.2 9.6
Dabrafenib 150 mg twice a day vs. dacarbazine	III	187 63	53 19	5.1 2.7	ND
Trametinib 2 mg daily vs. chemotherapy	III	214 108	24 7	4.8 1.5	ND
Dabraenib + trametenib	I/II	108	76	9.4	ND

TABLE 2 Key studies and summarized results in melanoma immunotherapy

Trial	Phase	Number of Patients	ORR (%)	PFS (months)	OS (months)
Ipilimumab 3 mg/kg ± gp100 vs. gp-100 vaccine	III	540 137	10.9 1.5	2.76 2.76	10.1 6.4
Ipilimumab 10 mg/kg + dacarbazine vs. dacarbazine + placebo	III	250 252	15.2 10.3	3 3	11.2 9.1
Anti-PD-1 antibody BMS936558	I	94	28 (19–38, depending on the dose level)	41% PFS rate at 24 weeks	ND

regard to the optimal dosing of ipilimumab. In the registration trial of ipilimumab, the dose of 3 mg/kg intravenously every 3 weeks for 4 total doses was used and this is the dose approved by the FDA. However, subsequent trials have used ipilimumab at a dose of 10 mg/kg, which has led to slightly higher response rates but also more toxicity (30,44). Therefore, a trial is ongoing comparing outcomes in patients treated with either the 3 or 10 mg/kg dosing to hopefully answer the question regarding ipilimumab dosing (NCT01515189). Similar questions remain with regard to "reinduction" at relapse and "maintenance therapy," and trials to address this are being developed.

One controversial area in targeted therapy is that in the United States, commercial use of vemurafenib is limited to patients who have a *BRAF* V600 mutation detected by the FDA-approved companion diagnostic known as the COBAS® assay. This assay has excellent sensitivity and specificity for *BRAF* V600E mutations and also detects approximately 66% of *BRAF* V600K variants. However, that leaves approximately 33% of V600K patients potentially unable to receive drug and there is data to suggest that V600K patients respond well to BRAF directed therapies. Likewise, patients with other less common variants of activating *BRAF* mutations may also respond and be denied access to drug. Therefore, there is an ongoing trial testing use of vemurafenib in patients with *BRAF* mutations other than V600E (NCT01586195).

It is also hypothesized that the use of targeted therapy and immunotherapy in combination may lead to longer duration of response than either therapy used alone. To explore this idea, there is an ongoing trial using ipilimumab with vemurafenib (NCT01400451) and planned studies using HDIL2 with vemurafenib in patients with *BRAF* mutated disease.

Ongoing and Awaited Melanoma Clinical Trials

There are a variety of ongoing and planned trials in the treatment of patients with advanced melanoma, as summarized in Table 3.

There is much work that needs to be done with regard to treating patients with no evidence of targetable mutations and in patients who have progressed through targeted therapy. Certainly, immunotherapy is the mainstay of treating patients with no targetable mutations, and there is much anticipation about the emerging data from the anti-PD-1/PD-L1 antibodies. Another fascinating area of ongoing research is using ERK inhibition. ERK is the last component of the MAPK pathway, and preclinical data have shown death of melanoma cell lines that are either BRAF mutated or wild type in response to ERK inhibition. In addition, preclinical data suggest responses in cell lines that have grown refractory to BRAF-directed therapy (49). ERK inhibitors are currently in early developmental stages, and there are plans for a trial using an ERK inhibitor in combination with anti-PD-1 antibody to initiate in the fall of 2012.

■ CONCLUSIONS

Management of patients with advanced melanoma has dramatically changed over the last few years with the FDA approval of ipilimumab and vemurafenib. All patients with advanced disease should have molecular characterization of their tumors with at least *BRAF* mutational analysis. Acral and mucosal primary melanomas should also be tested for *KIT* gene amplifications or activating mutations. If a patient has minimally symptomatic disease, initial management with immunotherapy, either in the form of HDIL2 or ipilimumab, may be preferred, even in the presence of *BRAF* or *KIT* mutations, because the probability of durable complete remission is greatest with immunotherapy. If patients are symptomatic of their disease and harbor a *BRAF* mutation, initiation of BRAF-directed therapies may be the

TABLE 3 Ongoing or upcoming immunotherapy clinical trials of interest in advanced/metastatic melanoma

Trial Description	Phase	Target Population	Clinicaltrials.gov Number
Stereotactic body radiation with ipilimumab	I/II	Unresectable stage IIIc/IV	NCT01497808 NCT01565837
Adoptive cell therapy using tumor-infiltrating lymphocytes; varying conditioning regimens	I/II	Unresectable stage IIIc/IV	NCT01236573 NCT01319565 NCT00287131
Ipilimumab 3 mg/kg vs. 10 mg/kg	III	Unresectable stage IIIc/IV	NCT01515189
Vemurafenib + Mek inhibitor GDC-0973	I	Unresectable stage IIIc/IV with BRAF V600E mutations	NCT01271803
Vemurafenib in BRAF mutations other than V600E	II	Unresectable stage IIIc/IV with any BRAF mutation	NCT01586195
Vemurafenib + ipilimumab	I/II	Unresectable stage IIIc/IV with BRAF V600E mutation	NCT01400451
Bevacizumab + ipilimumab	I	Unresectable stage IIIc/IV	NCT00790010
Dabrafenib + trametinib vs. vemurafenib	III	Unresectable stage IIIc/IV with BRAF V600E/K mutations	NCT01597908
Dabrafenib + trametinib vs. dabrafenib + placebo	III	Unresectable stage IIIc/IV with BRAF V600E/K mutations	NCT01584648
PD-1 antibody + peptide vaccine for resected stage IV	I	Completely resected stage IV	NCT01176474
PD-L1 antibody advanced solid tumors	I	Unresectable stage IIIc/IV melanoma and advanced, refractory solid tumors	NCT00729664

most effective in achieving rapid disease response. When possible, clinical trial to use BRAF-directed therapies in conjunction with either another targeted therapy or immunotherapy is preferable in attempting to avert the development of resistance seen with single-agent BRAF inhibition (Figure 3).

There are a variety of ongoing questions with regard to the optimal management of oligometastatic disease, CNS metastases, and in-transit metastases. There are emerging data that ipilimumab and BRAF-directed therapies can be efficacious in some patients with asymptomatic CNS disease, and further data are awaited. Surgical resection for select patients with oligometastatic disease does seem to confer a survival benefit in patients with relatively slowing growing disease that is amenable to complete resection. Hyperthermic limb perfusion and infusion therapies have been shown to be efficacious in select patients with in-transit metastases and remain a viable treatment option.

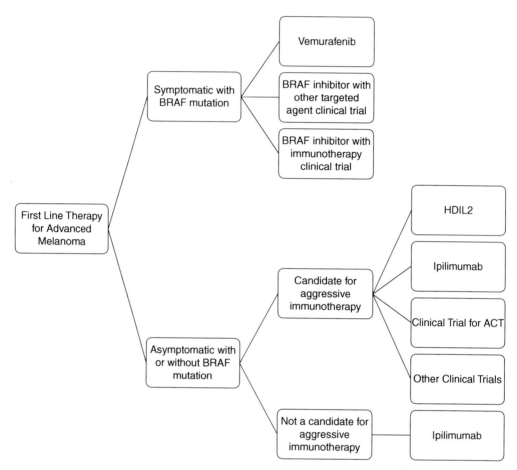

FIGURE 3
Flowchart depicting the initial management of advanced melanoma in patients with symptomatic or asymptomatic disease.

Although the last few years have brought great progress to the treatment of patients with advanced melanoma, there is much work yet to be done. Immunotherapy for melanoma remains an exciting area of research with the ongoing work in ACT and the encouraging results of the recently published phase I data of the anti-PD1 antibody. The success of BRAF-directed therapies has revolutionized the management of advanced melanoma, but the essentially universal emergence of resistance to these agents has prompted the next phase of research to include combination with other targeted therapies or immunotherapies. Emerging data in the next few years will likely greatly enhance our knowledge of the molecular and immunologic mechanisms that drive melanoma growth and will hopefully provide new treatment options for patients with advanced melanoma.

■ REFERENCES

1. Rigel DS. Trends in dermatology: melanoma incidence. *Arch Dermatol.* 2010;146(3):318.
2. Jemal A, Siegel R, Xu J, Ward E. Cancer statistics, 2010. *CA Cancer J Clin.* 2010;60(5):277–300.

3. Ekwueme DU, Guy GP Jr, Li C, Rim SH, Parelkar P, Chen SC. The health burden and economic costs of cutaneous melanoma mortality by race/ethnicity-United States, 2000 to 2006. *J Am Acad Dermatol*. 2011;65(5 Suppl 1):S133–S143.

4. Agarwala SS. Current systemic therapy for metastatic melanoma. *Expert Rev Anticancer Ther*. 2009;9(5):587–595.

5. Atkins MB, Lotze MT, Dutcher JP, et al. High-dose recombinant interleukin 2 therapy for patients with metastatic melanoma: analysis of 270 patients treated between 1985 and 1993. *J Clin Oncol*. 1999;17(7):2105–2116.

6. Davies H, Bignell GR, Cox C, et al. Mutations of the BRAF gene in human cancer. *Nature*. 2002;417(6892):949–954.

7. Long GV, Menzies AM, Nagrial AM, et al. Prognostic and clinicopathologic associations of oncogenic BRAF in metastatic melanoma. *J Clin Oncol*. 2011;29(10):1239–1246.

8. Woodman SE, Lazar AJ, Aldape KD, Davies MA. New strategies in melanoma: molecular testing in advanced disease. *Clin Cancer Res*. 2012;18(5):1195–1200.

9. Devitt BA, Liu W, Salemi R, et al. Clinical outcome and pathologic features associated with NRAS mutations in cutaneous melanoma. Presented at: the American Society of Clinical Oncology (ASCO) Annual Meeting: Collaborating to Conquer Cancer; June 1–5, 2012; Chicago, IL.

10. Postow MA, Carvajal RD. Therapeutic implications of KIT in melanoma. *Cancer J*. 2012;18(2):137–141.

11. Eisen T, Ahmad T, Flaherty KT, et al. Sorafenib in advanced melanoma: a Phase II randomised discontinuation trial analysis. *Br J Cancer*. 2006;95(5):581–586.

12. Tsai J, Lee JT, Wang W, et al. Discovery of a selective inhibitor of oncogenic B-Raf kinase with potent antimelanoma activity. *Proc Natl Acad Sci USA*. 2008;105(8):3041–3046.

13. Yang H, Higgins B, Kolinsky K, et al. RG7204 (PLX4032), a selective BRAFV600E inhibitor, displays potent antitumor activity in preclinical melanoma models. *Cancer Res*. 2010;70(13):5518–5527.

14. Flaherty KT, Puzanov I, Kim KB, et al. Inhibition of mutated, activated BRAF in metastatic melanoma. *N Engl J Med*. 2010;363(9):809–819.

15. Sosman JA, Kim KB, Schuchter L, et al. Survival in BRAF V600-mutant advanced melanoma treated with vemurafenib. *N Engl J Med*. 2012;366(8):707–714.

16. Chapman PB, Hauschild A, Robert C, et al.; BRIM-3 Study Group. Improved survival with vemurafenib in melanoma with BRAF V600E mutation. *N Engl J Med*. 2011;364(26):2507–2516.

17. Chapman PB, Hauschild A, Robert C, et al. Updated overall survival (OS) results for BRIM-3, a phase III randomized, open-label, multicenter trial comparing BRAF inhibitor vemurafenib (vem) with dacarbazine (DTIC) in previously untreated patients with BRAFV660E-mutated melanoma. Presented at: the American Society of Clinical Oncology (ASCO) Annual Meeting: Collaborating to Conquer Cancer; June 1–5, 2012; Chicago, IL.

18. Su F, Viros A, Milagre C, et al. RAS mutations in cutaneous squamous-cell carcinomas in patients treated with BRAF inhibitors. *N Engl J Med*. 2012;366(3):207–215.

19. Hauschild A, Grob JJ, Demidov LV, et al. Phase III, randomized, open-label, multicenter trial (BREAK-3) comparing the BRAF kinase inhibitor dabrafenib (GSK2118436) with dacarbazine (DTIC) in patients with BRAFV600E-mutated melanoma. Presented at: the American Society of Clinical Oncology (ASCO) Annual Meeting: Collaborating to Conquer Cancer; June 1–5, 2012; Chicago, IL.

20. Solit DB, Garraway LA, Pratilas CA, et al. BRAF mutation predicts sensitivity to MEK inhibition. *Nature*. 2006;439(7074):358–362.

21. Flaherty KT, Robert C, Hersey P, et al. Improved survival with MEK inhibition in BRAF-mutated melanoma. N Engl J Med. 2012;367:107–114.

22. Johannessen CM, Boehm JS, Kim SY, et al. COT drives resistance to RAF inhibition through MAP kinase pathway reactivation. *Nature*. 2010;468(7326):968–972.

23. Nazarian R, Shi H, Wang Q, et al. Melanomas acquire resistance to B-RAF(V600E) inhibition by RTK or N-RAS upregulation. *Nature*. 2010;468(7326):973–977.

24. Flaherty Kt, Infante JR, Daud A, et al. Combined BRAF and MEK inhibition in melanoma with BRAF V600 mutations. *N Engl J Med*. 2012; Epub Sept 29.

25. Ascierto PA, Berking C, Argarwala SS, et al. Efficacy and safety of oral MEK162 in patients with locally advanced and unresectable or metastatic cutaneous melanoma harboring

BRAFV600 or NRAS mutations. Presented at: the American Society of Clinical Oncology (ASCO) Annual Meeting: Collaborating to Conquer Cancer; June 1–5, 2012; Chicago, IL.

26. Ugurel S, Hildenbrand R, Zimpfer A, et al. Lack of clinical efficacy of imatinib in metastatic melanoma. *Br J Cancer.* 2005;92(8):1398–1405.

27. Guo J, Si L, Kong Y, et al. Phase II, open-label, single-arm trial of imatinib mesylate in patients with metastatic melanoma harboring c-Kit mutation or amplification. *J Clin Oncol.* 2011;29(21):2904–2909.

28. Peggs KS, Quezada SA, Korman AJ, Allison JP. Principles and use of anti-CTLA4 antibody in human cancer immunotherapy. *Curr Opin Immunol.* 2006;18(2):206–213.

29. Hodi FS, O'Day SJ, McDermott DF, et al. Improved survival with ipilimumab in patients with metastatic melanoma. *N Engl J Med.* 2010;363(8):711–723.

30. Robert C, Thomas L, Bondarenko I, et al. Ipilimumab plus dacarbazine for previously untreated metastatic melanoma. *N Engl J Med.* 2011;364(26):2517–2526.

31. Beck KE, Blansfield JA, Tran KQ, et al. Enterocolitis in patients with cancer after antibody blockade of cytotoxic T-lymphocyte-associated antigen 4. *J Clin Oncol.* 2006;24(15):2283–2289.

32. Flaherty L, Moon J, Atkins MB, et al. Phase III trial of high-dose interferon alpha-2b versus cisplatin, vinblastine, DTIC plus IL-2 and interferon in patients with high-risk melanoma (SWOG S0008): an intergroup study of CALGB, COG, ECOG and SWOG. Presented at: the American Society of Clinical Oncology (ASCO) Annual Meeting: Collaborating to Conquer Cancer; June 1–5, 2012; Chicago, IL.

33. Eton O, Legha SS, Bedikian AY, et al. Sequential biochemotherapy versus chemotherapy for metastatic melanoma: results from a phase III randomized trial. *J Clin Oncol.* 2002;20(8):2045–2052.

34. Ives NJ, Stowe RL, Lorigan P, Wheatley K. Chemotherapy compared with biochemotherapy for the treatment of metastatic melanoma: a meta-analysis of 18 trials involving 2,621 patients. *J Clin Oncol.* 2007; 25(34):5426–5434.

35. Topalian SL, Hodi FS, Brahmer JR, et al. Safety, activity, and immune correlates of anti-PD-1 antibody in cancer. *N Engl J Med.* 2012; 366(26):2443–2454.

36. Patnaik A, Lang SP, Tolcher AW, et al. Phase I study of MK-3475 (anti-PD-1 monoclonal antibody) in patients with advanced solid tumors. Presented at: the American Society of Clinical Oncology (ASCO) Annual Meeting: Collaborating to Conquer Cancer; June 1–5, 2012; Chicago, IL.

37. Rosenberg SA, Yang JC, Sherry RM, et al. Durable complete responses in heavily pre-treated patients with metastatic melanoma using T-cell transfer immunotherapy. *Clin Cancer Res.* 2011;17(13):4550–4557.

38. Essner R, Lee JH, Wanek LA, Itakura H, Morton DL. Contemporary surgical treatment of advanced-stage melanoma. *Arch Surg.* 2004;139(9):961–6; discussion 966.

39. Pennacchioli E, Gandini S, Verrecchia F, et al. Surgery in stage IV melanoma patients: results from a single institution. Presented at: the American Society of Clinical Oncology (ASCO) Annual Meeting: Collaborating to Conquer Cancer; June 1–5, 2012; Chicago, IL.

40. Carlino MS, Fogarty GB, Long GV. Treatment of melanoma brain metastases: a new paradigm. *Cancer J.* 2012;18(2):208–212.

41. Liew DN, Kano H, Kondziolka D, et al. Outcome predictors of Gamma Knife surgery for melanoma brain metastases. Clinical article. *J Neurosurg.* 2011;114(3):769–779.

42. Agarwala SS, Kirkwood JM, Gore M, et al. Temozolomide for the treatment of brain metastases associated with metastatic melanoma: a phase II study. *J Clin Oncol.* 2004; 22(11):2101–2107.

43. Siena S, Crinò L, Danova M, et al. Dose-dense temozolomide regimen for the treatment of brain metastases from melanoma, breast cancer, or lung cancer not amenable to surgery or radiosurgery: a multicenter phase II study. *Ann Oncol.* 2010;21(3):655–661.

44. Margolin K, Ernstoff MS, Hamid O, et al. Ipilimumab in patients with melanoma and brain metastases: an open-label, phase 2 trial. *Lancet Oncol.* 2012;13(5):459–465.

45. Rochet NM, Kottschade LA, Markovic SN. Vemurafenib for melanoma metastases to the brain. *N Engl J Med.* 2011;365(25):2439–2441.

46. Azer MWF, Menzies AM, Haydu L, et al. Patterns of progression in patients (pts) with B600 BRAF-mutated metastatic

melanoma to the brain treated with dabrafenib (GSK2118436). Presented at: the American Society of Clinical Oncology (ASCO) Annual Meeting: Collaborating to Conquer Cancer; June 1–5, 2012; Chicago, IL.

47. Testori A, Verhoef C, Kroon HM, et al. Treatment of melanoma metastases in a limb by isolated limb perfusion and isolated limb infusion. *J Surg Oncol.* 2011;104(4):397–404.

48. Raymond AK, Beasley GM, Broadwater G, et al. Current trends in regional therapy for melanoma: lessons learned from 225 regional chemotherapy treatments between 1995 and 2010 at a single institution. *J Am Coll Surg.* 2011;213(2):306–316.

49. Qin J, Xin H, Nickoloff BJ. Specifically targeting ERK1 or ERK2 kills melanoma cells. *J Transl Med.* 2012;10:15.

Index

Note: Page references with "*f*" and "*t*" denote figures and tables, respectively.